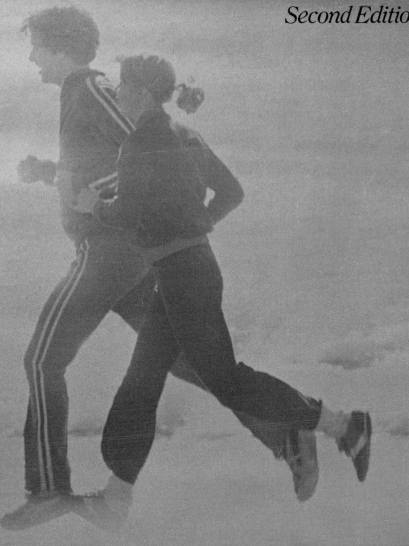

Nutrition, Weight Control, and Exercise

Frank I. Katch
William D. McArdle

Second Edition

Nutrition,
Weight Control,
and Exercise

Nutrition, Weight Control, and Exercise

FRANK I. KATCH
Professor and Chairman
Department of Exercise Science
University of Massachusetts
Amherst, Massachusetts

WILLIAM D. McARDLE
Professor
Department of Health and Physical Education
Queens College
City University of New York
Flushing, New York

SECOND EDITION

LEA & FEBIGER   PHILADELPHIA

LEA & FEBIGER
600 South Washington Square
Philadelphia, Pa. 19106
U.S.A.

Library of Congress Cataloging in Publication Data

Katch, Frank I.
  Nutrition, weight control, and exercise.

  Bibliography: p.
  Includes index.
  1. Nutrition. 2. Reducing. 3. Exercise—Physiological
aspects. 4. Food—Caloric content.
I. McArdle, William D. II. Title.
RA784.K32 1983   613.7   82-25873
ISBN 0-8121-0867-1

Printed in the United States of America

Print Number: 5 4 3 2

We dedicate this book to our parents, Roma Katch, and Claire and Harry McArdle, our wives Kerry and Kathy, and our children David, Kevin, and Ellen, and Kevin, Amy, Theresa, and Jennifer.

Preface

SINCE the publication of the first edition of Nutrition, Weight Control, and Exercise in 1977, the importance of total fitness to human well-being continues to become firmly established. Physical fitness courses such as aerobic conditioning, circuit training, jazznastics, figure control, and body movement are flourishing in the universities, public schools, health clubs, and Y's in this country and abroad—and recently, the corporate setting is gaining the full benefits from a properly devised fitness program.

Although opportunities for participation in vigorous physical activities had long been available to men, the involvement of women in such fitness-oriented programs was relatively new. In the past, activity for women was generally relegated to the figure salon and health spa where a woman could be passively exercised by machines and patronized by gadgetry. But this is no longer the case. Opportunities to engage in vigorous exercise for women and men is now commonplace—*and research shows that the training process for both sexes is essentially the same.* We have indeed come a long way, and we are encouraged by the public's response, enthusiasm, and desire for knowledge regarding the importance of regular, vigorous exercise in one's daily life. What is still amazing, however, is the proliferation of misinformation by self-serving zealots and others who make unwarranted claims about nutrition and diet, weight control, and exercise. We believe that providing information as to both the "why" and "how" of the multi-dimensional aspects of fitness can help stem the tide of the "Madison Avenue" approach which often exploits the admirable goals of good health and fitness. It is our hope that people will become intelligent and sophisticated consumers in the fitness marketplace.

In our initial experience in teaching conditioning courses for women and men we were faced with the dilemma of determining the specific relevant information to be included in our programs, and equally important, a level of sophistication at which this body of knowledge could be presented. We believed that any attempt at physiologic conditioning or weight control necessitated a general background in energy metabolism that was based on a basic understanding of human nutrition. Also, in order for students to appreciate the rationale underlying aerobic conditioning, we wanted them to understand the dynamics of ventilation and circulation. Because many students entered our classes with only minimal background in the natural sciences, we attempted to present the ancillary information related to exercise and weight control in a palatable, interesting, and accurate form that would be appealing to the neophyte as well as to the potential exercise scientist.

In the second edition of Nutrition, Weight Control, and Exercise, we have attempted to incorporate up-to-date and relevant information in each of the chapters. The book has been reorganized and includes two new chapters, and a questionnaire which can be used to generate an individualized computer nutrition and exercise plan. As with the first edition, no attempt was made to be all inclusive or to cover the numerous related topic areas as done in exercise physiology textbooks. We feel the content is appropriate for nutrition, weight control, exercise, and physical fitness courses at the university level, for the various exercise programs for men and women offered at health spas and clubs, as well as the professional preparation of exercise specialists in physical education, exercise science, and the health-related disciplines.

The book is divided into three main parts with chapter sub-divisions. The sequence of presentation is based on our belief that the understanding of a particular topic, although important in itself, also provides a foundation to understand more clearly the material presented in a succeeding section. For example, an understanding of the means by which the body generates energy is facilitated by the knowledge of the structure and function of the three categories of foodstuffs as well as the role of the various vitamins and minerals. Also, any intelligent approach to weight control must be predicated on an understanding of nutrition, energy metabolism, exercise, and the various components of body composition. Finally, the discussion of physiologic conditioning must be framed by a general understanding of the systems involved in oxygen transport and delivery. Part One discusses nutrients in food, optimum nutrition for exercise and sport (new chapter), energy and oxygen delivery systems for exercise, and energy value of food and physical activity. Part Two deals with the evaluation of body composition, obesity, weight control through exercise and diet, and the modification of eating and exercise behaviors. Part Three considers training for muscular strength and conditioning for anaerobic and aerobic power. A new chapter deals with aging, exercise, and cardiovascular health, and a final section is devoted to common questions and answers about nutrition, weight control, and exercise. The appendices contain the nutritive value of common foods, the energy expenditure of a wide variety of physical activities, and a questionnaire for a computer generated dietary and exercise program.

As with the first edition, we have continued to frame our discussion with the research findings of many of our colleagues in physical education, applied physiology, medicine, and nutrition. We have also included data from recent experiments in our laboratories in Massachusetts and New York, most of which were conducted with young adult men and women serving as subjects. We are particularly grateful to Dr. Albert Behnke for his helpful suggestions with Chapter 5, and to the many undergraduate and graduate students who provided input during many stages of the book's revision. We are also grateful to numerous people throughout the country who have provided constructive suggestions and helpful hints about the overall presentation of material. Appreciation is extended to M. Pollack and T. Jackson for providing body composition data on middle aged men and women, J. Hirsch, E.A. Simms, and George and Revea Orsten for providing original photographs, and Fitness Central, Inc., New York, for making arrangements to process the questionnaires for the computer dietary and exercise plan in Appendix C.

Amherst, Massachusetts

Flushing, New York

FRANK I. KATCH

WILLIAM D. McARDLE

Contents

I

Nutrition and Energy for Exercise

THE NUTRIENTS consumed in the daily diet provide the energy necessary to maintain bodily functions both at rest and during various forms of physical activity. Although the raw fuel for biologic work takes the form of carbohydrates, fats, and proteins, the efficient extraction and utilization of energy from these foods requires a delicate blending of other nutrients in the finely regulated watery medium of the cell. The different vitamins and minerals play important and highly specific roles in activating and facilitating energy transfer throughout the body. Fortunately, minute yet crucial quantities of these substances are readily obtained in the foods consumed in well-balanced meals. With proper nutrition, the need to consume vitamin or mineral supplements is both physiologically and economically wasteful.

In the transition from rest to more vigorous physical activity, the energy for muscular contraction is provided in several ways. Certain biochemical reactions can generate considerable energy quite rapidly for short periods of time without consuming oxygen. In sprint activities or all-out bursts of exercise, the body's capacity for this form of rapid energy production is critical in maintaining a high standard of performance. On the other hand, in performing exercise lasting longer than 2 minutes, energy must be extracted from food through reactions that do require oxygen. To be effective, the physiologic conditioning process necessitates a basic understanding of how energy is supplied as well as the energy requirements of a particular activity. This understanding is also fundamental in formulating an effective yet prudent program of weight control.

This section presents a broad overview of nutrition and energy transfer. Each group of nutrients is discussed in terms of its general structure, function, and source in specific foods in the diet. The concept of optimal nutrition is explored and practical recommendations and guidelines are provided for the active man and woman. Emphasis is placed on the importance of the food nutrients in sustaining physiologic function during moderate and more strenuous physical activity, as well as the energy value of foods and how energy is extracted from food and used to power various forms of physical activity.

1

Nutrients in Food

S IX CATEGORIES of nutrients compose the foods we eat: carbohydrates, fats, proteins, vitamins, minerals, and water. The nutrients are the basic substances the body uses for a variety of vital processes. These can be broadly classified as follows: (1) maintenance and repair of body tissues, (2) regulation of the thousands of complex chemical reactions that occur in cells, (3) provision of energy for muscle contraction, (4) conduction of nerve impulses, (5) secretion by glands, (6) synthesis of the various compounds that become part of the body's structures, (7) growth, and (8) reproduction. The sum of these processes in which the energy and nutrients from foods are made available to and utilized by the body is referred to as *metabolism*. A general understanding of the role of the nutrients in metabolism is important because proper nutrition not only affects the normal functioning of the body at rest, but also contributes to its efficient operation during the stress of physical activity.

Chemical Differences Between the Nutrients All the nutrients except water and minerals contain the element carbon. In fact, compounds containing carbon compose almost all the biologic substances within the body. Some of these compounds have relatively few carbon atoms while others contain hundreds or even thousands of carbon atoms joined together. One of the unique characteristics of a carbon atom is that it has four places to which other elements can be attached. These other elements are held in place by forces of attraction called *chemical bonds*. These bonds can be thought of as the chemical cement that helps to keep the atoms and molecules in a substance from coming apart readily.

In addition to carbon, atoms of hydrogen and oxygen also form the basic structural units for most of the biologically active substances within the body. Carbon, hydrogen, and oxygen atoms, organized in a specific way, form carbohydrates. Other combinations of the same elements make fats, while carbon, hydrogen, and oxygen, with the addition of nitrogen and other mineral substances, bind together to form proteins. These four elements—carbon, hydrogen, oxygen, and nitrogen—are the *organic* building blocks from which the nutrients are made. Each nutrient can be distinguished by the type of bonding within the nutrient substance as well as by the size and complexity of the basic molecule.

3

WHERE DO CARBOHYDRATES COME FROM?

The diagram in Figure 1-2 illustrates the general process of *photosynthesis*, by which carbohydrates are manufactured in green plants. The roots of plants and trees take up water in the soil. Carbon dioxide in the air comes into contact with the leaves, while the solar energy from visible sunlight is absorbed by the leaves' green pigment, *chlorophyll*. The interaction of carbon dioxide in the atmosphere, water, sunlight, and chlorophyll provides the necessary ingredients for the synthesis of the carbohydrate molecule. When a carbohydrate molecule is formed, oxygen is released into the atmosphere to be used by animals in the life-sustaining process of energy metabolism.

FUNCTIONS OF CARBOHYDRATES

The major function of carbohydrates is to provide a continuous energy supply to the trillions of cells within the body. Glucose is essential for the proper functioning of the nervous system. The symptoms of lowered blood glucose or *hypoglycemia*, include feelings of weakness, hunger, and dizziness. This condition impairs exercise performance and may partially explain the fatigue associated with prolonged exercise such as marathon running.

The carbohydrates in food, whether in the form of a disaccharide like table sugar or a more complex polysaccharide like starch in potatoes or rice, must eventually break down in digestion into simple 6-carbon sugar molecules before the bloodstream can absorb them from the intestines. Sugar is then transported in the blood to individual cells throughout the body. In the cell the bonds of the glucose molecule are broken through specific chemical reactions. As a result energy is provided to power the cell's vital functions. If the amount of glucose is inadequate to meet the cell's energy needs, the reserve glucose stored as glycogen is recruited as an energy source. The level of sugar in the blood is elevated immedi-

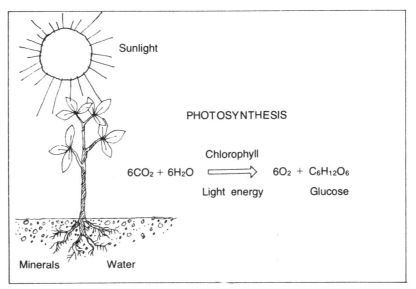

PHOTOSYNTHESIS

$$6CO_2 + 6H_2O \xrightarrow[\text{Light energy}]{\text{Chlorophyll}} 6O_2 + C_6H_{12}O_6$$

Glucose

Sunlight

Minerals   Water

Figure 1-2. *The process of photosynthesis to make sugars from CO_2, H_2O, sunlight, and chlorophyll.*

ately following a meal, however, increasing the transport of glucose into the cell. This excess sugar is then converted to glycogen and stored for later use. Once the capacity of the cell for glycogen storage is reached, the excess sugars are readily converted into fat and stored in the adipose (fat) tissue beneath the skin. This helps to explain how the body's fat content can increase when a person consumes excess calories, even though the diet is high in carbohydrates.

Because comparatively little glycogen is stored in the body, it it important that adequate amounts of carbohydrate be consumed routinely. The quantity of liver and muscle glycogen can be modified considerably through the diet. For example, a 24-hour fast results in a large reduction in liver and muscle glycogen reserves. On the other hand, maintaining a carbohydrate-rich diet for several days enhances the body's carbohydrate stores to a level almost twice that obtained with a normal, well-balanced diet. The effect of enhanced carbohydrate storage on exercise performance is discussed in the next chapter.

CARBOHYDRATES IN FOODS

Approximately 50% of the food consumed in the typical American diet consists of carbohydrates. Interestingly, the percentage of starch consumed has decreased by about 30% since the turn of the century, while the consumption of sugars has correspondingly increased from 31% to over 50% during the same period. Some clinical nutritionists have suggested that this change in carbohydrate sources is associated with the increasing prevalence of dental caries, adult diabetes, and coronary heart disease.

Figure 1-3 graphically displays the percentage of carbohydrates in some common foods. As can be seen, cookies, candies, cakes, and white bread consist predominantly of carbohydrates. Because the values in Figure 1-3 are based on carbohydrate percentage in relation to total food weight, including water content, fruits and vegetables appear to be less valuable carbohydrate sources. However, the dried portion of these foods is almost pure carbohydrates.

WHAT IS A FAT?

A molecule of fat, like a carbohydrate molecule, is composed of carbon, oxygen, and hydrogen atoms linked together in a specific and unique way. Essentially, a fat consists of two different clusters of atoms. One cluster, *glycerol*, which is the basic building block, is composed of 3 atoms of carbon combined with three hydroxyl (OH) groups. The second cluster, known as a *fatty acid*, is attached to glycerol. The most common fatty acids contain between 16 and 18 atoms of carbon in each molecule. When glycerol and fatty acid molecules are joined chemically they produce a molecule of "neutral fat" or *triglyceride*. The triglyceride represents the most plentiful fat in the body as more than 95% of body fat is of this form.

There are two types of fatty acids, saturated and unsaturated. Figure 1-4 illustrates the general differences in bonding and arrangement of hydrogens in saturated and unsaturated fatty acids. For simplification, the symbol R represents the rest of the molecule. For saturated fatty acids, only single bonds link the carbon atoms; therefore at least two hydrogen atoms can attach to each of the carbon atoms of the main chain. This interconnected chain of carbon atoms holds as many hydrogens as is chemically possible. The molecule is said to be saturated with hydrogen atoms and is called a *saturated* fatty acid such as the predominant fatty

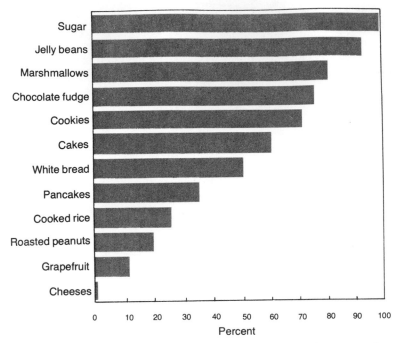

Figure 1-3. *Percentage of carbohydrates in common foods as served. (Adapted from Handbook No. 8: Composition of Foods, United States Department of Agriculture, Washington, D.C., 1963.)*

acids in butter. In contrast, a fatty acid is *unsaturated* if it contains one or more double bonds along the main carbon chain. Each double bond in the chain takes the place of two hydrogen atoms. If the fatty acid has only one such double bond, it is *monounsaturated* as in olive or peanut oil. If it has two or more double bonds, the molecule is *polyunsaturated* as in corn or safflower oil. Regardless of the degree of saturation, all fats have the same number of calories.

Aside from the triglycerides, several other fats are present in the body. One such group, the *phospholipids*, combines fat and phosphorous and nitrogen compounds. These fats form in all cells. In addition to helping maintain the structural integrity of the cell, phospholipids are important in blood clotting. Other compound fats are the *glucolipids*, fatty acids bound with carbohydrate and nitrogen, and the *lipoproteins*, formed primarily in the liver from the union of either triglycerides, phospholipids, or cholesterol with protein (see below). *The lipoproteins are important because they constitute the main form of transport for fat in the blood.* If blood lipids (Greek: lipos meaning fat) were not bound to protein or some other substance they would float to the top like cream in milk that was not homogenized.

Specifically, the *high density lipoproteins* (HDL) contain the largest amount of protein and, correspondingly, the smallest amount of cholesterol. *Low* and *very low density lipoproteins* (LDL and VLDL, respectively) contain the greatest fat and least protein components. The LDL have the greatest affinity for the arterial wall as they help carry cholesterol into the cell. They are intimately involved in the process of arterial narrowing in coronary heart disease. The HDL may operate to *protect against heart disease* in two ways: (1) to carry cholesterol away from the

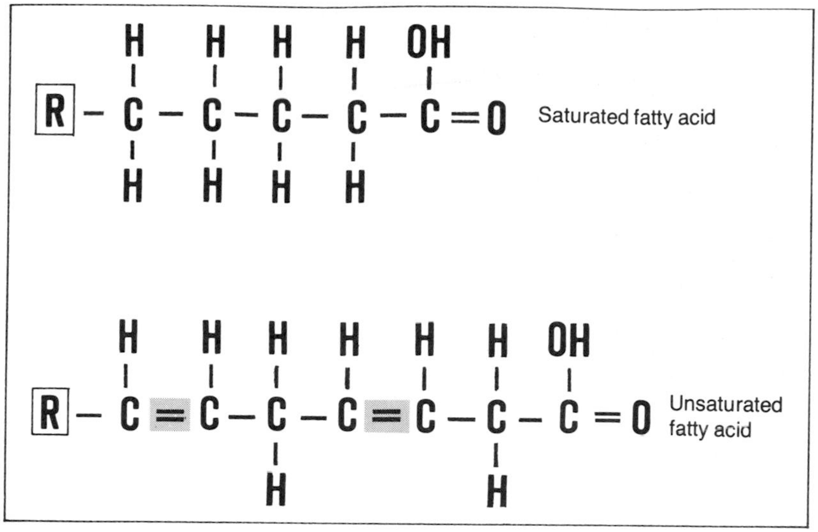

Figure 1-4. *The major structural difference between saturated and unsaturated fatty acids is the presence or absence of double bonds between the carbon atoms.*

arterial wall to the liver to be broken down to bile and excreted via the intestines, and (2) to compete with the LDL fragment for receptor sites on the arterial wall.

The quantity of LDL and HDL as well as the specific ratio of these blood lipoproteins may provide a more meaningful signal than cholesterol per se in predicting the probability of contracting coronary heart disease. This ratio is improved with a low calorie-low saturated fat diet. It also appears that regular aerobic exercise increases the HDL level and favorably affects the LDL/HDL ratio. This will be discussed more fully in Chapter 11.

Another perhaps more widely known fatty substance is *cholesterol,* present in all cells, which is either consumed in foods (*exogenous cholesterol*) or synthesized within the body (*endogenous cholesterol*). Cholesterol is *not* contained in vegetable food sources and is negligible in egg whites and skimmed milk. Cholesterol is an important nutrient that is normally required in many of the complex functions of the body. It is utilized in the manufacture of bile (for digestion and absorption of fats) as well as the hormones estrogen, androgen, and progesterone, which are responsible for the development of male and female secondary sex characteristics.

Because cholesterol and triglycerides have been implicated as a possible associative factor in the development of heart disease, many people have attempted to reduce or eliminate these fats from their diets. Although the diet-heart disease controversy still rages, recent descriptive research suggests that a long term reduction in overall fat consumption and cholesterol intake has a lowering effect on blood lipids and on the incidence of coronary heart disease. It also appears that certain people are sensitive to high cholesterol intake and the subsequent development of heart disease, while others may be protected from high dietary levels of cholesterol and saturated fats. However, there is still insufficient proof from well-designed, carefully controlled experiments that diet can significantly lower serum cholesterol in humans in their natural setting or that lowering the serum cholesterol actually reduces a heart disease risk. With this in mind, however, it is still prudent to replace a portion of saturated fats and cholesterol (less than 300 milligrams (mg) daily) in the diet with polyunsaturated fats. It should be pointed out, however, that even on a cholesterol-free diet the body will still produce about 1.0 to 2.0 grams (g) of endogenous cholesterol each day.

There is also suggestive evidence that a diet high in animal fat may be directly or indirectly related to the development of cancer of the colon, stomach, esophagus, breast, liver, and uterus. It is believed that these substances may enhance the activity of cancer-producing agents, or act as carriers of these agents to their site of action. Further research is being conducted to determine if cancer can be prevented by making certain modifications in the diet.

WHERE DO FATS COME FROM?

Both plants and animals provide ready sources of fat. Plants manufacture fat by the same process of photosynthesis they use to make carbohydrates. Animals will use or store the fat they ingest, or synthesize fat from the carbon, hydrogen, and oxygen atoms present in the excess quantities of ingested carbohydrates and proteins.

One of the distinguishing properties of an unsaturated fat is its relatively low melting point. These fats tend to liquefy easily and generally take liquid form at room temperature. Because the body is unable to synthesize unsaturated fats they must be consumed in the diet. Unsaturated fats present as liquids are called *oils*. The more common vegetable oils are corn oil, cottonseed oil, and soybean oil. Unsaturated oils can be changed to semisolid compounds by a chemical process called *hydrogenation*. This process reduces a double bond in the unsaturated fat to a single bond, thereby allowing more hydrogen atoms to attach to the carbon atoms in the chain thus causing the fat to behave as a saturated fat. The most common hydrogenated fats include lard substitutes and margarine.

Saturated fats are derived mainly from animal sources and include the fat in meats such as beef, lamb, pork, and chicken, and in dairy products like egg yolk, cream, milk, and cheese. Shellfish such as lobster, shrimp, and crab also contain a large amount of saturated fat and cholesterol. In the United States, the fat consumed in the diet represents approximately 40 to 50% of the total calorie intake. This amounts to about 115 pounds of fat consumed per person each year, of which over 50 pounds or 16% of the total calories are saturated fat.

FUNCTIONS OF FAT
Energy Source

During a light or moderate muscular exercise such as jogging, energy is derived in approximately equal amounts from the body's stores of carbohydrates and fats. In prolonged exercise of an hour or more there is a significant increase in the amount of fat utilized to supply energy, and, if exercise is continued, the body's fat stores may supply nearly 90% of the total energy required for exercise. On the other hand, in intense but short-term exercise such as all-out running or swimming, essentially all the energy is generated from the glycogen stored in the specific muscles used in the activity.

In terms of its capability for energy storage, fat is remarkably efficient in that more than twice the energy is stored in a pound of body fat as in an equal weight of carbohydrate. This high energy density is due mainly to the amount of hydrogen in the fat molecule, which is larger than the amount of hydrogen in the carbohydrate molecule. Humans would be considerably larger if their energy reserves depended predominantly on carbohydrate storage. In addition, when the union of glycerol and fatty acid makes a fat molecule, it produces three molecules of water. In contrast, when glucose is stored as glycogen, 2.7 g of water are retained for each gram of dried glycogen. Thus fat exists in a relatively concentrated form, whereas the addition of water to glycogen makes this a heavy fuel. If birds and insects had to depend on glycogen as the main fuel during long flights, it would either be impossible to fly or the glycogen load would severely limit their flying time.

The preceding discussion is in no way intended to minimize the role of carbohydrate in energy metabolism for prolonged work. Although significantly less carbohydrate is used in long-term exercise than fat, a minimum amount must be available for energy if exercise is to continue. We will discuss the function of carbohydrates in both short- and long-term exercise more fully in Chapter 3.

Protection of Vital Organs

Approximately 4% of the total amount of fat in the body serves as a shock absorber and protective shield against internal and external trauma to vital organs such as the heart, liver, kidneys, spleen, brain, and spinal cord. Even during semistarvation for as long as a year or more, the protective layer of fat around these organs is reduced only slightly compared to the reduction in fat stored in the subcutaneous tissue just below the skin.

Insulation

Fat stored in the subcutaneous tissues also acts as an insulator to protect the body against the thermal stress of a cold environment. Although this benefit may provide a comfortable rationalization for many of us who are exquisite insulators, it probably is of value to relatively few people, such as ocean or channel swimmers or occupational deep sea divers, who must work while submerged in water for prolonged periods. In fact, the insulation provided by excess body fat generally serves as a liability in temperature regulation. This is especially true in warm environments, where fat people are at a disadvantage in terms of dissipating body heat to the environment. It is common to observe that fat people sweat easily on warm days, while those who are relatively lean and possess less insulation can maintain body temperature for some time before relying on the cooling benefits of the sweat mechanism. This problem of heat regulation for fat people is magnified during physical activity, where the body's heat production can increase 20 times or more above the resting levels.

Other Functions

The fat consumed in the diet serves several functions besides protection, insulation, and energy storage. Dietary fat acts as the carrier of four vitamins, A, D, E, and K. These vitamins are fat soluble and are transported to the cells in conjunction with fat. As the amount of fat consumed in the diet is reduced, the availability and utilization of these important vitamins is also reduced. Thus diets consistently low in fat content may ultimately lead to a deficiency of one or more of the fat-soluble vitamins.

Another function of fat is that its presence in the small intestines stimulates the release of a substance that has the effect of depressing "hunger pangs." These sensations frequently occur when there is a long interval between meals. Because fats are not completely absorbed from the small intestines for up to four hours after a meal, it has been suggested that dietary fats may retard the feeling of hunger. This is one of the reasons why a limited amount of fat is often recommended in some reducing diets.

FATS IN FOOD

The approximate percentage contribution of some of the common food groups to the total fat content of the American diet is illustrated in Figure 1-5. About 30 to 40% of the total dietary fat is present in the "visible fats" in butter, lard, mayonnaise, cooking oils, and the fat you see in meat, while the remainder is derived from "invisible fats" in eggs, milk, cheese, nuts, vegetables, and cereals. For every 10 pounds of fat consumed, about 3.4 pounds come from vegetable fat, while the remaining 6.6 pounds are supplied from animal sources. The common vegetable oils are 100% fat, whereas margarine and mayonnaise possess about 80% fat. Most foods from animal sources range between 4 to 80% in fat content.

Protein

WHAT IS A PROTEIN?

The structure of proteins is similar in one respect to that of carbohydrates and fats. Each molecule contains atoms of carbon, oxygen, and hydrogen. The major difference is that proteins also contain nitrogen, which makes up approximately 16% of the molecule. The basic units or "building blocks" of protein are *amino acids.* Amino acids are small organic compounds that contain at least one amino group and one group called an *organic acid.* The amino radical, which forms the backbone of the amino acid, consists of two hydrogen atoms attached to a nitrogen atom (NH_2), while the organic acid is made up of one carbon atom, two oxygen atoms, and one hydrogen atom (COOH). The chemical structure of the simple amino acid alanine is illustrated in Figure 1-6.

There are 20 different amino acids present in proteins, although tens of thousands of the same amino acids may be present in a single protein. In the formation

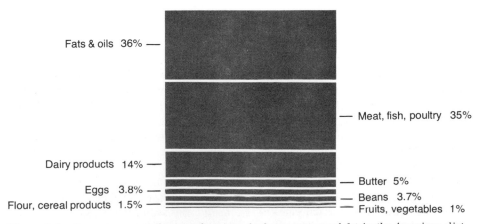

Fats & oils 36%

Meat, fish, poultry 35%

Dairy products 14%

Butter 5%

Eggs 3.8%

Beans 3.7%

Flour, cereal products 1.5%

Fruits, vegetables 1%

Figure 1-5. *Percentage contribution of various food groups to total fat in the American diet.*

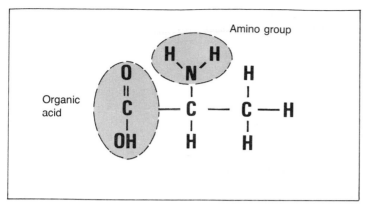

Figure 1-6. *Structural arrangement of the amino acid alanine.*

of protein, the number of possible combinations of amino acids and associated structures becomes almost infinite. Of the different amino acids, 8 (9 in children and stressed older adults) cannot be synthesized in the body at a sufficient rate to prevent an impairment in normal cellular function. These amino acids are called *essential* because they must be obtained through foods. The 12 amino acids that can be manufactured within the body are termed *nonessential.* This does not mean they are unimportant, but simply that the body can synthesize nonessential amino acids from ingested nutrients in the diet.

WHERE DO PROTEINS COME FROM?

Proteins are found in the cells of all animals and plants. Plants make their own special kinds of proteins by incorporating nitrogen contained in the soil. Of the remaining elements, carbon is obtained from the air, while oxygen and hydrogen are available from water absorbed directly by the roots. Animals, on the other hand, do not have the broad capability for amino-acid synthesis possessed by plants. In many instances, animals must rely on ingested protein sources such as the fruits and vegetables that grow from plants, or the animal protein in meat and in animal by-products such as eggs and milk.

FUNCTIONS OF PROTEINS

The amount of protein an average living cell contains is approximately 15% of its total weight. However, the amount of protein contained in different cells varies considerably. For example, a brain cell is only about 10% protein, whereas protein constitutes 20% of the weight of the muscles, heart, liver, and glands. Furthermore, the protein contained in muscles strengthened through frequent weight-lifting exercise is significantly greater than the protein in unexercised muscles. This increase in protein content contributes to an increase in muscle size, which is readily apparent following a strength training program, especially in men. However, large amounts of dietary protein do not *cause* a muscle to become larger. The procedure for increasing the strength and size of muscles is discussed in Chapter 9.

Protein usually takes the shape of either a long, threadlike molecule or a more globular molecule. The long chain protein molecules are often referred to as *struc-*

tural proteins, since their function is literally to hold the cell together. Structural proteins are present in the membranes that surround both the cell and its nucleus, as well as in the specific structures contained within the cell. The globular forms of protein make up the *enzymes*, which are substances that speed up the chemical reactions within the cell. As many as 1000 different enzymes are present in the fluids of a single cell and are in contact with surfaces of structures within the cell. One of the unique characteristics of an enzyme is that it interacts with one specific substance to perform one specific function. When a protein molecule in food is split into amino acid units, the enzymes initiate and accelerate the breakdown process. Similarly, in order to extract energy from carbohydrates and fats, specific enzymes must interact with these foods during the complex course of their breakdown and subsequent energy release. The process by which energy is extracted from food for use by the body is discussed in Chapter 3.

The importance of protein is further illustrated in a variety of other tissues. Hair, fingernails, and the protective outer layer of skin are composed of the protein *keratin*. The specialized cells that form bone, the *osteoblasts*, secrete a protein substance that ultimately forms the major portion of new bone. Specialized proteins, *thrombin, fibrin*, and *fibrinogen* are intimately involved in the clotting of blood. In muscles, the structural proteins *actin* and *myosin* "slide" past each other during muscular contraction. *Hemoglobin*, which carries oxygen and carbon dioxide in the red blood cells, consists of an iron-containing compound *heme*, and a large protein molecule *globin*. The *hormones* are protein substances secreted into the body from the endocrine glands, which control and regulate the function of various processes. For example, the front portion of the small pituitary gland located under the brain secretes six different hormones. Underproduction of hormones from this part of the gland will retard growth, slow metabolic rate, and influence electrolyte balance, fertility, and the metabolism of carbohydrates, fats, and proteins.

Contrary to the beliefs of many coaches and exercise enthusiasts, the contribution of protein to the energy requirements for muscular work is relatively small, even in events as grueling as marathon running. It has been estimated that only about 5 to 15% of the total energy in well-nourished individuals is supplied from the breakdown of protein. Thus consuming an excessive amount of protein is unwarranted from the standpoint of energy metabolism.

PROTEIN IN FOOD

The proteins contained in food are classified as complete or incomplete, depending on their content of amino acids. A *complete* or *high quality* protein contains all the essential amino acids in both quantity and correct proportion required to promote normal growth. An *incomplete* or *lower quality* protein lacks one or more of the essential amino acids. Consequently diets containing predominantly incomplete protein may eventually hamper the ability of various cells to carry out their normal functions.

Figure 1-7 depicts the percentage contribution of the various food groups to the total protein in the American diet. As can be seen, the major sources of protein are meat, fish, and poultry, whereas only 5% of the daily protein intake of Americans is in the form of peas, beans, or nuts. Generally, more than two-thirds of the protein in the American diet comes from animal sources compared to about one-half 70 years ago. Figure 1-8 illustrates the percentage of protein contained per 100 grams of some common foods.

Meat, fish,
poultry, eggs 44%

Dairy products 24%

Cereals 19%

Beans, peas, nuts 5%

Fruits & vegetables 7%

Fats & oils 1%

Figure 1-7. *Percentage contribution of various food groups to total protein in the American diet.*

The recommended daily protein requirement has been established by the National Research Council in the United States. Table 1-1 shows the protein intake recommendations for adolescent and adult men and women. *On the average, the daily recommended intake is about 0.8 gram of protein per kilogram (g/kg) of body weight.* (To determine your protein requirement, multiply your body weight in pounds by 0.36.) Thus, a woman of 50 kg (110 lbs) would require about 40 g of protein per day. Heavier people require a greater intake. For an average-sized man who weighs 70 kg (154 lbs), the daily protein intake should be approximately

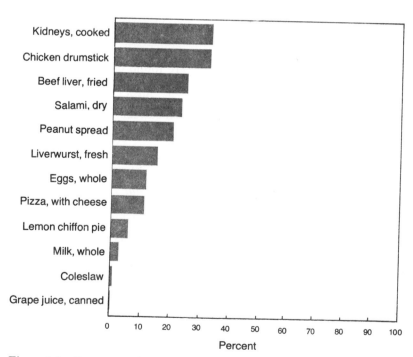

Kidneys, cooked
Chicken drumstick
Beef liver, fried
Salami, dry
Peanut spread
Liverwurst, fresh
Eggs, whole
Pizza, with cheese
Lemon chiffon pie
Milk, whole
Coleslaw
Grape juice, canned

0 10 20 30 40 50 60 70 80 90 100

Percent

Figure 1-8. *Percentage of protein in common foods as served. (Adapted from Handbook No. 8: Composition of Foods, United States Department of Agriculture, Washington, D.C., 1963.)*

In adults, symptoms can include nausea, headaches, drowsiness, loss of hair, diarrhea, and loss of calcium from bones, causing brittleness. Discontinuing such high intakes of vitamin A reverses these symptoms. Large dosages of two other fat-soluble vitamins, D and K, may also produce undesirable toxic side effects, and they should not be consumed in excess without proper medical supervision.

The other group of vitamins is classified as *water soluble* because they are transported in the watery medium of tissues and cells. Because of their solubility in water, these vitamins are not stored in the body to any appreciable extent and are normally voided in the urine. Thus the water-soluble vitamins must be consumed in the daily diet, or at least within a several day period. The 10 water-soluble vitamins include vitamin C (ascorbic acid) and what are commonly referred to as the *B-complex vitamins*. Included in this group are thiamine (B_1), riboflavin (B_2), niacin, pyridoxine (B_6), folacin, pantothenic acid, biotin, choline, and cobalamin (B_{12}). These vitamins act as part of *coenzymes* which are small protein molecules that can combine with another protein to make it an active enzyme.

Any excess of the water-soluble vitamins is usually excreted in the urine on a daily basis. An excess intake of the fat-soluble vitamins is maintained within the body tissues and in some instances produces a toxic "vitamin overdose." Thus ingesting more vitamins than recommended will be of little or no benefit.

WHERE DO VITAMINS COME FROM?

With the exception of vitamin B_{12}, which is synthesized *only* in animals, vitamins are manufactured in the green leaves and roots of plants by the process of photosynthesis, which we have already discussed. The synthesis of vitamins involves the integration of the energy from sunlight with carbon dioxide, water, and minerals in the soil. Animals obtain their vitamins from the plants, seeds, grains, and fruits they eat, or from the meat of other animals that have previously consumed these foods. There is essentially no difference between a vitamin synthesized in the laboratory and a so-called "natural" vitamin pre-formed from a plant or animal source.

Most animals are able to manufacture some of the vitamins within their own cells. Vitamin C, for example, can be synthesized by all animals with the exception of humans, monkeys, guinea pigs, and several species of birds. Several of the vitamins, notably vitamins A, niacin, and folacin, are converted to an activated form in the body from precursor substances known as *provitamins*. The most well known of the provitamins are the *carotenes*, the yellow and yellow-orange pigments that give color to vegetables and fruits such as carrots, squash, corn, pumpkins, sweet potatoes, apricots, peaches, and melons. Carotenes, which are the precursors of vitamin A, are also present in all green plants, but the green pigment chlorophyll masks their color. They are converted to vitamin A in the walls of the intestines and in the liver. Besides playing an important role in the prevention of night blindness and other eye diseases, this vitamin prevents some digestive and urogenital tract diseases and, in carotene form, may provide protection against several forms of cancer. Another provitamin substance in the skin is converted to vitamin D when the skin is exposed to the ultraviolet rays of the sun or to artificial ultraviolet light. Niacin, the B-complex vitamin that prevents pellagra (a skin disease), is converted to an active form by its precursor, the essential amino acid tryptophan.

FUNCTIONS OF VITAMINS

Vitamins perform many different functions. They generally serve as essential links and regulators in the chain of metabolic reactions within cells. If there is a dietary deficiency in either the vitamin or its precursor, the resulting defect in cellular function manifests itself in a variety of symptoms. The more important functions of the vitamins and the symptoms resulting from vitamin deficiencies are summarized in a general way in Table 1-2.

VITAMINS AND EXERCISE PERFORMANCE

Contrary to popular belief, vitamins themselves contain *no* usable energy. However, it is well established that five or six vitamins of the B-complex group interact with various enzymes that are important in the energy-yielding reactions during the metabolism of fats and carbohydrates. This has led many coaches, athletes, and fitness enthusiasts to believe that supplements of these vitamins will enhance or "supercharge" energy production, and consequently lead to improved physical performance. However, there is little experimental evidence to support this practice.

This is also the case for vitamins other than the B-complex group such as vitamins C and E. While there is some indication that the vitamin C requirement is increased in humans in times of stress, *it has yet to be demonstrated that an excess of this vitamin is needed during physical training.* Studies have shown that supplements of vitamin C had negligible effects on endurance performance and on the rate, severity, and duration of injuries compared to treatment with a placebo. In addition, the combined findings from several well-controlled studies showed only a slight reduction in frequency, duration, and severity of colds in individuals on vitamin C supplementation compared to counterparts taking a placebo. Its major effect may be to act as an antihistamine to reduce cold symptoms. It has never been firmly established with careful research that a deficiency state for vitamin E exists, let alone that vitamin E supplements are beneficial to stamina, circulatory function, energy metabolism, aging, the effects of air pollution, or sexual potency.

VITAMIN SUPPLEMENTATION

Only in rare instances do healthy people who eat well-balanced meals require vitamin supplements. It has been estimated that the American consumer spends between $300 million and $500 million annually on unnecessary vitamin supplements. While most nutritionists feel that taking a daily multivitamin capsule of the recommended dosage will do no harm (the psychologic effects may even be beneficial), it is of great concern that some men and women resort to taking *megavitamins,* or doses of at least *tenfold* and up to 1,000 times the *Recommended Dietary Allowance,* in the hope of improving health or exercise performance. Except in cases of specific serious medical illness, this practice can be harmful. Once the enzyme systems that are catalyzed by specific vitamins are saturated, the excess vitamins in the megadose function as chemicals in the body.

Generally, an excess of the water soluble vitamins will be excreted in the urine on a daily basis. However, there may be specific and serious exceptions to this general rule. For example, a megadose of the water soluble vitamin C can raise serum uric levels and precipitate gout in people predisposed to this disease. Also,

Table 1-2. *Vitamins—their functions and symptoms of their deficiency.*

A (Retinol)	Vision, growth	Poor vision (night blindness), failure of bones to grow in length, skin and respiratory infections, failure of tooth enamel
D	Bone calcification	Bone diseases
E (Tocopherol)	Not clear in humans	Unclear, possibly anemia
K	Blood clotting and coagulation and energy metabolism of the cell	Prolonged blood-clotting or coagulation time
B-1 (Thiamine)	Metabolism of nutrients in cells	Beriberi—the degeneration of nerves and muscles, loss of appetite, mental depression, and neurological dysfunction
B-2 (Riboflavin)	Reactions that release energy in the cells	Lesions of the skin, eye, mouth, and retardation of growth
Niacin	Release of energy from the breakdown and synthesis of carbohydrate, fat, and protein	Diseases of the skin, gastrointestinal tract, and nervous system, resulting in dermatitis, diarrhea and depression
B_6 (Pyridoxine)	Synthesis and breakdown of amino acids	Usually no deficiency because this vitamin is so readily available in foods
Pantothenic acid	Metabolism of carbohydrates, fats, and proteins, important in the formation of cholesterol	Subclinical symptoms such as irritability, restlessness, easy fatigue, muscle cramps
Folacin	Formation of normal red blood cells and of DNA and RNA	Toxemia of pregnancy and anemia and retarded production of white blood cells
B_{12}	Normal growth, maintenance of neural tissue, and formation of blood	Pernicious anemia (sore tongue, weight loss, mental and nervous disorders, degeneration of the spinal cord)
Biotin	Removal or addition of carbon dioxide in chemical reactions and metabolism of carbohydrate and protein	Dermatitis, such as scaling or hardening of skin, loss of appetite, nausea, muscle pains, high blood cholesterol levels

Table 1-2 (*continued*)

C (Ascorbic acid)	Important for collagen formation that acts as "cement" to bind connective tissue cells together, tooth formation	Scurvy, sore joints, poor healing of wounds

some American blacks, Asians and Sephardic Jews have a genetic metabolic deficiency that can be activated to hemolytic anemia by excesses of vitamin C. In individuals who are iron-deficient, megadoses of vitamin C destroy significant amounts of vitamin B_{12} in the diet. In healthy people, vitamin C supplements frequently irritate the bowel and cause diarrhea. It is now believed that an excessive intake of vitamin B_6 may produce liver disease, whereas a megadose of nicotinc acid inhibits the uptake of fatty acids by cardiac muscle during exercise.

An excess intake of the fat soluble vitamins is maintained within the body tissues and, in some instances, produces a toxic "vitamin overdose." Possible side effects of vitamin E megadose include headache, fatigue, blurred vision, gastrointestinal disturbances, muscular weakness, and low blood sugar. This is ironic because it is not known whether a lack of vitamin E per se is seriously harmful to humans. Because vitamin E is usually found associated with unsaturated fats, it is difficult even to "construct" a vitamin E-deficient diet. The toxicity to the nervous system of megadoses of vitamin A and the damaging effects to the kidneys of excess vitamin D have been well demonstrated.

Perhaps the misuse and abuse of vitamins by individuals hoping to improve athletic performance can be put in proper perspective by the following quotation: "The sale of vitamins is probably the biggest rip-off in our society today. Their only effect would appear to be a highly enriched sewage around athletic training or competition sites."

Minerals

WHAT IS A MINERAL?

The body is composed of at least 31 known chemical elements, of which 24 are considered to be essential for sustaining life. These essential elements are combined in thousands of different ways to form the various structures within the body. The most abundant nonmetal, chemical element is oxygen, which amounts to 65% of a person's body weight. Three other nonmetal elements constitute 31% of the body mass; these are carbon (18%), hydrogen (10%), and nitrogen (3%). In addition to the organic elements oxygen, carbon, hydrogen, and nitrogen, the remaining 4%, which would amount to about 5 pounds for a 125-pound woman, is composed of a group of 22 metallic elements called *minerals*. Although the total quantity of minerals present in the body is relatively small, each of them is vital for proper cell functioning. For example, minerals are part of enzymes, hormones, and vitamins. They are also found in muscles, connective tissues, and the various body fluids. Calcium and phosphorus in teeth and bones account for 58 to 85% of the total percentage of minerals in the body, while sodium, potassium, chlorine, sulphur, and magnesium average 24%. The remaining minerals include trace amounts of iron, zinc, selenium, manganese, iodine, copper, fluorine, and chromium. The body even contains small quantities of aluminum, silver, tin, lead, barium, and gold. If purchased in a store, the total worth of the body's minerals would be only about ten cents!

WHERE DO MINERALS COME FROM?

Minerals occur freely in nature and are found mainly in the waters of rivers, lakes, and oceans, in topsoil, and beneath the earth's surface. Small amounts of minerals are absorbed into the root systems of plants and trees, where they become incorporated into the natural foods, the carbohydrates, fats, and proteins. Minerals then become part of the body structure of animals who must consume food and water in order to survive. Similarly, the human supply of minerals is obtained almost exclusively from water and food.

MINERALS IN FOOD

As with vitamins, healthy people who eat well-balanced meals consume enough of the essential mineral elements to maintain normal physiologic functioning and health. Mineral supplements may be necessary, however, in some geographic regions where mineral elements in the soil or water supply are relatively scarce. The mineral iodine, for example, is stored mainly in the thyroid gland and becomes part of *thyroxin*, a hormone that influences the rate of energy metabolism in cells. A diet deficient in iodine results in the over-enlargement of the thyroid gland as the gland attempts to produce an adequate supply of thyroxin. This disease, *goiter*, is one of the most prevalent nutrient deficiency diseases in the world. Iodine added to most common table salts (iodized salt) is an inexpensive, easily obtained iodine supplement.

Another common mineral deficiency results from lack of iron in the diet. About 5 g or one-sixth of an ounce of iron is normally contained within the body. Two-thirds of this amount is combined with hemoglobin, the iron-protein compound manufactured in the marrow of long bones. This compound is found in red blood cells and increases the oxygen carrying capacity of the blood about 65 times. Trace amounts of the mineral element copper are also involved in the synthesis of hemoglobin. People who do not take in enough iron or have limited rates of iron absorption or high rates of iron loss can develop anemia, a condition that reduces the concentration of hemoglobin as well as the size of red blood cells. This condition, commonly referred to as *iron-deficiency anemia*, is characterized by general sluggishness, fatigue, and loss of appetite. Nutritionists estimate that between 30 to 50% of American women of childbearing age suffer some form of iron insufficiency. This is due to the fact that women usually lose between 5 and 45 mg of iron during the menstrual cycle. This increases the iron requirement of females to almost twice that of males (18 versus 10 mg). Because the typical Western diet contains about 6 mg of iron per 1000 calories of food ingested, it is difficult for the average woman who consumes 2100 calories a day to obtain the required iron. A moderate iron deficiency is common during pregnancy when there is a greater demand for iron for both the mother and fetus.

Iron deficiency is corrected in most cases with a diet rich in iron-containing foods such as liver, nuts, legumes, dried uncooked fruits, oysters, shellfish, leafy green vegetables, egg yolk, and meats, especially kidney and heart. Iron supplements can also be obtained in tablet or liquid form or in foods specifically fortified with iron. The Food and Nutrition Board's recommendations for daily intakes of iron for both men and women of different ages are listed in Table 1-3. Physical training does not appear to increase the iron requirement or aggravate existing iron deficiencies.

Recent experiments have shown that individuals who suffer from iron deficiency anemia have a reduced capacity for sustaining even mild exercise. This occurs because a lowered iron content in the red blood cell results in an inadequate supply of oxygen to the exercising muscles. This was illustrated in one experiment in which 29 iron-deficient, anemic men and women with low hemoglobin levels were placed into one of two groups: one group received intramuscular injections of iron over an 80-day period, while the other group received intramuscular injections of colored saline solution. Both groups were tested for exercise capacity before receiving iron or placebo 4 to 6 days after receiving the first iron supplement or placebo, and after 80 days of treatment. The results in Table 1-4 clearly showed that the group given the iron supplement improved significantly in exercise response. Peak heart rate measured during a 5-minute stepping performance decreased from 155 to 113 beats per minute for men and from 152 to 123 beats per minute for the women. This translates into an average of 15% more oxygen delivered per heart beat. The heart rate and hemoglobin levels showed no change for the group receiving the placebo treatment.

FUNCTIONS OF MINERALS

Minerals are present in all living cells. They are part of the cell membranes, cell nucleus, and various cellular structures such as the "powerhouse" of the cell, the *mitochondrion*, which converts food nutrients to energy. They are intimately involved in *catabolism* which refers to the breakdown of the nutrient substances glucose, fatty acids, and amino acids to their end products, carbon dioxide and

Table 1-3. *Recommended daily allowances for iron.*

	AGE	IRON (MG)
Children	1–3	15
	4–10	10
Males	11–18	18
	19+	10
Females	11–50	18
	51+	10
	Pregnant	18+[a]
	Lactating	18

Source: Food and Nutrition Board, *Recommended Dietary Allowances*, 8th ed., National Academy of Sciences, Washington, D.C., Revised, 1980.

[a]Ordinary diets cannot meet this increased requirement; therefore the use of 30 to 60 mg of supplemental iron is recommended.

Table 1-4. *Hemoglobin (Hb) and exercise heart rate responses of anemic subjects to iron treatment.*

SUBJECTS	Hb (G PER 100 ML BLOOD) (AVERAGE)	PEAK EXERCISE HEART RATE (AVERAGE)
Normal		
Men	14.3	119
Women	13.9	142
Iron-Deficient Men		
Pre-treatment	7.1	155
Post-treatment	14.0	113
Iron-Deficient Women		
Pre-treatment	7.7	155
Post-treatment	12.4	123
Iron-Deficient Men		
Pre-placebo	7.7	146
Post-placebo	7.4	137
Iron-Deficient Women		
Pre-placebo	8.1	154
Post-placebo	8.4	144

[a]From Gardner, G.W., et al.: Cardiorespiratory, hematological, and physical performance responses of anemic subjects to iron treatment. *American Journal of Clinical Nutrition, 28:*982, 1975.

water. In this process considerable energy is extracted from the food and used to maintain the body's energy supply. Minerals are also required for the reverse process, *anabolism,* which refers to the synthesis of glycogen from glucose, fat from fatty acids and glycerol, and protein from amino acids.

Minerals also serve as important parts of the structure of various hormones, enzymes, and other substances that help to regulate the chemical reactions within cells. For example, in the previous section we mentioned that the mineral iodine was necessary for the synthesis of thyroxin, the hormone that accelerates the rate of energy metabolism in cells. Underproduction of thyroxin causes a decreased metabolic rate that could result in the development of obesity. Iron was shown to be an important structural component of hemoglobin, the oxygen-carrying compound in red blood cells. In addition, iron is a structural component of *myoglobin,* a compound similar to hemoglobin, which aids in the transport of oxygen within muscle cells. Iron is also present in very small amounts in specialized substances called *cytochromes* that function as catalysts in the energy transfer system operations within the cell.

Calcium, the body's most abundant mineral combines with the mineral phosphorus to form the bones and teeth. Calcium is also essential in maintaining the normal function of muscles, as well as for blood clotting, and the transport of fluid across cell membranes. Phosphorus is an essential component of the high energy compounds *adenosine triphosphate* (ATP) and *creatine phosphate* (CP). As we will show in Chapter 3, these compounds are crucial in supplying the energy for all forms of biologic work. Phosphorus also combines with substances in the blood and acts to buffer the acid end products of energy metabolism. Because it can regulate the acid content of the blood, some coaches and trainers recommend that their athletes consume special "phosphate drinks" three to four hours prior to competition to improve their subsequent performance. Although some people have attributed enhanced performance to these drinks, scientific evidence in support of this practice is lacking. It is also possible that an excess intake of phosphorus, plentiful in red meats and diet soft drinks, can accelerate the rate of bone loss (*osteoporosis*) in athletic women who are relatively thin with a low percentage of body fat.

Magnesium plays a vital role in glucose metabolism by facilitating the reactions that synthesize glucose to glycogen in the liver and muscles. Magnesium is also involved in the breakdown of glucose, fatty acids, and amino acids to provide cellular energy. Furthermore, magnesium is important in bone formation, in maintaining normal muscle function, in the conduction of nerve impulses, and in the synthesis of fats and proteins from fatty acids and amino acids.

The minerals sodium, potassium, and chlorine have quite similar functions. Sodium and chlorine are present mainly in the fluids outside the cells, while potassium is found predominantly in the intracellular fluids. Collectively these three elements are called *electrolytes*, because they are present in the body as electrically charged particles called *ions*. The major function of electrolytes is to control and maintain the correct rate of fluid exchange within various fluid compartments of the body. In this way the constant flow of dissolved nutrients into the cell and waste products from the cell is properly regulated. The proper maintenance of both fluid and electrolyte balance is also of critical importance, especially during exercise in warm environments. When sweating excessively, the body loses the electrolytes present in sweat. These conditions impair heat tolerance and exercise performance. If electrolytes, and especially water, are not replaced, severe dysfunction in the form of heat cramps and heat stroke can occur. The yearly toll of heat-related deaths during spring and summer football practice provides a tragic illustration of the importance of both fluid and electrolyte replacement. Thus it is common for athletes, tunnel and mine workers, and others who sweat profusely during work to increase their normal salt and fluid intake automatically, independent of their thirst, to offset the effects of dehydration. *The crucial and immediate need is to replace the water lost through sweating.*

A 1 liter or 2.2 pound sweat loss is accompanied by a loss of about 1.5 g of salt. These electrolytes can easily be replenished by adding a slight amount of table salt to the fluids ingested or to the normal daily food intake. Thus, ingesting the so-called athletic drinks is of no special benefit in replacing the minerals lost through sweating. In fact, research indicates that most individuals unconsciously consume more salt when the need exists. For fluid losses in excess of 9 to 10 pounds and for prolonged periods of work in the heat, salt supplements may be necessary and can be achieved by adding about ⅓ teaspoon of table salt per quart of water. Although a potassium deficiency may occur with intense exercise in the heat, the appropriate potassium level is generally assured by consuming a diet containing normal amounts of the mineral or eating potassium-rich foods such as citrus fruits and bananas. A glass of orange or tomato juice replaces almost all of the calcium, potassium, and magnesium lost in about 3 quarts (6 lb) of sweat.

Water

WATER CONTENT OF THE BODY

Water is the most important environmental substance essential to human life. It makes up about 80% of the liquid substance of all cells. Aside from its excellent temperature stabilizing properties, it dissolves more substances than any other known solvent. Food and oxygen are always supplied in an aqueous solution to the cells and waste products always leave the cell via this medium. Water is remarkably inert and most substances remain unchanged when dissolved in water. In solution they may remain unaltered within the body until they are needed.

From 40 to 60% of a person's body weight consists of water. Because water makes up about 72% of the weight of muscle tissue and only 20 to 25% of the weight of fat, the differences between individuals in terms of total body water are determined largely by differences in body composition. Therefore for two individuals of the same body weight the total body water will be larger for the individual with the greater muscle mass. On the average, men contain relatively less body fat than women. This explains why approximately 55% of men's body weight is water, while only 50% of women's body weight is water. This would come to 93 pounds of water for a 154-pound man and 72 pounds of water for a 130-pound woman. Expressed in terms of volume it would amount to approximately 42 liters of water for the average-sized man and 35 liters for the average-sized woman.

The distribution of water in the body is usually described in terms of its location. There are two main water "compartments." One is *intracellular*, referring to fluid inside each cell. The other compartment is *extracellular*, referring to the fluids outside the cells. These include the fluids that make up the plasma of blood and lymph, and a variety of other fluids like saliva, fluids in the eyes, fluids secreted by glands and the intestines, fluids that bathe the nerves of the spinal cord, and fluids excreted from the skin and kidneys. Of the total body water, about 62% is intracellular and 38% is extracellular.

NORMAL WATER BALANCE IN THE BODY

Because a delicate balance is maintained between the body's water intake (gain of water) and water output (loss of water), its water content remains fairly stable from day to day and from month to month (Fig. 1-9).

Water Intake

The water needs of the body are supplied from three sources: (1) from fluids, (2) in foods, and (3) during metabolism.

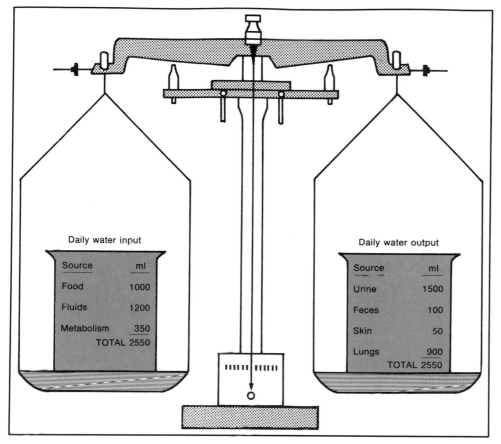

Daily water input	
Source	ml
Food	1000
Fluids	1200
Metabolism	350
TOTAL	2550

Daily water output	
Source	ml
Urine	1500
Feces	100
Skin	50
Lungs	900
TOTAL	2550

Figure 1-9. *Water balance in humans. (McArdle, W.D., Katch, F. I., and Katch, V. L.: Exercise Physiology, Lea & Febiger, 1981.)*

FROM FLUIDS   This source includes the normal intake of drinking water as well as the water contained in beverages and soups. The adult fluid intake ranges from about 800 to 1600 ml of water each day, with an average of approximately 1200 ml. This amount will vary considerably under certain conditions, especially during exercise and thermal stress, where fluid intake can increase 5 or 6 times above normal. One of the more interesting examples of fluid depletion occurred during a 2-day, 17-hour run across Death Valley, California. A highly conditioned runner ran 55 miles of the 110-mile distance in 125°F heat. The runner lost 30 pounds in body weight during the 2 days. However, with the fluid replacement (salt solution and glucose, including soft drinks and fruit juices), the final body weight loss was only 3 pounds. In terms of fluid depletion, the runner had lost between 3½ and 4 gallons of fluid.

IN FOODS   The second source of water is food, especially fruits and vegetables which have a surprisingly large water content. On the other hand the amount of water contained in honey, candy, and butter is relatively low.

DURING METABOLISM   This is the water produced during energy-yielding chemical reactions. For example, when a molecule of sugar is metabolized, energy is released and carbon dioxide and water are produced. The metabolism of 100 g of carbohydrate produces 55 g of water, while 100 g of protein and fat yields 42 and 107 g of water, respectively.

Water Output

There are four ways in which water is lost from the body: (1) in urine, (2) through the skin, (3) as water vapor in expired air, and (4) in feces.

IN URINE   Urine is formed in the kidneys, the two organs located toward the back in the lower abdominal area. The major function of the kidneys is to filter the fluid of the blood and reabsorb essential nutrient materials—such as proteins, minerals, and electrolytes—that otherwise would be lost in the urine. Urine is approximately 96% water. Under normal conditions, urine is continuously formed in the kidneys and is passed to the bladder for storage at the rate of about 1 milliliter per minute. For an adult, the volume of urine excreted each day ranges from 1000 to 1500 ml (about 1 to 1½ quarts). This volume will vary considerably, however, depending on such factors as temperature, humidity, fluid intake, diet, and level of physical activity.

THROUGH THE SKIN   Water is lost through the skin in the form of sweat produced from specialized glands. These sweat glands are very small structures located beneath the skin, and are primarily found on the palms of the hands, soles of the feet, forehead, and underneath the arms. The body's capacity for sweat production is demonstrated by the fact that there are about 3000 individual sweat glands in 1 square inch of skin on the palm. In total there are about 2.5 million sweat glands distributed throughout the surface of the body. Under normal environmental conditions (not too hot, cold, or humid) approximately 500 to 700 ml of sweat are secreted each day. The volume of sweat secreted through the skin increases dramatically during exercise to help dissipate heat that builds up in the muscles from the energy-producing metabolic reactions.

When the sweat comes into contact with the skin, a cooling effect occurs *only* as the sweat evaporates. The cooled skin in turn serves to cool the blood which has been shunted from the interior toward the surface of the body. The evaporative cooling effect can be demonstrated by placing a few drops of rubbing alcohol on the skin. Because alcohol evaporates more rapidly than water or sweat, the cooling sensation is more pronounced. The process of sweat production and subsequent evaporation provides a refrigeration mechanism to help cool the body and keep body temperature from rising too high. From 8 to 12 liters, or about 25 pounds, of sweat can be produced during prolonged exercise performed in a hot, humid environment. Marathon runners frequently experience fluid losses in excess of 6 quarts (10 to 12 lbs) during competition, a loss that represents between 6 to 10% of body weight.

The relative humidity of the surrounding air is an important factor affecting the efficiency of the sweating mechanism in temperature regulation. The term *relative humidity* refers to the water content of the air. During conditions of 100% relative humidity, the air is completely saturated with water vapor. Thus evaporation of fluid from the skin to the air is impossible and this important avenue for body cooling is closed. Under such conditions sweat beads on the skin and eventually rolls off. On the other hand, on a dry day the air can hold considerable moisture, the evaporation of fluid from the skin is quite rapid, and body temperature is more easily controlled.

AS WATER VAPOR   Small droplets of water are contained in the expired air during each breath. As a result about 250 to 300 ml of water are eliminated daily as a result of breathing. In furry animals who cannot make use of evaporative cooling from the skin, the evaporation of water from the respiratory passages provides the important means of temperature regulation. This evaporative cooling effect can be increased considerably in these animals by means of the rapid, shallow breathing called *panting*.

IN FECES   Approximately 70% of fecal matter is composed of water, the remainder being nondigestible material, bacteria from the digestive process, and the residues of digestive juices from the intestines, stomach, and pancreas. The daily amount of water eliminated in feces is about 100 ml. Under abnormal conditions like diarrhea or vomiting, water losses may be considerable, ranging from 1500 to 5000 ml.

WATER REPLACEMENT

The most serious consequence of profuse sweating is the loss of body water. The amount of water lost through sweating depends on the severity of physical activity as well as on the environmental temperature and humidity. The most effective defense against the heat is adequate hydration, which is achieved by balancing water loss with water intake.

Adequacy of Rehydration

Changes in body weight before and after exercise should be used to indicate water loss in exercise and the adequacy of rehydration during the subsequent exercise. Coaches often have their athletes "weigh-in" before and after practice and insist that weight loss be minimized by periodic water breaks during activity. In fact, if rehydration were left entirely to the person's thirst, it could take several days to reestablish fluid balance, even after severe dehydration!

Practical Recommendations for Fluid Replacement

Ingestion of "extra" water prior to exercise in the heat provides some protection because it increases sweating during exercise and brings about a significant decrease in body temperature. In this regard, it would be wise to consume 400 to 600 ml (13 to 20 oz) of water 10 to 20 minutes before exercising in the heat. This procedure, however, does not eliminate the need for continual fluid replacement *during* the exercise. A volume of about 250 ml (8.5 oz) ingested at 10- to 15-minute intervals is probably a realistic goal because larger volumes tend to produce feelings of a "full stomach."

Studies of fluid absorption indicate that cold fluids (5°C; 41°F) are emptied from the stomach at a *significantly faster rate* than fluids at body temperature. Of considerable importance is the observation that gastric emptying is retarded when the ingested fluid contains sugar, whether in the form of glucose, fructose, or sucrose! With intense exercise, even a small amount of carbohydrate blocks fluid movement from the stomach into the intestinal tract. From a practical standpoint, during exercise in the heat, when the need for water greatly exceeds the need for carbohydrate supplementation, glucose in solution hinders water replenishment. Certainly, drinking commercial preparations such as Gatorade, Instant Replay, or Take-Five which contain 5% glucose, would significantly *retard* the replacement of lost fluid during exercise in the heat. In terms of survival, fluid replacement is *primary* during prolonged exercise in the heat.

Summary

The three major categories of foods are composed of the organic elements carbon, hydrogen, and oxygen. The addition of a fourth element, nitrogen, distinguishes the proteins from carbohydrates and fats. These nutrients differ in form and structure depending on the way their atoms are linked or bonded together. In the carbohydrate molecule, atoms of hydrogen and oxygen are bonded to a chain of 6 carbon atoms in a ratio of 2 hydrogen and 1 oxygen for every carbon. Essentially, the more complex carbohydrates, such as starch and the body's carbohydrate store, glycogen, are formed by the union of numerous simple sugar molecules like glucose. In the body, carbohydrates function as fuel to power the vital functions of all cells. This food is manufactured in plants and consumed in the diet in the form of cereals, fruits, potatoes, and breads. With fat, relatively large numbers of carbon and hydrogen atoms are packed within the molecule, with only a small number of oxygen atoms. As with carbohydrates, a major function of dietary fat is to supply energy. This energy is especially important during long-term exercise when the available stores of carbohydrates (glycogen) are reduced. However, various forms of fat serve additional important biologic and health-related functions. These include blood clotting, hormone synthesis, the protection of vital organs, insulation, and the transport of four important vitamins. Fats are found in meats, fish, poultry, and numerous plants; the greatest portion of fat in the American diet comes from animal sources.

Protein is crucial to the normal growth and function of the body, although the energy derived from this food is minimal in relation to the body's total energy needs, even during a vigorous and prolonged activity such as marathon running. Protein compounds make up the contractile elements of the muscle fiber. Other proteins provide structural integrity to bones, skin, and the membranes surrounding cells, as well as to the specific structures within cells, while other protein compounds provide the basic materials for synthesizing hormones, enzymes, and the oxygen-carrying compounds contained within the blood and muscles. The protein within animal and plant cells provides the crucial amino acid building blocks necessary for constructing the body's life-sustaining compounds.

Vitamins are relatively simple organic compounds needed in minute quantities if the normal operation of the body is to proceed smoothly. These substances serve as crucial links in many metabolic reactions. A vitamin deficiency over a period of time can cause serious symptoms, including a variety of skin defects, night blindness, stunted growth, bleeding, metabolic disorders, and eventually death. Vitamins are usually classified according to their solubility; vitamins A, D, E, and K are soluble in fats and oils and vitamins B-complex and C are soluble in water. Generally, eating a balanced diet provides adequate quantities of *all* vitamins. This requirement does not appear to be increased with exercise.

About 4% of a person's body weight is composed of a group of 22 metallic elements called minerals. These minerals form integral parts of hormones, enzymes, and vitamins as well as providing the major hardening constituents of bones and teeth. Minerals provide for the movement of adequate water between the fluid compartments of the body and are also responsible for the development of electrical gradients across membranes of nerves to permit neural communication. The mineral iron is a crucial constituent of the oxygen-carrying compound hemoglobin and also, with the mineral copper, serves important functions in the metabolic reactions that generate energy within the cells. As is the case with vitamins, adequate mineral intake is assured with a well-balanced diet. In most cases the minerals lost through sweating can be replaced in the diet and specific supplementation is not required.

Water provides the medium in which all the body processes occur. A delicate balance in the volume and salinity of body fluids is maintained through the regulation of thirst and the output of urine by the kidneys. Normally, an adult drinks about 1.2 liters of water each day. In warm environments, however, water is lost in sweat, requiring an increase in fluid intake. This is especially critical during exercise performed in hot, humid environments where the quantity of fluid lost through sweating can increase to one liter an hour or more. Under these conditions, if adequate water is not replenished, the body's ability to regulate temperature will fail and serious injury or death will occur. Cool, plain water, consumed both prior to and at frequent intervals during exercise, is the most effective defense against dehydration.

2

Optimal Nutrition for Exercise and Sport

A**N OPTIMAL** *diet may be defined as one in which the supply of required nutrients is adequate for tissue maintenance, repair and growth.* The general consensus among nutritionists is that active, exercising men and women do *not* require additional nutrients beyond those obtained in a balanced diet. For example, people who eat well-balanced meals of meats, cereals, vegetables, fruits, and milk consume more than an adequate supply of vitamins to meet daily needs. Because vitamins can be used repeatedly in metabolic reactions, the vitamin needs of athletes and other active people are generally no greater than the requirements of sedentary people. Also, as the level of energy expenditure increases significantly, the amount of food required increases in order to maintain body weight. Competitive marathon runners, for example, will consume as much as 5,000 calories daily simply to supply the energy required for their daily training. This increase in food intake in itself will usually increase the intake of vitamins and minerals provided the person maintains a well-balanced diet. *In essence, sound nutrition for an active person is sound human nutrition.* The extra calories required for exercise can be obtained from a variety of nutritious foods of the individual's choice. However, sound nutritional guidelines must be followed in planning and evaluating food intake.

Recommended Nutrient Intake

Figure 2-1 illustrates the caloric contributions of the major food components in a balanced diet recommended for active people.

PROTEIN

As we discussed in Chapter 1, the standard recommendation for protein intake is 0.8 g of protein per kg of body weight. This amounts to approximately 12%

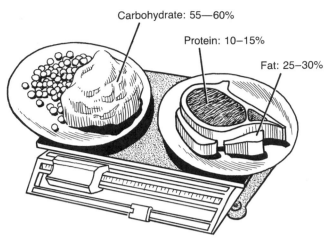

Carbohydrate: 55—60%

Protein: 10–15%

Fat: 25–30%

Figure 2-1. *Recommended caloric contributions of major food components in a balanced diet for active men and women.*

of the total calories in the average American diet. A person who weighs 170 lb (77.1 kg) would therefore require about 62 g or 2.19 oz of protein daily.

The average American consumes more than twice the protein requirement. For athletes, many of whom consume considerable quantities of food, the diet may contain more than three times the protein requirement! There is no benefit from eating excessive protein. Muscle mass is *not* increased simply by eating high-protein foods. Additional calories in the form of protein are converted to fat and stored in the subcutaneous depots. In fact, excessive protein may be harmful because the metabolism of large quantities of this nutrient may place an inordinate strain on liver and renal function.

FAT

Standards for optimal fat intake have not been firmly established because relatively little is known about the human requirement for this nutrient. The amount of dietary fat varies widely according to personal taste, money spent on food, and the availability of fat-rich foods. For example, only about 10% of the energy in the average diet of people living in Asia is furnished by fat, whereas in the United States, Canada, Scandinavia, Germany, and France, fat accounts for 40 to 50% of the caloric intake. Many nutritionists believe that in order to promote optimal health, fat intake should not exceed more than 30% of the energy content of the diet. Of this, at least 50% should be in the form of unsaturated fats. Even this quantity of dietary fat may be too high, especially for individuals suffering from gallbladder disease and certain diseases of the cardiovascular system.

To attempt to eliminate "all" fat from the diet, however, may be unwise and detrimental in terms of exercise performance. With low-fat diets, it is difficult to increase one's intake of carbohydrate and protein to furnish sufficient energy to maintain a stable body weight during strenuous training. Also, because the major essential fatty acid, *linoleic acid*, and many vitamins gain entrance to the body through dietary fat, a "fat free" diet could eventually result in a relative state of malnutrition.

CARBOHYDRATE

At this time it is difficult to state precisely how much carbohydrate should be consumed in the diet. Like fat, the prominence of carbohydrates in the diet varies widely throughout the world, depending upon factors such as the availability and relative cost of fat and protein-rich foods. Carbohydrate-rich foods such as grains, starchy roots, and dried peas and beans are usually the cheapest foods in relation to their energy value. In the Far East, carbohydrates (rice) contribute 80% of the total caloric intake, whereas in the United States only about 40 to 50% of the energy requirement comes from carbohydrates. For a sedentary 70 kg person, for example, this amounts to approximately 147 g of carbohydrate per day.

Most evidence suggests that there is no health hazard in subsisting chiefly on carbohydrates (starches), provided that the essential amino acids, minerals, and vitamins are also present in the diet. In fact, the diet of the relatively primitive Tarahumara Indians of Mexico is high in complex carbohydrates (75% of calories) and fiber (19 mg/day) and correspondingly low in cholesterol (71 mg/day), fat (12% of calories), and saturated fat (2% of calories). These people are noted for their remarkable physical endurance; they reportedly run distances of up to 200 miles in competitive soccer-type sports events that often last several days! This type of diet may offer health benefits to those who partake of it. Particularly notable among the Tarahumaras is the virtual absence of hypertension, obesity, and death from cardiac and circulatory complications.

If the individual is physically active, the "prudent" diet should contain at least 50 to 60% of its calories in the form of carbohydrates, predominantly starches. In training for specific sports and prior to competition, the carbohydrate intake may even be increased above this recommended level to ensure adequate glycogen stores. The specific dietary-exercise techniques for facilitating glycogen storage will be discussed in a following section.

The Four-Food-Group Plan: The Essentials of Good Nutrition

A practical approach to sound nutrition is to categorize foods that make similar nutrient contributions and then provide servings from each category in the daily diet. A key word is *variety*. This can be readily achieved by use of the *Four-Food-Group Plan* (Table 2-1). As long as the recommended number of servings from the variety provided in each group is supplied, and cooking and handling are proper, adequate nutrition is assured. More of these and other foods can be used as needed for growth, for activity, and for desirable weight. For those individuals on meatless diets, a small amount of milk, milk products, or eggs should be included because vitamin B_{12} is only available in foods of animal origin. In fact, if milk and

Table 2-1. *The Four-Food-Group Plan—the foundation for a good diet. (McArdle, W.D., Katch, F.I. and Katch, V.L.: Exercise Physiology, Lea & Febiger, 1981)*

FOOD CATEGORY	EXAMPLES	RECOMMENDED DAILY SERVINGS[c]
1. Milk and milk products[a]	Milk, cheese, ice cream, sour cream, yogurt	2
2. Meat and high-protein[b]	meat, fish, poultry, eggs—with dried beans, peas, nuts, or peanut butter as alternatives	2
3. Vegetables and fruits	Dark green or yellow vegetables; citrus fruits or tomatoes	4
4. Cereal and grain food	Enriched breads, cereals, flour, baked goods, or whole-grain products	4

[a] If large quantities of milk are normally consumed, *fortified* skimmed milk should be substituted to reduce the quantity of saturated fats.

[b] Fish, chicken, and high-protein vegetables contain significantly less saturated fats than other protein sources.

[c] A basic serving of meat or fish is usually 100 g or 3.5 oz of edible food; 1 cup (8 oz) milk; 1 oz cheese; ½ cup fruit, vegetables, juice; 1 slice bread; ½ cup cooked cereal or 1 cup ready-to-eat cereal.

eggs are included in a vegetarian diet ("lacto-ovovegetarian" diet), nutritional quality will be every bit as good as the typical recommended diet that contains meat, fish, and poultry.

The Four-Food-Group Plan guidelines provide for the necessary vitamin, mineral, and protein requirements even though the energy content of this food intake amounts to only about 1200 calories per day. In terms of average values for adult Americans, the total daily energy requirement is about 2100 and 2700 calories for women and men, respectively. *Thus, once the basic nutrient requirements are met, the extra energy needs of the active person can be supplied from a variety of food sources based on individual preference.*

Table 2-2 presents examples of three daily menus formulated from the guidelines of the basic diet plan shown in Table 2-1. These menus provide *all* essential nutrients, even though the energy value of each is considerably below the average adult requirement. In fact, these menus serve as excellent nutritional models for reducing diets. For active individual whose daily energy requirements may be as large as 5000 calories, all that need be done once the essentials are provided is to increase the quantity of food consumed; this is achieved either by increasing the size of portions, the frequency of meals or snacks, or the variety of nutritious food consumed at each meal.

Table 2-2. *Four daily menus formulated from guidelines established by the Four-Food-Group Plan[a]. (McArdle, W.D., Katch, F.I. and Katch, V.L.: Exercise Physiology, Lea & Febiger, 1981.)*

3 MEALS A DAY	5 MEALS A DAY	6 SMALL MEALS A DAY	3 MEALS, 3 SNACKS
Breakfast	**Breakfast**	**Breakfast**	**Breakfast**
½ cup unsweetened grapefruit juice	½ grapefruit	½ cup orange juice	½ small grapefruit
1 poached egg 1 slice toast	⅔ cup bran flakes	¾ cup ready-to-eat cereal	1 cup cereal, such as Wheaties
1 teaspoon butter or margarine	1 cup skim or low-fat milk or	½ cup skim milk	1 cup skim milk
½ cup skim milk	other beverage	tea or coffee, black	3 teaspoons sugar
tea or coffee, black			2 slices toast
	Snack	**Mid-Morning Snack**	2 pats butter
Lunch	1 small package raisins	⅓ cup low fat cottage cheese	1 tablespoon jelly, coffee or
2 ounces lean roast beef*	½ bologna sandwich		tea
½ cup cooked summer squash		**Lunch**	
1 slice rye bread	**Lunch**	2 ounces sliced turkey on	**Lunch**
1 teaspoon butter or margarine	1 slice pizza	1 slice white toast	3 ounces hamburger*
1 cup skim milk	carrot sticks	1 teaspoon butter or margarine	1 bun
10 grapes	1 apple	2 canned drained peach halves	slice lettuce & tomato
	1 cup skim or low-fat milk	½ cup skim milk	20 french fries
Dinner			1 medium banana
3 ounces poached haddock*	**Snack**	**Mid-Afternoon Snack**	1 cup milk
½ cup cooked spinach	1 banana	1 cup fresh spinach and lettuce salad	
tomato and lettuce salad		2 teaspoons oil + vinegar or lemon	**Dinner**
1 teaspoon oil + vinegar or lemon	**Dinner**	3 saltines	6 ounces baked chicken (no skin)*
1 small biscuit	baked fish with		1 medium baked potato
1 teaspoon butter or margarine	mushrooms (3 oz.)*	**Dinner**	½ cup cooked carrots
½ cup canned drained	baked potato	1 cup clear broth	2 dinner rolls
fruit cocktail	2 teaspoons margarine	3 ounces broiled chicken breast*	2 pats butter
½ cup skim milk	½ cup broccoli	⅓ cup cooked rice with	1 cup fresh fruit cup
	1 cup tomato juice or skim or	1 teaspoon butter or margarine	1 cup milk
	low-fat milk	¼ cup cooked mushrooms	coffee or tea
		½ cup cooked broccoli	
		½ cup skim milk	**Snacks:** (morning,
			afternoon, evening)
		Evening Snack	1 sweet roll or doughnut
		1 medium apple	1 cup fruit juice
		½ cup skim milk	sandwich
			2 slices bread, whole wheat
			1 slice ham
			mustard
			1 cup milk
Total Calories: about 1200	Total Calories: about 1400	Total Calories: about 1200	Total Calories: about 3000[b]

*Cooked weight.

[a]Each menu provides *all* essential nutrients; the energy or caloric value of the diet can be easily increased by increasing the size of the portions, the frequency of meals, or the variety of foods consumed at each sitting.

[b]3000 kcal diet from *Food in Training*, General Mills, Inc., Minneapolis.

Computerized Meal Plans

Nutritionists and exercise specialists have applied computer technology in the formulation of well-balanced meals and exercise programs for weight control. The formulation of daily menus is based on the Four Food Group Plan and dietary exchange method developed by the American Dietetic Association. Rather than prescribing a particular food plan, the computerized dietary plan allows the person to select the *specific* foods he or she will eat from a basic list of the most common foods. Combined with age, weight, height, weight loss desired, and current level of physical activity, the computer prepares three nutritious meals for breakfast, lunch, and dinner for a 14-day period. The menu varies from day to day. The meals are balanced for nutrient intake of carbohydrate, fat, protein, vitamins and minerals and are designed so the individual can reduce excess weight (fat) at a safe but steady level. The 15-18 page printout includes a weight loss curve, daily meal plans, and a beginner, intermediate, or advanced aerobic walk/jog/run, cycle, or swim program. Appendix C shows examples of the nutrition and exercise computer printout, as well as the questionnaire which can be completed and mailed for your own personal use.

Diet and Endurance Performance

The specific nutrient fuel for muscular contraction depends not only on exercise intensity, but also on the duration of the activity and, to some degree, on the diet of the individual. During continuous, moderate exercise the energy for muscular contraction is provided predominantly from the body's fat and carbohydrate reserves. If this exercise continues and glycogen stores in the liver and muscles are reduced, an even greater percentage of the energy for exercise must be supplied by the breakdown of fat. This food nutrient is mobilized from storage sites such as adipose tissue and the liver and delivered via the circulation to the working muscles. However, if exercise is performed to the point where the glycogen stored in specific muscles is severely lowered, the performer may tire easily. Interestingly, however, glycogen is reduced only in the muscles that are actively involved in performing the exercise. Because enzymes are not present to aid the transfer of glycogen between muscles, the relatively inactive muscles retain their glycogen supply.

Fatigue can occur during prolonged exercise even though sufficient oxygen is available to the muscles and the potential energy from stored fat remains almost unlimited. This is because the relatively small amount of glycogen stored in the muscles becomes depleted. If a solution of glucose and water is ingested at the point of fatigue, exercise may be prolonged for an additional period of time, but for all practical purposes the muscles' "fuel tank" will read empty and continued energy production is severely limited.

CARBOHYDRATE NEEDS IN INTENSE TRAINING

Strenuous endurance training for activities such as distance running, swimming, cross-country skiing, or cycling can bring on a state of fatigue in which successive days of hard training become exceedingly more difficult. This "staleness" may be related to gradual depletion of the body's carbohydrate reserves with repeated strenuous training, even though the person's diet contains the recommended percentage of carbohydrate. As shown in Figure 2-2, after three successive days of running 16.1 km (10 miles) a day, the glycogen in the thigh muscle was nearly depleted. This occurred despite the fact that the runners' daily food intake contained 40 to 60% carbohydrates. In addition, by the third day, the quantity of glycogen used during the run was much less than on the first day with the energy for work being supplied predominantly by the body's fat reserves.

Even if the diet is high in carbohydrates, muscle glycogen is not rapidly restored to the preexercise level. Although liver glycogen is restored rapidly, at least 48 hours are required to restore muscle glycogen levels after prolonged, exhaustive exercise. From the values in Figure 2-2, some individuals may require more than 5 days to reestablish muscle glycogen levels if the diet contains only moderate amounts of carbohydrates. Unmistakably, if a person performs long-term, strenuous exercise on successive days, daily allowances must be adjusted to permit optimal glycogen resynthesis. In addition, *at least 2 days of rest and high carbohydrate intake must be provided to establish the preexercise muscle glycogen levels.*

DIET, GLYCOGEN STORES, AND ENDURANCE

In the late 1930s scientists observed that endurance performance was markedly improved simply by consuming a carbohydrate-rich diet for 3 days. Con-

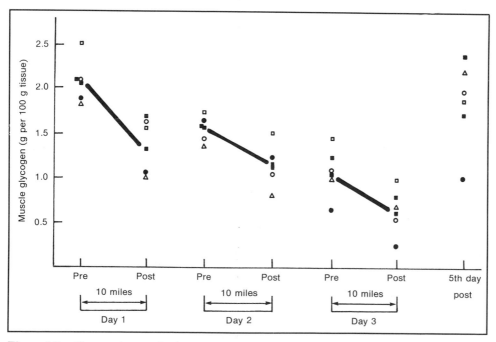

Figure 2-2. *Changes in muscle glycogen concentration for 6 male subjects before and after each 16.1-km run performed on 3 successive days. Muscle glycogen was measured 5 days after the last run and is referred to as "fifth day post." (From Costill, D.L. et al.: Muscle glycogen utilization during prolonged exercise on successive days. J. Appl. Physiol., 31:835, 1971.)*

versely, if the diet consisted predominantly of fat, endurance capability was drastically reduced. Because of this important relationship between diet and physical performance, researchers have evaluated several possible ways of increasing the glycogen content of muscle. In one series of experiments subjects consumed three different diets. One diet maintained the normal caloric intake but supplied the major quantity of calories in the form of fat. The second diet was normal and contained the recommended daily percentages of carbohydrates, fats, and proteins. The third diet provided 82% of the calories in the form of carbohydrates. The results showed that the glycogen content sampled from the leg muscles of subjects fed the high-fat diet, the normal diet, and the high-carbohydrate diet averaged 0.6, 1.75, and 3.75 g of glycogen per 100 g of muscle, respectively. In addition, the endurance capacity of the subjects varied considerably depending on the diet each consumed in the days prior to the endurance test. The endurance capacity of the subjects fed the high-carbohydrate diet was more than three times greater than the endurance capacity of these same subjects on the high-fat diet. Clearly, these findings emphasize the important role of nutrition in establishing the appropriate energy reserves. A simple modification of the diet can alter significantly the body's stores of carbohydrates, as well as effect subsequent performance in prolonged submaximal exercise. These observations are especially important not only for the endurance athlete but also for people who have modified their diets so that the normal, recommended percentage of carbohydrates is reduced.

Reliance on starvation diets or on other potentially harmful diets such as high-fat, low-carbohydrate diets, "liquid-protein" diets, or water diets, is counterproductive for weight control, exercise performance, optimal nutrition, and good health. *Such low carbohydrate diets make it extremely difficult from the standpoint of energy supply to participate in vigorous physical activity or training.*

Carbohydrate Loading: A Way to Increase Glycogen Reserves

Research has shown that a particular combination of diet and exercise can result in a significant "packing" of muscle glycogen. This procedure is termed *carbohydrate loading* and is commonly "in vogue" among endurance athletes. The end result of this specific dietary modification is an even greater increase in muscle glycogen than would occur with a carbohydrate-rich diet. This procedure outlined in Table 2-3 is accomplished as follows: First reduce the glycogen stores with a period of relatively long, moderate, continuous, exercise. Second, deplete muscle glycogen further by maintaining a high-fat diet for several days while continuing an exercise program. Third, reduce the activity level for the next several days and at the same time switch to a carbohydrate-rich diet. The muscle glycogen will increase to a new, higher level. Of course, adequate daily protein, minerals and vitamins, and abundant water must also be part of the daily diet.

Because glycogen supercompensation occurs *only* in those specific muscles exercised, the person must engage the muscles involved in his or her sport. In preparation for a marathon, a 15- or 20-mile run is usually necessary, whereas for

Table 2-3. *Two-stage dietary plan for increasing muscle glycogen storage. (McArdle, W.D., Katch, F.I. and Katch, V.L.: Exercise Physiology, Lea & Febiger, 1981.)*

Stage 1—Depletion

> Day 1: Exhausting exercise performed to deplete muscle glycogen in specific muscles

> Days 2, 3, 4: Low carbohydrate food intake (high percentage of protein and fat in the daily diet)

Stage 2—Carbohydrate Loading

> Days 5, 6, 7: High carbohydrate food intake (normal percentage of protein and fat in the daily diet)

Competition Day

> Follow high-carbohydrate pre-event meal

swimming and bicycling, moderately intense submaximal exercise, also for 90 minutes, is required.

The combination of diet and exercise to produce glycogen packing or "supercompensation" should be of considerable interest to the endurance athlete, especially the marathon runner and long distance swimmer, whose success depends in part on the magnitude of the body's carbohydrate reserves. *However, for those who are not endurance athletes, normal levels of muscle glycogen are more than adequate to provide the energy to sustain exercise.* Normal levels of glycogen can be assured by ingesting approximately 50 to 60% of the daily caloric intake as carbohydrates. If the energy demands of daily exercise are high, as in an intensive exercise-training program, increase the carbohydrate content of the diet. Many endurance athletes consume so-called spaghetti and rice diets to achieve a high level of carbohydrate intake. A week before the actual competition, they use the preceding three-step exercise and dietary modification program to assure the desired glycogen supercompensation.

It should be noted that the wisdom of repeated bouts of carbohydrate loading has yet to be verified. A severe carbohydrate overload interspersed with periods of high fat or protein intake could pose problems to people susceptible to adult diabetes or heart or kidney disease.

SAMPLE DIETS FOR CARBOHYDRATE LOADING

Table 2-4 provides an example of meal plans that can be used during carbohydrate depletion (stage 1) and carbohydrate loading (stage 2) preceding the endurance event.

The Precompetition Meal

The main purpose of the precompetition or pregame meal is to provide the athlete with adequate food energy and assure optimal hydration. As a general rule, foods that are high in fat content should be eliminated from the diet on the day of competition because these foods are digested slowly and remain in the digestive tract for a longer time than foods containing similar amounts of energy in the form of carbohydrates.

The time at which the precompetition meal is eaten does not appear to be an important consideration, at least in terms of exercise performance. However, because the main function of the pregame meal is to provide food energy and water,

Table 2-4. *Sample meal plan for carbohydrate depletion and carbohydrate loading diets preceding the endurance event.*[a] *(McArdle W.D., Katch, F.I. and Katch, V.L: Exercise Physiology, Lea & Febiger, 1981.)*

MEAL	STAGE 1 DEPLETION	STAGE 2 CARBOHYDRATE LOADING
Breakfast:	½ cup fruit juice 2 eggs 1 slice whole-wheat toast 1 glass whole milk	1 cup fruit juice, hot or cold cereal 1 to 2 muffins 1 tbsp. butter coffee (cream/sugar)
Lunch:	6-oz hamburger* 2 slices bread salad 1 tbsp. mayonnaise & salad dressing 1 glass whole milk	2–3-oz hamburger* with bun 1 cup juice 1 orange 1 tbsp. mayonnaise pie or cake
Snack:	1 cup yogurt	1 cup yogurt, fruit or cookies
Dinner:	2 to 3 pieces chicken, fried 1 baked potato with sour cream ½ cup vegetable iced tea (no sugar) 2 tbsp. butter	1–1 ½ pieces chicken, baked 1 baked potato with sour cream 1 cup vegetable ½ cup sweetened pineapple iced tea (sugar) 1 tbsp. butter
Snack:	1 glass whole milk	1 glass chocolate milk with 4 cookies

*Cooked weight
[a]During stage 1, the intake of carbohydrate is approximately 100 grams or 400 calories; in stage 2, the carbohydrate intake is increased to 400 to 625 grams or about 1600 to 2500 calories.

a 3-hour period should be allowed for the meal to be digested and absorbed by the body.

43
*Optimal
Nutrition for
Exercise
and Sport*

Many athletes are psychologically accustomed and even dependent on the "classic" pregame meal, which usually consists of steak and eggs. Although this meal may be satisfying to the athlete, coach, and restauranteur, its benefits in terms of exercise performance have yet to be demonstrated. In fact, such a meal, which is actually low in carbohydrates, may be detrimental to optimal performance. For one thing, carbohydrates are digested and absorbed more rapidly than either proteins or fats. Thus, this food is available for energy faster and may also reduce the feeling of fullness following a meal. Furthermore, a high-protein meal elevates the resting metabolism more than a high-carbohydrate meal. This heat places an additional strain on the body's temperature-regulating ability which could be detrimental to exercise performance in hot weather. Concurrently, the breakdown of protein for energy facilitates dehydration because the by-products of amino acid breakdown demand large amounts of water for urinary excretion.

Equally important for favoring carbohydrate intake is the fact that this is the main nutrient energy source for intense exercise and is also of crucial importance in prolonged exercise. The precompetition meal must provide adequate quantities of this nutrient, to assure a normal level of blood glucose and sufficient glycogen "energy reserves" for most activities, *provided that the person has maintained a nutritionally sound diet throughout training.*

Summary

Many dietary options are available for obtaining the required nutrients for tissue maintenance, repair, and growth. Within rather broad limits, the nutrient requirements of active individuals engaged in training programs can be achieved with a balanced diet. With well-planned menus, the necessary vitamin, mineral, and protein requirements can be achieved with a food intake of about 1200 calories a day. Additional food can then be consumed to meet the energy needs that fluctuate, depending on the daily level of physical activity. The use of a computer to prepare nutritious meals, based on individual food choices, can play an important role in weight management and dietary control programs designed to reduce excess body fat.

The recommended protein intake is 0.8 g of protein per kg of body weight. For the average man and woman, this is a liberal requirement and represents about 12 to 15% of the daily total caloric intake. Athletes generally consume three times the recommended protein intake. This is because the proportionately greater caloric intake of physically active people usually provides proportionately more protein.

Precise recommendations for fat and carbohydrate intake have not been established. A prudent recommendation is that 25 to 30% of the daily calories be obtained from fats; of this, at least 70% should be in the form of unsaturated fatty acids because excessive intake of saturated fats is related to various diseases, especially coronary heart disease. For people who are physically active, 50 to 60% of the calories should come from carbohydrates, particularly unrefined complex carbohydrates. Successive days of prolonged, hard training may gradually deplete the body's carbohydrate reserves, even if the recommended carbohydrate intake is maintained. This could lead to a training "staleness" because muscle glycogen may take several days to return to normal levels following a single session of prolonged exercise.

The precompetition meal should include foods that are readily digested and contribute to the energy and fluid requirements of exercise. For this reason, the meal should be high in carbohydrate and relatively low in fat and protein. Clearly, the typical low-carbohydrate "steak-and-eggs diet" does not meet the requirements for optimal pre-event nutrition. Two or three hours should be sufficient time to permit digestion and absorption of the pre-event meal.

3

Energy Systems for Exercise

Part 1.   Energy for Exercise

N AN AUTOMOBILE ENGINE, the proper mixture of gasoline with oxygen ignites to provide the necessary energy to drive the pistons. Various gears and linkages harness this energy to turn the wheels. *Within this framework energy can be viewed as the capacity or ability to do work.* Increasing or decreasing the energy supply either slows down or speeds up the engine. Similarly, the human body must continuously be supplied with its own form of energy to perform its many complex functions. Aside from the energy required for muscle contraction, people expend considerable energy for other forms of biologic work. This includes the energy required for the digestion, absorption, and assimilation of the food nutrients, for the functioning of various glands that secrete special hormones at rest and during exercise, for the establishment of the proper electrochemical gradients along the cell membrane to permit transmission of signals from the brain via the nerves to the muscles, and for the synthesis of new chemical compounds, such as the protein in muscle tissue that becomes enlarged from specialized strength training. The story of how the body maintains its continuous supply of energy begins with the energy currency, ATP.

The Energy Currency, Adenosine Triphosphate (ATP)

The cells do not use the nutrients consumed in the diet for their immediate supply of energy. Instead, an energy-rich compound called *adenosine triphosphate,* or simply *ATP,* is the "fuel" used for *all* the energy-requiring processes within the cell. In turn, the energy in food is extracted to rebuild more ATP. The potential energy stored in the ATP molecule represents chemical energy made in the body as it is needed. As discussed in Chapter 1, molecules are composed of

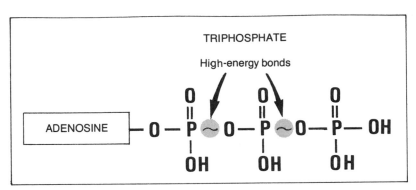

Figure 3-1. *Simplified structure of ATP, the energy currency of the cell. The symbol ~ represents the high-energy bonds.*

atoms held together by bonds. It is the breaking of these bonds that releases energy. Figure 3-1 illustrates a simplified structure of an ATP molecule.

ATP consists of one molecule of adenine and ribose, called *adenosine*, combined with three phosphates, each consisting of phosphorus and oxygen atoms. A considerable quantity of energy is stored in the ATP molecule at the bonds that link the two outermost phosphate groups with the remainder of the molecule. These bonds, symbolized ~, represent the high-energy phosphate bonds. When the outermost bond is broken, it releases an amount of energy equivalent to approximately 7000 calories. The remaining molecule with one high-energy bond is known as *adenosine diphosphate*, or *ADP*.

The energy released from the breakdown of ATP activates other energy-requiring molecules. For example, the energy from ATP is transferred to the molecules that make up the contractile elements in muscle tissue. Once activated, these elements slide past each other and cause the muscle to shorten. Because the energy released from ATP is harnessed to power *all* forms of biologic work, ATP is considered the "energy currency" of the cell (Figure 3-2).

Energy-releasing reactions that are dependent on a constant supply of oxygen are *aerobic*. For example, if the flow of oxygen through the carburetor of an automobile engine is restricted, the energy supply will be reduced and the engine will lose power and ultimately stall. This is not the case, however, with the breakdown of ATP. Instead, the ATP molecule releases its energy in the absence of oxygen. This is an *anaerobic* energy-releasing reaction. It is this capacity to provide energy anaerobically that enables the cell to generate energy for immediate use. This immediate energy would not be available if oxygen was required at all times. For this reason we can sprint for a bus, lift considerable weight without taking a breath, and survive submersion under water for more than one minute.

The Energy Reservoir, Creatine Phosphate (CP)

Although ATP serves as the energy currency for all cells, its quantity is limited. In fact, only about three ounces of ATP are stored in the body at any one time. This would provide only enough energy for running as fast as possible for several seconds. Therefore ATP must constantly be resynthesized to provide a continuous

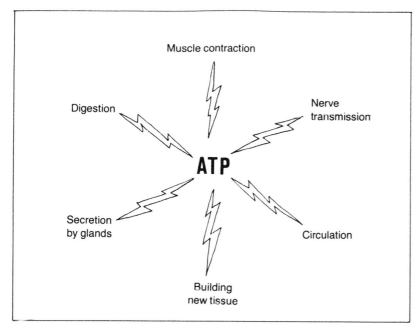

Figure 3-2. *ATP is the energy currency for all forms of biologic work.*

supply of energy. Some of the energy for ATP resynthesis is supplied directly and rapidly by the anaerobic splitting of a phosphate molecule from another energy-rich compound called *creatine phosphate,* or *CP.* This molecule is somewhat similar to ATP in that a large amount of energy is released when the bond between the creatine and phosphate molecules is split. Figure 3-3 presents a schematic illustration of the release and use of phosphate-bond energy in ATP and CP.

The arrows pointing in opposite directions indicate that the reactions are reversible. That is, creatine (C) and phosphate (P) can be joined again to form CP. The same is true for ATP, shown in the top reaction where the union of ADP and P reforms ATP. The resynthesis of ATP is possible if sufficient energy is available to rejoin an ADP molecule with one P molecule. The breakdown of CP can supply this energy, as illustrated in the bottom reaction. Cells store creatine phosphate in considerably larger quantities than ATP. Its mobilization for energy is almost instantaneous and does not require oxygen. For this reason, CP is considered the "reservoir" of high energy phosphate.

The energy released from the breakdown of the energy-rich phosphates ATP and CP will sustain all-out exercise such as running or swimming for approximately 5 to 8 seconds. In an activity like the 100-yard dash, the body cannot maintain maximum speed for longer than this. During the last few seconds of this sprint race, the runners are actually slowing down, and the winner is the one who slows down least! Thus the mobilization of energy from the phosphate pool (ATP + CP) and the size of the pool may be important factors in determining a person's ability to maintain maximum speed over a short distance.

To gain an appreciation of the relative importance of the high-energy phosphates in exercise, you need only list the activities in which short but intense bursts of energy are crucial to successful performance. Football, tennis, track and

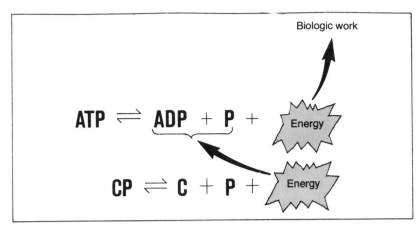

Figure 3-3. *ATP and CP are anaerobic sources of phosphate bond energy. The energy from the breakdown of CP is used to rebond ADP and P to form ATP.*

field, golf, volleyball, karate, baseball, weightlifting, and wood chopping are but a few activities that may require a maximal effort for up to 8 seconds during the performance (Figure 3-4).

In almost all sports the capacity of the ATP-CP energy system can play an important role in the success or failure of some phase of the performance. However, if the all-out effort must continue longer than eight seconds or if moderate exercise is to continue for much longer periods, an additional source of energy must be provided for the resynthesis of ATP. If this does not happen, our "fuel tanks" would read "empty" and all movement would cease. *The foods we eat and store in ready access within the body provide the energy to recharge the supply of ATP and CP.*

The identification of the predominant sources of energy required for a particular sport or activity provides the basis for an effective physiological conditioning program. If you desire an improved capacity for sustained effort such as hiking or distance swimming, it would be unprofitable to train specifically to increase the ATP-CP reserves. On the other hand, a highly conditioned ATP-CP energy system is of considerable importance in sports like football and baseball.

Energy from Food

As shown in Figure 3-5, the body extracts the potential energy stored within the structure of the carbohydrate, fat, and protein molecules consumed in the diet or stored within the body. This energy is harnessed for one major purpose—to combine ADP and phosphate to reform the energy-rich compound ATP.

A flaming steak on an open barbecue is a good illustration of the potential energy stored in food. The heat from the flame ignites the fat in the meat, causing it to suddenly release its stored energy in the form of heat. In the cells of the body, however, the energy is not released suddenly at some kindling temperature and then dissipated as heat. The energy produced by the breaking of chemical bonds is released gradually, at a constant, fairly low temperature through a series of chemical reactions controlled by special enzymes. These enzymes regulate the rate or speed at which the reactions occur by helping to bring different molecules together so they will interact and bond to one another. Thousands of such chemical reactions take place simultaneously within the cell, each governed by a specific enzyme. The end product of the breakdown of foods is the liberation of energy, approximately 40% of which is captured and stored for later use as chemical energy in the bonds of ATP. The remaining energy is dissipated in the form of heat. This is an incredible efficiency compared with machines like the steam engine, which transforms its fuel into useful energy with an efficiency of only about 30%.

ATP is made available from food in several ways. The metabolism of glucose illustrates the way the cells extract and capture the chemical energy contained in foods. This example is used for several reasons. First, carbohydrates are the *only* food that can provide energy anaerobically for the formation of ATP. During heavy, fatiguing exercise where anaerobic reactions must supply a large amount of energy rapidly, carbohydrates are the main contributor to the energy supply. Second, under conditions of rest and low to moderate levels of exercise in well-nourished individuals, carbohydrates supply between 40 and 50% of the body's energy re-

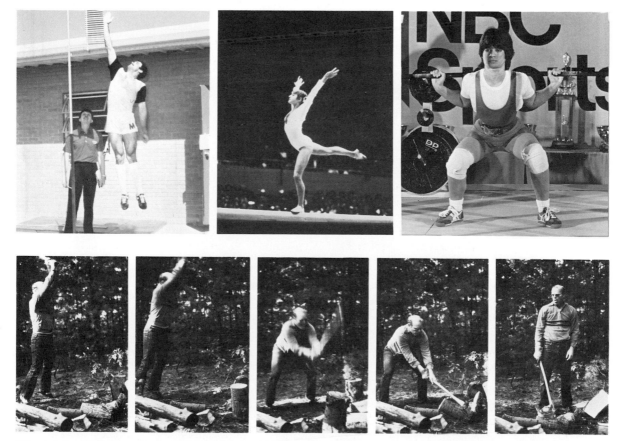

Figure 3-4. *Importance of the high energy phosphates ATP and CP during physical activity. Photo of power lifter Pam Meister. (Courtesy of Muscle and Fitness and Shape Magazines.)*

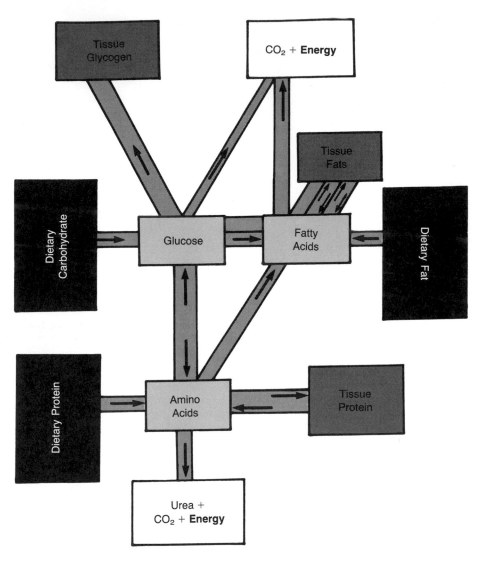

Most carbohydrates from food are hydrolyzed to glucose which can be used for energy immediately, or resynthesized to and stored as glycogen or fat. Digestion occurs primarily in the intestine from which the simple sugars are absorbed. Absorption of glucose is rapid . . . glucose being an obligatory energy source for the nervous system, and a primary energy source for tissues.

Fats are hydrolyzed to glycerol and fatty acids which can be used immediately for energy or stored as fat to be used later for energy.

Amino acids from protein are used for building and repairing body tissues . . . but only if overall energy requirements are being met with enough fat and carbohydrate. If these are lacking, protein is diverted and used for energy. Excess protein is always used for energy or converted to fat. It is important to note that certain amino acids can be converted to glucose . . . an important defense mechanism that assures the brain of sufficient glucose to keep functioning.

Figure 3-5. *An illustration of the interlocking pathways by which the body generates the energy it needs either from the foods ingested or from the body's own resources. (Modified from This Medicine Called Nutrition. Best Foods, Englewood Cliffs, N.J., 1979.)*

quirements. Third, during the breakdown of carbohydrates certain chemical compounds are formed that are necessary in order that the fat and protein food nutrients can also be broken down or metabolized to supply energy.

ANAEROBIC ENERGY FROM FOOD

When a molecule of glucose enters a cell to be used for energy, it immediately undergoes a series of chemical reactions collectively referred to as *glycolysis*. These reactions *do not* require oxygen. As the result of enzyme action, the original 6-carbon glucose molecule is transformed into two 3-carbon molecules of pyruvic acid. This breakdown of glucose to pyruvic acid occurs in the intracellular, watery medium of the cell. Three important aspects to the breakdown of glucose to pyruvic acid occur during glycolysis. First, the bonds that chemically bind the glucose molecule together are broken; second, hydrogen atoms are stripped away from the glucose molecule; and third, two new molecules of ATP are produced.

The extraction of usable energy in the form of two ATP molecules during the anaerobic reactions of glycolysis represents only about 5% of the total number of ATPs that can be produced when the glucose molecule is completely degraded to carbon dioxide and water during subsequent aerobic reactions. Nevertheless, *the ATP produced during glycolysis is important because it provides a rapid, though limited, source of energy for muscular activity.* The cells' capacity to maintain glycolysis is crucial during physical activities that require a sustained, all out effort for periods of up to about 60 seconds. The anaerobic energy from glucose can be thought of as a reserve of "rapid" food energy for the resynthesis of ATP. This energy reserve is utilized by the athlete "kicking" the last part of a 1- or 2-mile race, or the basketball team that employs a full-court press during the final minutes of a close game. In other short-duration but high-intensity activities such as a 440-yard run or 100-yard swim, the predominant supply of energy for ATP production also comes from the anaerobic reactions of glycolysis during carbohydrate metabolism.

AEROBIC ENERGY FROM FOOD

Because the anaerobic reactions of glycolysis release only about 5% of the energy contained within the glucose molecule, an additional means for extracting the remaining energy must be available. It is extracted when the pyruvic acid molecules are converted to a form of acetic acid, *acetyl Co-A*. This process releases hydrogen atoms and carbon dioxide gas. Acetyl Co-A then passes into highly specialized structures within the cell, the *mitochondria*. Think of these structures as the cell's "powerhouses," or "energy factories," where over 90% of the total ATP is produced. Figure 3-6 shows a simplified diagram of the release of hydrogen atoms during the complete breakdown of glucose. In the cell fluid, hydrogen atoms are released as the glucose molecule is degraded to pyruvic acid during glycolysis and during pyruvic acid's subsequent transformation to acetyl Co-A. In the reactions within the mitochondria, carbon and hydrogen atoms are stripped from the molecules of acetyl Co-A. As a result, 2 molecules of ATP are regenerated, 16 additional hydrogen atoms are set free, and 4 molecules of carbon dioxide gas are formed. This "metabolic mill" also extracts hydrogen from fragments of fat and protein (amino acid) metabolism in similar fashion. This aspect of the chemical breakdown of acetyl Co-A is known as the *Krebs cycle*. It was named after the chemist Hans Krebs, who was awarded the Nobel Prize in 1953 for his pioneering studies of these vital metabolic processes.

Oxygen Consumption During Exercise

Although the energy released from anaerobic metabolism is very rapid and does not require oxygen, the total amount of ATP resynthesized in this manner is relatively small. However, during the aerobic reactions of the Krebs cycle, considerable chemical energy stored in the molecules of carbohydrates, fats, and to a lesser degree in proteins can be released and used effectively to provide a constant supply of ATP. These aerobic reactions provide by far the major supply of energy to the body.

STEADY STATE

The curve in Figure 3-8 illustrates the amount of oxygen consumed by the cells of the body during each minute of a relatively slow jog continued at the same pace for 20 minutes. This usage of oxygen by the cells is referred to as *oxygen consumption*.

During the first 3 minutes there is a steep rise in the amount of oxygen consumed above the resting level. Then the curve begins to flatten out during minutes 4 and 5 and remains essentially unchanged during the last 14 minutes of jogging. The horizontal or flat part of the curve is referred to as *steady state*. This steady state or plateau in oxygen consumption represents a balance between the energy required by the working muscles and the aerobic energy-releasing reactions. The energy for steady-state exercise is generated predominantly in the slow-twitch muscle fibers. Theoretically, once a steady state is attained, exercise could go on indefinitely if the individual had the will power to continue. However, factors other

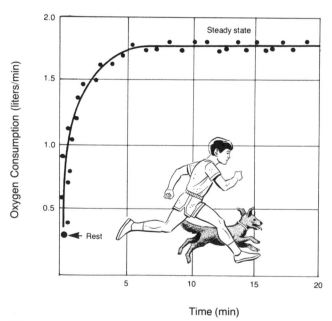

Figure 3-8. *Time course of oxygen consumption during a continuous jog at a relatively slow pace for 20 minutes.*

than motivation play an important role in determining the duration of steady-state work. These factors include the loss of important body fluids in sweat due to an increase in body temperature and the depletion of essential nutrients, especially blood glucose and glycogen stored in the liver and muscles.

There are many levels of steady state. Steady-state exercise for the athlete might be exhausting for the untrained. For some of us, lying in bed, working around the house, and playing an occasional round of golf represent the spectrum of activity for which adequate oxygen can be supplied to maintain a steady state. The champion marathon runner, on the other hand, can run 26 miles in slightly more than 2 hours and still be in steady state. This 5-minute-per-mile pace is a magnificent accomplishment from the point of view of the many physiologic functions involved. One of the most important of these functions is delivering an adequate supply of oxygen to the exercising muscles. Because the delivery and utilization of oxygen are so crucial with respect to energy metabolism, they are especially important during activities of relatively long duration. Therefore the emphasis of physiologic conditioning programs to develop endurance must be to improve the transport and utilization of oxygen. How this is accomplished is discussed in Chapter 10.

MAXIMAL OXYGEN CONSUMPTION

Consider from the previous example of steady-state exercise that the individual continues to jog at a comfortable pace until a series of six hills is encountered, each steeper than the next. The jogger's goal is to run up each of the hills without slowing down, although it is obvious that with each succeeding hill the task will become more strenuous. Thus the amount of energy required, as well as that expended, will increase progressively. In terms of oxygen consumption, the amount of energy released from aerobic reactions will increase in proportion to the severity of the exercise. As the hills become steeper, the exercise becomes more severe. Accompanying this increase in exercise intensity is a proportionate and linear increase in oxygen consumption up to a certain limit.

Figure 3-9 illustrates what the curve for oxygen consumption would look like if the jogger were able to run up each hill without slowing down. Oxygen consumption increases and then levels off as the jogger runs up each of the first three hills. This leveling-off of oxygen consumption while running up the first three hills indicates that the runner has reached a progressively higher level of steady state. On the next two hills, however, the oxygen consumption does not increase by the same amount as it did on the first three hills. In fact, the oxygen consumption does not increase at all during the run up the steepest hill, even though the jogger was just able to make it to the top! What has occurred is that the runner has attained his or her maximum capacity to generate energy aerobically and cannot increase it further. This region where the work continues to grow more difficult, yet the oxygen consumption fails to increase, is referred to as the *maximal oxygen consumption*. When this point is reached, the runner has attained the maximum capacity to deliver oxygen to the exercising muscles.

If a person exercises at a work intensity above maximal oxygen consumption, as occurred when the jogger ran up the last hill, anaerobic energy-generating reactions must supply the additional energy for this work. This mechanism for energy metabolism predominates because the energy from aerobic reactions is insufficient to meet the total energy demands of the exercise. Because energy can only be

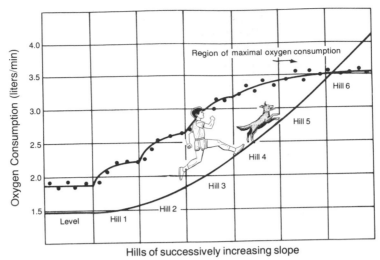

Figure 3-9. *Oxygen consumption during exercise of increasing intensity up to the maximal oxygen consumption. This occurs in the region where a further increase in work is not accompanied by an additional increase in oxygen consumption.*

supplied maximally from anaerobic sources for only about 60 seconds, the runner will soon become exhausted and will be unable to continue.

Maximal oxygen consumption is one of the most important factors that determine a person's capacity to sustain high-intensity exercise for longer than 4 to 5 minutes. Figure 3-10 compares the maximal oxygen consumption of male and female athletes with untrained, sedentary persons. The results show that the endurance athletes have nearly twice the aerobic capacity of the sedentary group. The values for aerobic capacity represented by Figure 3-10 have been expressed in terms of body weight as milliliters of oxygen per kilogram of body weight per minute, or ml/kg · min. Some physiologists have used this means of expressing aerobic capacity in an attempt to adjust for individual variations in body size.

The finding that women have lower maximal aerobic capacities than men of an essentially equal training status can be attributed to a large extent to the fact that women possess more body fat (and less muscle mass) than men. In fact, if the maximal oxygen consumptions of women are expressed in relation to "fat-free" or lean body weight, the difference between the sexes is minimal. This extra fat, although serving important biologic purposes, is not metabolically as active as the same quantity of muscle, and actually acts as "dead weight" in most physical activities.

Lactic Acid

During moderate levels of exercise such as jogging or slow swimming, the energy demands are adequately met by reactions that use oxygen. In biochemical terms, a sufficient amount of ATP for muscular contraction is made available through energy released via the oxidation of hydrogen, mainly in the slow-twitch

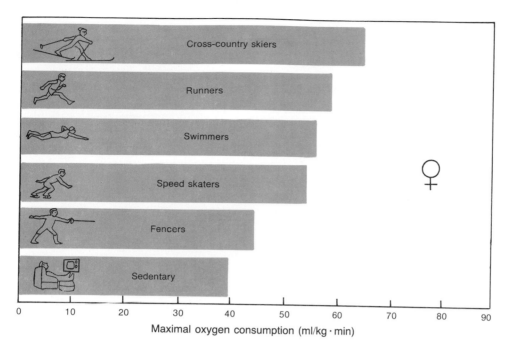

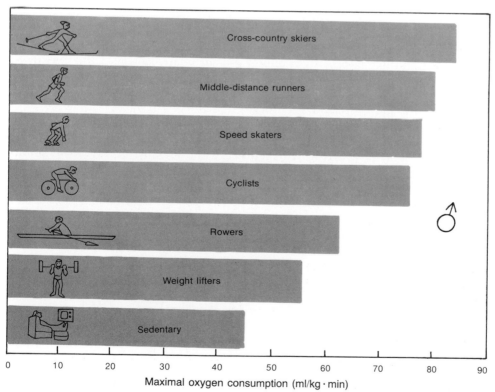

Figure 3-10. *Maximal oxygen consumption of male and female olympic-caliber athletes and healthy sedentary subjects. (Adapted from Saltin, B., and Åstrand, P.O.: Maximal oxygen uptake in athletes. Journal of Applied Physiology, 23:353, 1967.)*

muscle fibers. Under these conditions a steady rate of aerobic metabolism (steady state) can be maintained for a relatively long time as illustrated in Figure 3-8. However, as the demands for energy become more severe the supply of oxygen to the working muscles must increase. During strenuous work, as shown in Figure 3-9, the oxygen consumption reaches a maximum value because the aerobic energy-transferring reactions can no longer increase their energy output. Increasing exercise intensity demands more anaerobic energy and activates a larger number of fast-twitch fibers. *At about 50 to 55% of the maximal oxygen consumption the resynthesis of ATP through the anaerobic energy released from CP and glycolysis begins to exceed the energy supplied from aerobic metabolic reactions.* When this occurs, it is impossible to maintain a steady state because more hydrogen is produced than can combine with oxygen to form water. The excess hydrogen begins to accumulate in the working muscles. However, the concentration of hydrogen does not build up significantly because the excess hydrogen atoms combine temporarily with pyruvic acid. This temporary storage of hydrogen with pyruvic acid is a unique aspect of energy metabolism because it allows special carrier molecules to continue to transport hydrogen to combine with the available oxygen. When two excess hydrogen atoms are joined to pyruvic acid a new chemical is formed called *lactic acid.* Figure 3-11 shows two hydrogen atoms being joined with pyruvic acid to form lactic acid.

The advantage of converting pyruvic acid to lactic acid is that a ready "sump" is provided so the end products of glycolysis can disappear. Once lactic acid is formed it diffuses rapidly from the muscle into the bloodstream and away from the site of the energy-releasing reactions. In this way glycolysis can proceed to supply additional energy anaerobically to resynthesize ATP. Consequently exercise can continue even though the oxygen supply is inadequate. However, this avenue for extra energy release is only temporary because as the level of lactic acid in the blood and muscles increases and the ceiling for aerobic resynthesis is reached, fatigue sets in and exercise must stop.

Figure 3-12 illustrates the relationship between oxygen consumption expressed as a percentage of maximal oxygen consumption and lactic acid formation during light, moderate, and heavy exercise in untrained subjects and endurance athletes.

As illustrated, during light to moderate levels of energy expenditure the lactic acid level in the blood remains fairly constant for both groups despite an increas-

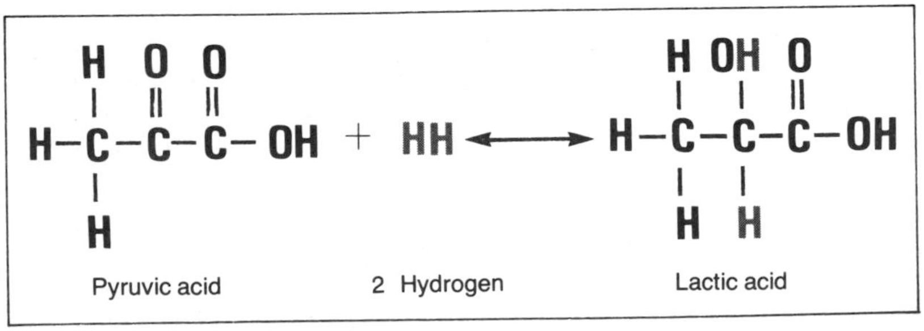

Figure 3-11. *Excess hydrogen molecules unable to combine with oxygen are passed by special carrier molecules to temporarily combine with pyruvic acid. This forms a new chemical, lactic acid.*

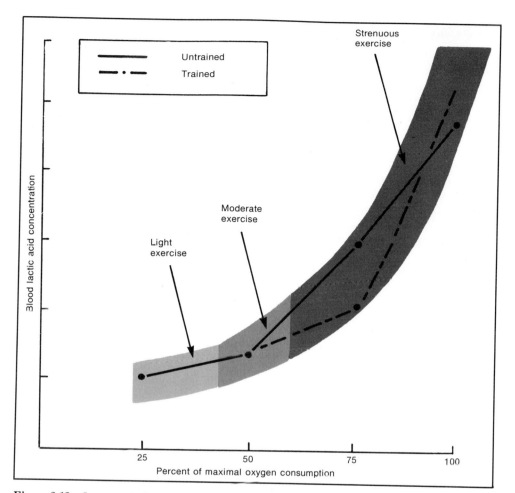

Figure 3-12. *Increases in blood lactic acid concentration at different levels of exercise expressed as a percentage of maximal oxygen consumption for trained and untrained subjects. (McArdle, W.D., Katch, F.I., and Katch, V.L.: Exercise Physiology, Lea & Febiger, 1981.)*

ing level of oxygen consumption. Each of these two exercise intensities is maintained in steady state as the ATP for muscular contraction is made available via aerobic metabolism. During exercise that involves approximately 55% of the untrained subjects' maximal oxygen consumption, however, the lactic acid level in the blood begins to rise. The increase in lactic acid becomes even greater as the exercise grows more intense and the body cannot meet the additional energy demands aerobically. This pattern is essentially similar for the trained athletes except that the threshold for lactic acid buildup, termed *anaerobic threshold,* occurs at a higher percentage of the athletes' aerobic capacity.

Studies of well-trained athletes have shown that when they are exhausted after strenuous exercise the blood lactic acid level is 20 to 30% higher than in untrained subjects under similar circumstances. An athlete's ability to tolerate a high level of lactic acid in the blood during competition may account in part for a superior performance, especially in relatively short and intense physical activities.

Recovery Oxygen Consumption (Oxygen Debt)

After exercise stops, the breathing, pulse rate, and bodily processes do not immediately return to their resting levels. If the exercise is not too strenuous, the recovery period is fast and proceeds unnoticed. If the activity is stressful, like sprinting for a bus or trying to swim 100 yards as fast as possible, the body requires considerable time to return to resting conditions. Recovery from each form of activity is associated to a large extent with the specific metabolic processes involved in that particular form of exercise.

Figure 3-13 shows two curves for oxygen consumption during exercise and recovery. The exercise portion of the top curve is similar to the curve in Figure 3-8 and illustrates the change in oxygen consumption during the transition from rest to moderate, steady-state exercise.

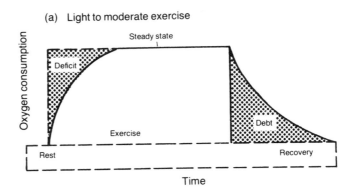

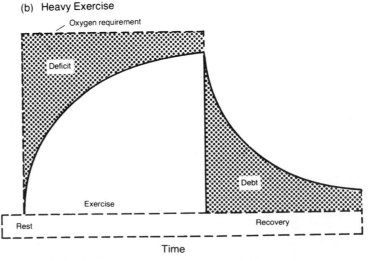

Figure 3-13. *Oxygen consumption during and in recovery from (a) light to moderate exercise, steady-state exercise, and (b) heavy exercise.*

During the first 3 minutes of exercise the oxygen consumption increases progressively until the body reaches a steady state. At this point oxygen-consuming reactions supply the energy requirements for exercise. Under these aerobic conditions the accumulation of lactic acid in the muscles is minimal. Not surprisingly, the oxygen consumption does not increase instantaneously to the steady-state level because the immediate energy for muscular work is always provided directly by the anaerobic breakdown of ATP. Oxygen is used only in subsequent reactions when it combines with the hydrogen atoms released during glycolysis and the reactions of the Krebs cycle. Thus a temporary "deficit" in oxygen consumption exists during the first few minutes of exercise. The amount of this deficit is shown to the left of the oxygen consumption curve. Quantitatively this deficit represents the difference between the oxygen consumption at steady state and the amount of oxygen that would have been consumed if oxygen consumption had reached steady state immediately. The anaerobic energy provided during the deficit phase of exercise represents energy that was "borrowed," so to speak, until the steady state was reached. Once exercise stops the deficit is "repaid" at the expense of an elevated oxygen consumption during recovery. During light exercise when steady state is reached quickly this payoff is relatively small and rapid. During heavy exercise, on the other hand, the oxygen deficit can be quite large. During the exhaustive exercise illustrated in the bottom curve, a steady state cannot be reached and anaerobic reactions provide considerable energy with an accumulation of lactic acid. The oxygen in excess of the resting value consumed during recovery from exercise, whether it be small from light exercise or large from heavy exercise, is called the *oxygen debt* or more precisely, the *recovery oxygen consumption.* In Figure 3-13 the recovery oxygen consumption is indicated by the shaded area under the recovery curves.

The curves of recovery illustrate several important characteristics of oxygen debt. During recovery from light and moderate exercise oxygen consumption declines rapidly to resting values as soon as exercise stops. One-half the total oxygen debt is repaid within the first 25 to 30 seconds during this "fast" repayment. Within 1 to 2 minutes the oxygen consumption has returned to the resting level. *The extra oxygen consumed in recovery from moderate exercise is associated with the restoration of the ATP and CP high-energy phosphates that were depleted and not resynthesized during the exercise.* A small amount of oxygen is also used to reload the blood with oxygen and to supply the slightly elevated oxygen demands of the heart and breathing musculature.

Recovery from strenuous exercise in which there is a large lactic acid accumulation and increase in body temperature presents a somewhat different picture. In addition to the fast component of the recovery curve of oxygen consumption, there is a second and slower phase termed the "slow" component. In this phase of recovery lactic acid is reconverted to pyruvic acid and metabolized for energy through the Krebs cycle. It is also believed that some lactic acid is synthesized back to glycogen in the liver. A precise biochemical explanation of the recovery oxygen consumption, especially the role of lactic acid, has not yet been made because the specific chemical dynamics of oxygen debt are still unclear. It is known, however, that the oxygen debt following strenuous exercise becomes larger than the deficit because a considerable amount of oxygen consumed during recovery is *not* directly related to the level of anaerobic metabolism during exercise. For example, the respiratory muscles require considerably more oxygen for the work of breathing during recovery than they normally require at rest. In intense exercise the volume of air moved into and out of the lungs can increase 8 to 10 times above rest, yet still remain elevated for some time in recovery. The heart also works harder and requires a greater oxygen supply during recovery. Body temperature, which is elevated during exercise, has a direct stimulating effect on metabolic reactions, and hence a significant effect on the recovery oxygen consumption. In addition, the blood must be reloaded with oxygen as it returns from the exercised muscles. In fact, all physiologic systems activated to meet the demands of exercise increase their own particular need for oxygen during recovery.

Some books dealing with exercise imply that lactic acid is a metabolic "waste product." On the contrary, lactic acid is not treated as an unwanted chemical and then excreted from the body. It is a valuable potential source of chemical energy that is retained at relatively high concentrations within the body during heavy physical exercise. When sufficient oxygen is present during the recovery period, lactic acid is readily converted back to pyruvic acid and used for energy. In this way the body preserves about 90% of the energy in the original glucose molecule for later use as an energy source.

It is important to understand the distinguishing features of the fast and slow components of the recovery oxygen consumption. If exercise is not too strenuous, so that it can be performed in steady state, or if it is heavy exercise but of short duration (10 to 15 seconds), lactic acid will not accumulate to any appreciable extent. In this case recovery is rapid (fast component) and exercise can begin again without the hindering effects of fatigue. If intense exercise must continue beyond a 20-second period—as can occur in sports like basketball, soccer, or hockey—the energy is supplied predominantly from the anaerobic reactions of glycolysis. This occurs at the expense of a build-up in lactic acid in the blood and exercising muscles. Under these circumstances recovery will take much longer (slow component) and may not be complete with short rest periods such as times-out, or even with longer rest periods such as half-time breaks.

The Energy Spectrum of Exercise

The relative contributions of the anaerobic and aerobic energy systems may differ markedly depending on the type of exercise performed. Performances of short duration and high intensity such as the 100-yard dash, 25-yard swim, high jump, volleyball spike, golf swing, or weight lifting, require an immediate supply of energy. This energy is provided exclusively from anaerobic sources, specifically the high-energy phosphate compounds ATP and CP stored within the specific muscles activated in the activity. In strenuous exercise lasting several minutes the major source of energy comes from the anaerobic process of glycolysis with the resulting formation of lactic acid. Intense exercise of an intermediate duration performed for 5 to 10 minutes as in middle-distance running, swimming, basketball, or soccer, represents a blend of metabolic energy demands. Under these conditions, it is desirable to possess a high capacity for both aerobic and anaerobic metabolism. Performances of long duration such as marathon running, distance swimming, cycling, recreational jogging, or hiking require a fairly constant aerobic energy supply with little or no reliance on the mechanism of lactic acid production.

Figure 3-14 illustrates the relative contribution of the anaerobic and aerobic energy sources during maximal physical activities of various durations. These data

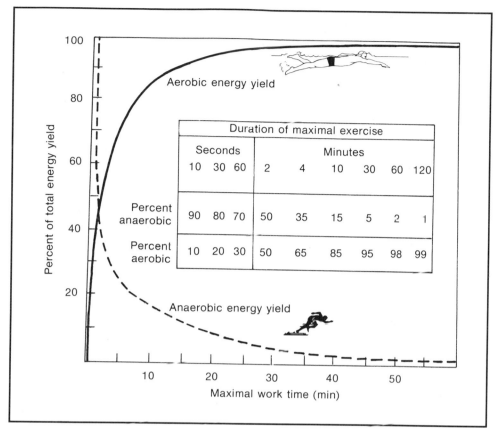

Figure 3-14. *Relative contribution of aerobic and anaerobic energy during maximal physical activity of various durations. It should be noted that 1½ to 2 minutes of maximal effort requires 50 percent of the energy from aerobic and anaerobic processes. (Adapted from Åstrand, P.O., and Rodahl, K.: Textbook of Work Physiology. New York, McGraw-Hill Book Company, © 1977. Used with permission of McGraw-Hill Book Company).*

were originally obtained from running and cycling experiments, although they can easily be applied to other activities that involve large muscle groups. For example, a 40- to 60-yard sprint of 5 to 8 seconds would closely approximate a long pass pattern in football, while a 440-yard run of 60 to 70 seconds would be similar in duration to a 100-yard swim.

At one extreme the total energy for exercise would be supplied entirely by anaerobic sources. In middle-distance events or in other intense activities lasting from 2 to 4 minutes, the ATP-CP and lactic acid energy systems generate approximately 50% of the energy, while reactions requiring oxygen supply the remainder. A world-class marathon runner, on the other hand, derives essentially all his or her energy from aerobic metabolism.

An understanding of the energy requirements of various activities provides some explanation why a world record-holder in the one-mile run is not necessarily a noted distance runner. Conversely, premier marathoners are generally unable to run a mile in less than 4 minutes. *The scientific approach to training is to identify the predominant energy system or systems involved in a given activity and then to gear training toward the improvement of the energy capacity of that system. Improved capability for energy metabolism will assure improvement in performance.*

Part 2. Ventilation and Circulation: The Oxygen Delivery Systems

Most sport, recreational, and occupational activities require a relatively constant and sustained supply of energy. Under such conditions the energy for the resynthesis of ATP is provided by the aerobic metabolism of carbohydrates and fat, and to a minor degree, protein. Unless a steady state can be achieved between aerobic energy-yielding reactions and the energy requirement of the activity, an anaerobic-aerobic metabolic energy imbalance develops, lactic acid accumulates and fatigue quickly ensues. The ability to sustain physical activity, therefore, depends to a large degree on the capacity and integration of the body's two major oxygen delivery systems, the *ventilatory* and *circulatory* systems.

Lung Ventilation

LUNG STRUCTURE AND FUNCTION

The lungs provide the surface across which oxygen moves from the external environment into the body and carbon dioxide produced in the tissues exits to the outside. The volume of the lungs of an average-sized adult varies from 4 to 6 liters, or about the amount of air contained in a basketball. If this tissue were spread out like a carpet it would cover a surface about 35 times greater than the surface area of the person, and would cover half a tennis court! This provides a tremendous interface for the aeration of blood with the environment.

A general view of the structure of the ventilatory system is presented in Figure 3-15. As air is brought into the lungs through the nose and mouth, it is filtered, humidified, and adjusted to body temperature. This air conditioning process continues as the inspired air passes down the trachea into the *bronchi*, two large tubes that serve as the primary conduits into each of the two lungs. The bronchi further subdivide into many smaller *bronchioles*, which conduct the air into the respiratory tract's terminal branches, or *alveoli*. These are the microscopic, thin-walled elastic sacs that serve as the surface across which gas exchange between the lungs and the blood takes place. Millions of tiny, thin-walled blood vessels called *capillaries* lie side-by-side with the alveoli, with air moving on one side and blood on the other. Thus when air is breathed into the lungs only two thin membranes, that of the alveolus and that of the capillary, provide the barrier to the movement of gases between the internal and external environments.

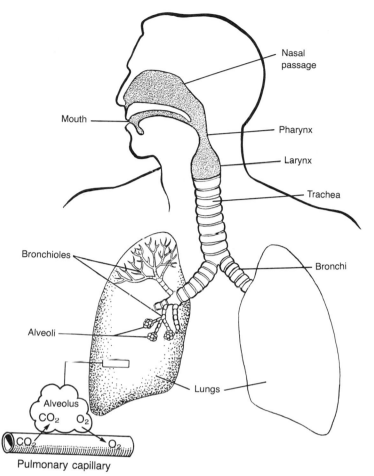

Figure 3-15. *A general view of the ventilatory system showing respiratory passages, the alveoli, and the function of an alveolus in gaseous exchange.*

MECHANICS OF BREATHING

A large, dome-shaped sheet of muscle called the *diaphragm* serves the same purpose as the rubber membrane attached to the bottom of the jar illustrated in Figure 3-16. This muscle makes an airtight seal that separates the lower chest from the upper abdominal cavity. When we breathe air into the lungs, a process known as *inspiration*, the diaphragm contracts, flattens out, and moves downward toward the abdominal cavity. As a result the chest cavity enlarges and air rushes in through the nose and mouth and the lungs inflate. In contrast to the balloons, which are attached to the jar, the lungs are not merely suspended in the chest cavity. Rather, surface tension created by moisture within the chest cavity causes the lungs to adhere to the chest wall and literally to follow its every movement. This occurs mainly as a result of the recoil provided by the relaxation of the inspiratory muscles. The action causes the size of the chest cavity to decrease and air moves out of the lungs. In well-conditioned endurance athletes pulmonary ventila-

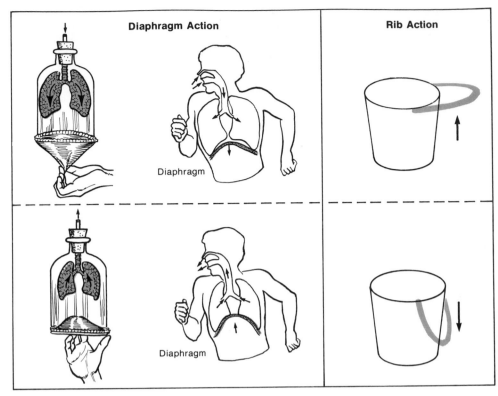

Figure 3-16. *Mechanics of breathing. During inspiration, the chest cavity increases in size due to the raising of the ribs and the lowering of the muscular diaphragm. During exhalation, the ribs swing down and the diaphragm returns to the relaxed position. This reduces the volume of the thoracic cavity and air rushes out. The movement of the rubber bottom of the jar simulates the action of the diaphragm and causes air to enter and leave the two balloons; the movement of the bucket handle simulates the action of the ribs. (McArdle, W.D., Katch, F.I., and Katch, V.L.: Exercise Physiology, Lea & Febiger, 1981.)*

tion may increase to 160 to 220 liters of air per minute in response to maximum metabolic demands. Even such strenuous exercise does not tax maximally the athlete's ability to breathe, so a breathing reserve still remains.

GAS EXCHANGE IN THE LUNGS

The movement of gas molecules as they enter or leave the lungs and body tissues occurs by the process of *diffusion,* as the gas moves from an area of higher concentration to an area of lower concentration. The exchange of oxygen and carbon dioxide molecules between the lungs and the blood and the subsequent diffusion of these gases at the tissue level, as shown in Figure 3-17, is due entirely to the pressure differentials between the gases in various parts of the body. Because the pressure exerted by the oxygen molecules in the alveoli is considerably greater than that in the returning venous blood, oxygen is "forced" through the alveolar membrane into the blood. Carbon dioxide, on the other hand, exists under greater pressure in returning venous blood than it does in the alveoli. Consequently

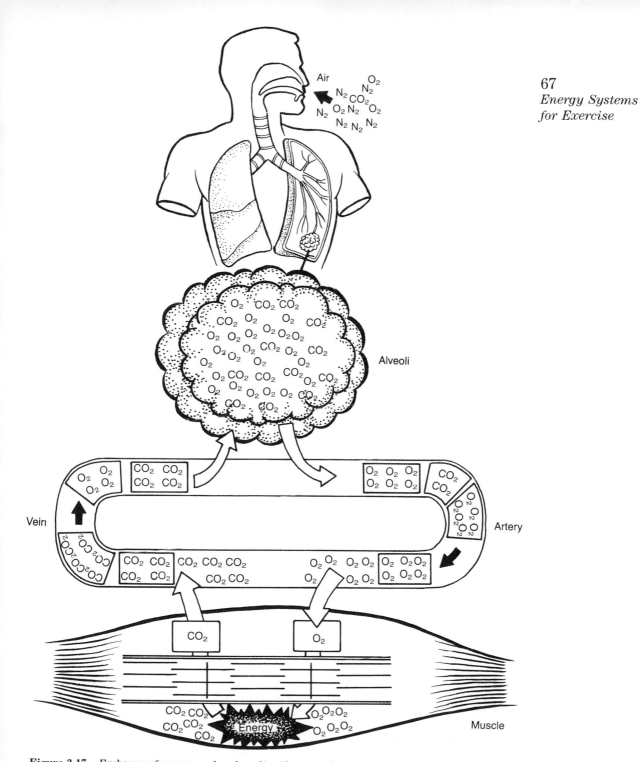

Figure 3-17. *Exchange of oxygen and carbon dioxide at rest between alveoli and the blood and the blood and tissues. During exercise both alveolar and arterial oxygen and carbon dioxide values remain almost the same as when at rest. In the muscles, however, the increased demands for energy cause the oxygen values to drop precipitously with a corresponding increase in carbon dioxide. Therefore venous blood will vary considerably in oxygen and carbon dioxide content, depending on the person's level of physical activity.*

the carbon dioxide is driven into the lungs. The process of gas diffusion in the healthy lung is so rapid that an equilibrium of blood gas with alveolar gas takes less than 1 second.

The pressure of oxygen and carbon dioxide gas in the arterial blood differs considerably from the pressure of these gases in the trillions of cells in the body. This is because at the tissue level oxygen is continuously used during aerobic metabolism, producing an almost equal quantity of carbon dioxide gas. This results in a rapid diffusion of gas between the blood and tissues. Oxygen leaves the blood and moves toward the metabolizing cell while carbon dioxide flows from the cell to the blood. After leaving the tissues the blood travels in the veins, where it is returned to the heart and subsequently pumped to the lungs where diffusion again takes place.

As the demands for energy increase during exercise, large amounts of oxygen diffuse from the alveoli of the lungs into the deoxygenated blood returning from the exercising muscles. Simultaneously, considerable quantities of carbon dioxide produced in the muscles and carried in the blood move into the lungs. To maintain the proper concentrations of alveolar gases to meet the increased need for oxygen and removal of carbon dioxide, lung ventilation must increase. With the proper adjustment of ventilation to the body's metabolic demands, the composition of alveolar air is kept remarkably constant, even during the most strenuous physical activity.

OXYGEN TRANSPORT

By far, the greatest quantity of oxygen in the blood is carried in "piggyback" fashion by combining with *hemoglobin*, the iron-containing protein compound in the red blood cells. Hemoglobin increases the oxygen-carrying capacity of blood some 65 times above that normally dissolved in the plasma. The iron atoms in each hemoglobin molecule "capture" oxygen molecules loosely and temporarily, thus enabling oxygen to be released in response to the needs of the active tissues. It is this oxygenation of hemoglobin that gives arterial blood its characteristic red color. When the content of the red blood cell decreases significantly, as in certain types of anemia, the quantity of oxygen carried by the blood decreases correspondingly. As discussed in Chapter 1, such a condition could result in reduced performance and early fatigue in activities that depend on a high oxygen supply.

LUNG VENTILATION DURING EXERCISE

Significant increases in the ventilation of the lungs result from an increase in the depth or in the rate of breathing, or both. The curve in Figure 3-18 illustrates the relationship between oxygen consumption and lung ventilation during various levels of exercise.

During moderate exercise ventilation volume increases linearly with oxygen consumption, averaging between 20 and 25 liters of air breathed for each liter of oxygen consumed by the tissues. Because of this increase in ventilation, the pressures of oxygen and carbon dioxide in the aveoli remain at near resting values and the oxygenation of the blood flowing through the lungs is complete. In more vigorous exercise ventilation volume compared with oxygen consumption increases disproportionately. In other words the amount of air breathed for each liter of oxygen consumed is greater than it is during more moderate exercise. If the ability

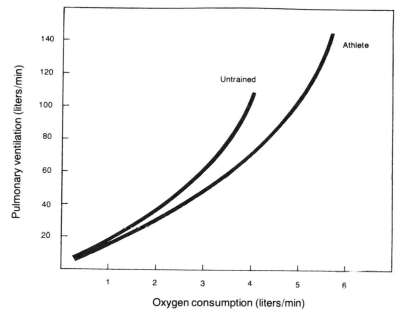

Figure 3-18. *Relationship between pulmonary ventilation and oxygen consumption for trained athletes and untrained subjects.*

to breathe were inadequate for the metabolic demands, the line relating lung ventilation and oxygen consumption would curve in the opposite direction. Such a curve would indicate a failure of ventilation to keep pace with the oxygen consumption. If such was the case in exercise, we would truly "run out of air." But this does not occur, and people actually overbreathe during heavy exercise. The lungs of healthy people are more than adequate to maintain proper alveolar gas pressures, even during the most severe exercise when the circulation is stressed to its maximum. For most people, the blood leaving the lungs to flow throughout the body during exercise is loaded with virtually the *same amount* of oxygen it carries during rest. *The capacity to breathe and ventilate the lungs will not limit a healthy's person's performance during physical activity.*

Circulation

The highly efficient ventilatory system is complemented by a rapid transport and delivery system consisting of the blood, the heart, and over 60,000 miles of blood vessels, which serve to integrate the body as a unit. The circulatory system serves three important functions during physical activity: (1) to deliver blood to the exercising muscles, where oxygen is exchanged for almost equal amounts of carbon dioxide; (2) to return blood to the lungs where the metabolic gases are exchanged with the ambient environment; and (3) to transport heat, a by-product of cellular metabolism, from the body's core to the skin where it then dissipates to the environment.

THE CARDIOVASCULAR SYSTEM

Figure 3-19 presents a schematic view of the circulatory system. Within the confines of this closed system the force for blood flow is provided by a four-chambered *heart*. The heart, a fist-sized pump, beats about 70 times a minute, or more than 100,000 times a day. When this remarkable organ pumps at its maximum capacity during exercise, it puts out more blood than the fluid coming from a household faucet turned wide open!

Figure 3-20 shows the details of the heart as a pump. The two hollow chambers that make up the right side of the heart serve two important functions: (1) to receive oxygen-depleted blood returning from all parts of the body, and (2) to pump the blood to the lungs for aeration. The left side of the heart receives oxygen-rich blood from the lungs and pumps it into the *aorta*, which is the main conduit of the arterial system. From it branch other main arterial channels that route oxygen-rich blood to the body's organs and tissues.

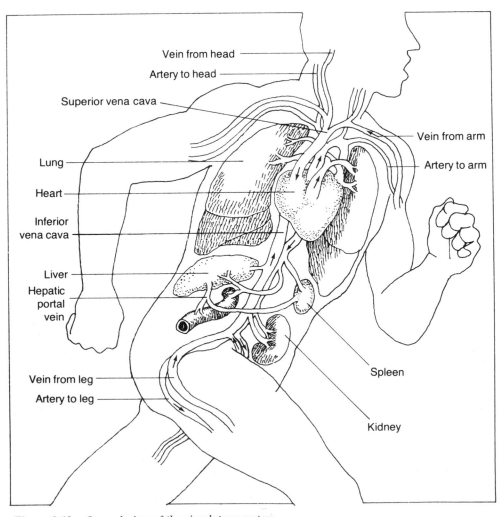

Figure 3-19. *General view of the circulatory system.*

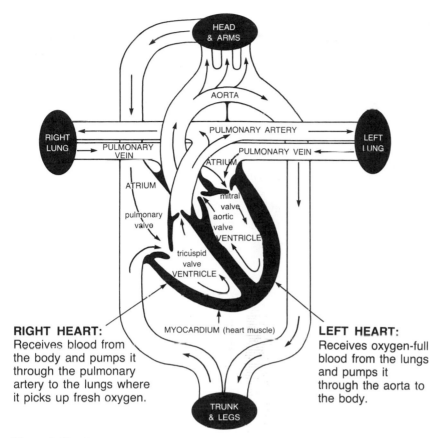

Figure 3-20. *The structure of the heart pump. (From Heart Facts 1981. © American
Heart Association, Dallas, 1980. Reproduced with permission.)*

RIGHT HEART:
Receives blood from
the body and pumps it
through the pulmonary
artery to the lungs where
it picks up fresh oxygen.

LEFT HEART:
Receives oxygen-full
blood from the lungs
and pumps it
through the aorta to
the body.

The arterial system eventually branches into smaller blood vessels called *arterioles*. Nerves and local metabolic conditions act on the smooth muscular bands in the arteriole walls and enable these vessels to alter their internal diameter. The dilation and constriction of arterioles allow for the rapid redistribution of blood to and from various regions of the body. The arterioles end in a network of small blood vessels, called *capillaries*, with microscopically thin walls. It is only at the capillary level that the exchange of gases and nutrients takes place between the slow-moving blood and the tissues.

The deoxygenated blood leaves the capillaries at almost a trickle to enter the *venules* or small veins, and eventually into the *veins* which return the blood to the heart. Spaced at short intervals within the veins are thin, membranous, flaplike *valves* (Figure 3-21), which permit the one-way flow of blood back to the heart. Because the blood in these veins is under relatively little pressure, they are easily compressed by the smallest muscular contractions or even by minor pressure changes within the chest cavity during the act of breathing. This alternate compression and relaxation of the veins and the one-way action of the valves provides a "milking" action for the steady flow of blood from the capillaries into the veins and back to the heart.

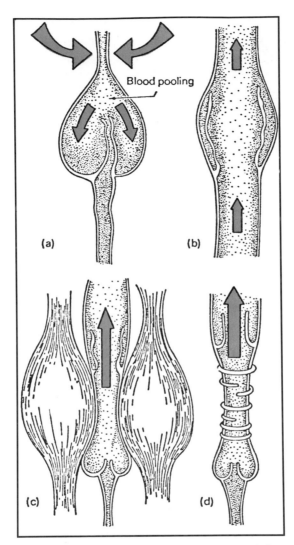

Figure 3-21. *Valves in the veins (a) prevent back flow of returning flow but (b) do not hinder the normal flow very much. Blood can be pushed through veins (c) by nearby active muscle, or (d) by the action of smooth muscle bands. (From Elias, H., and Pauly, J.E.: Human Microanatomy. Philadelphia, F.A. Davis, 1966.)*

During heavy weightlifting or other activities that involve sustained, non-rhythmic muscular contractions, neither the muscle nor ventilatory pumps contribute significantly to venous return. In such situations blood flow to the heart may actually be impaired to a degree where dizziness and even fainting occur as blood flow to the brain is reduced. Aside from diminishing venous return, such "static" activities also result in a significant but transient increase in arterial blood pressure. *This poses an additional workload for the heart which could be dangerous for people with existing high blood pressure or heart disease.*

BLOOD PRESSURE

With each contraction of the left ventricle a surge of blood enters the aorta, distending it and creating pressure within it. The stretch and subsequent recoil of the vascular wall travels as a wave through the entire system. This wave of pressure can readily be felt as the characteristic pulse in the superficial radial artery on the thumb side of the wrist or temporal artery (side of head at temple) or at the carotid artery along the side of the trachea ("Adam's apple") in the neck. Each site is convenient for determining the heart rate at rest and following exercise because the pulse rate and heart rate are identical in healthy persons. Figure 3-22 illustrates the pulse being taken at these three convenient locations.

At rest, the highest pressure generated by the heart to move blood through a healthy, resilient vascular system is usually about 120 mm Hg during the contraction or *systole* of the left ventricle. As the heart relaxes the natural elastic recoil of the aorta and other arteries provides a continuous head of pressure to maintain an even blood flow in the arterial system until the next surge of blood is received from the contraction of the heart. During this relaxation phase, or *diastole* of the cardiac cycle, the blood pressure in the arterial system decreases to about 70 or 80 mm Hg. This blood pressure, which represents the forces exerted by the blood against the walls of the arteries during a cardiac cycle, would be written as 120/80 mm Hg. In people with arteries "hardened" by deposits of minerals and fatty materials within the walls, or with an excessive resistance to blood flow in the periphery resulting from kidney malfunction or nervous strain, systolic pressure may increase from 120 to 250 to 300 mm Hg. This high blood pressure or hypertension imposes a chronic and excessive strain on the normal function of the cardiovascular system. If chronic hypertension is not corrected, it can eventually lead to *heart failure*, where the heart is unable to maintain its pumping ability, or *stroke*, a condition in which brittle vessels burst and cut off the blood supply to vital organs. More will be said about hypertension in Chapter 11.

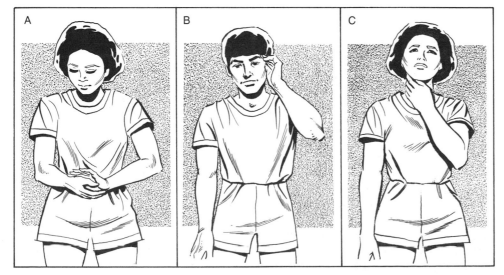

Figure 3-22. *Pulse rate taken at the (A) radial, (B) temporal, and (c) carotid artery.*

EFFECTS OF TRAINING ON CIRCULATORY FUNCTION

The output of the heart pump, referred to as *cardiac output*, is one of the most important indicators of the functional capacity of the circulation to meet the demands of aerobic physical activity. It is determined by two factors: (1) the rate of the pump's stroke or *heart rate*, and (2) the quantity of fluid ejected with each stroke or *stroke volume*. Thus

Cardiac Output = Heart Rate × Stroke Volume.

The demand for blood flow to the muscles increases in proportion to the severity of the exercise. In relatively sedentary, college-aged males the cardiac output during strenuous exercise increases about 4 times the resting level to an average maximum of 20 liters or 20,000 ml of blood pumped per minute. Maximal heart rates at this age usually average 195 beats per minute. Consequently the "untrained" heart will pump about 103 ml of blood with each beat during maximum exercise. This is in contrast to world-class endurance athletes who have maximum cardiac outputs of 35 to 40 liters of blood per minute. For these athletes, maximum heart rate is not appreciably different from the maximum heart rate of sedentary people of similar age. Thus, the stroke volume of the athlete's heart is about 180 ml of blood per beat. *The key factor enabling the endurance athlete to pump more blood each minute than an untrained counterpart is a significantly larger stroke volume.*

Cardiac Output = Heart Rate × Stroke Volume.

At Rest

Sedentary	5,000 ml	=	70 beats/min ×	71.4 ml
Trained	5,000 ml	=	50 beats/min ×	100.0 ml

Maximum Exercise

Sedentary	20,000 ml	=	195 beats/min ×	102.6 ml
Trained	35,000 ml	=	195 beats/min ×	179.5 ml

Figure 3-23 (a and b) illustrates the response of heart rate and stroke volume in relation to oxygen consumption during exercise of increasing severity. The subjects were two groups of men; one group was highly trained endurance athletes, while the other group was made up of sedentary college students measured before and after a 55-day training program designed to improve aerobic fitness.

The researchers observed several important physiologic responses. First, the stroke volume of the athletes' hearts was considerably larger than the untrained students' both at rest and during exercise. Second, the response pattern of the stroke volume in both groups during exercise was similar. The increase in stroke volume was greatest when going from rest to light exercise. Thereafter the increase in stroke volume was quite small. Third, stroke volume increased only slightly from rest to exercise in the untrained men. Thus the major increase in cardiac output for the untrained subjects was brought about by an increase in heart rate. For the trained athletes, on the other hand, both heart rate *and* stroke volume increased to augment blood flow to the muscles during exercise. Following

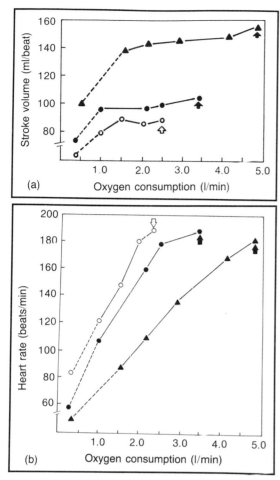

(a)

(b)

Figure 3-23. *Stroke volume (a) and heart rate (b) in relation to oxygen consumption during upright exercise in endurance athletes (▲) and sedentary college students prior to (○) and following (●) 55 days of aerobic training; (⬁, ♠ = maximal values). (From Saltin, B.: Physiological effects of physical conditioning. Medicine Science Sports, 1:50, 1969. Copyright 1969, the American College of Sports Medicine. Reprinted by Permission.)*

55 days of training, the students' stroke volume (and maximum cardiac output) had increased substantially, but the values were still considerably lower than the stroke volume of the athletes. The degree to which both training and genetic factors account for the exceptionally large stroke volumes of successful endurance athletes during maximal exercise is still not clearly understood. Scientists generally agree, however, that the ability of the heart trained by exercise to maintain a high stroke volume both at rest and during exercise is due to a more forceful contraction, which empties the ventricle almost completely with each beat. *Numerous studies have documented that the ability of the heart to increase its*

Energy Value of Food and Physical Activity

T HE GREATEST DEMAND for energy occurs during physical activity. The energy trapped within the chemical bonds of carbohydrates, fats, and proteins is extracted during a series of complex chemical reactions and made available to the cells in the form of the energy currency, ATP. Because the three major food nutrients contain energy and because all bodily functions both at rest and during exercise require energy, it is possible to classify both food and physical activity in terms of a common denominator, *energy*.

Energy Contained in Food—Calories

A *calorie* is a unit of heat used to express the energy value of food. Although the term is widely used in the popular literature, it has a precise scientific meaning. One *Calorie* (spelled with a capital C), represents the amount of heat necessary to increase the temperature of 1 kg of water, which is slightly more than a quart, by 1°C. A Calorie—or more accurately, a kilocalorie—is abbreviated *kcal*. For example, two scoops of "Rocky Road" ice cream on a sugar cone contain about 408 kcal and thus the energy to raise the temperature of about 408 quarts or 102 gallons of water by 1°C. This is indeed a relatively large amount of energy. On the other hand, a small glass of cranberry juice contains only 60 kcal, or enough energy to increase the temperature of about 60 quarts of water by 1°C.

Measurement of Calories

The energy or kcal value of any food can be measured directly by the amount of heat released from the food when it is burned in an apparatus called a *bomb calorimeter*. This method of directly measuring the energy content of foods is known as *direct calorimetry*.

The bomb calorimeter illustrated in Figure 4-1 works as follows. A weighed portion of food is placed inside a small chamber filled with oxygen. The food is

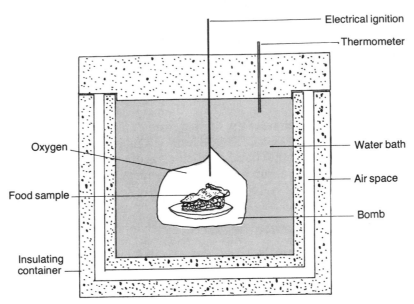

Figure 4-1. *Determining the caloric value of foods in a bomb calorimeter.*

literally exploded and burned in the chamber when an electric current ignites a fuse inside the bomb. The heat released as the food burns is absorbed by a surrounding water bath. Because the calorimeter is fully insulated, no heat escapes to the outside. The precise amount of heat absorbed by the water is determined by measuring the increase in water temperature with a sensitive thermometer. For example, when one 4.7 ounce, 4-inch sector of apple pie is completely burned in the calorimeter, 350 kcal of heat energy are released. This is enough to raise 3.5 kilograms or 7.7 pounds of ice water to the boiling point.

Caloric Value of Foods

Many laboratories throughout the world have used the bomb calorimeter to determine the energy value of foods. The burning of 1 g of pure carbohydrate yields 4.10 kcal, 1 g of pure protein releases 5.65 kcal, and 1 g of pure fat yields 9.45 kcal. Because most foods in the normal diet consist of various proportions of these three nutrients, the caloric value of a given food such as hamburger or french fries is determined by the amount of carbohydrate, fat or protein in an average serving. It is evident from the caloric values for a gram of each nutrient that the energy content of food that contains a considerable amount of fat will be greater than food which is relatively fat-free. As an example, the number of calories in 1 cup of whole milk is 160 kcal, whereas the same amount of skimmed milk contains 90 kcal. If someone who normally consumes 1 quart of milk each day switches to skimmed milk, the quantity of calories ingested each year would be reduced by an amount equal to about 25 pounds of body fat!

When 1 g of carbohydrate or fat is "burned" or metabolized in the cell's energy factory, the body obtains the same value of 4.10 kcal for carbohydrate and

9.45 kcal for fat as did the bomb calorimeter. The energy yield from fat is more than twice that of carbohydrate because of the differences in the structural composition between the two nutrients. As noted in Chapter 1, the chemical formula for a simple carbohydrate is $C_6H_{12}O_6$. There is always a ratio of two hydrogen atoms for each oxygen atom. Fat molecules, on the other hand, contain significantly more hydrogen than oxygen. Palmitic acid, one of the constituents of a fat, has the structural formula $C_{16}H_{30}O_2$. Consequently, there are more hydrogen atoms that can be cleaved away during the breakdown of a fat to combine eventually with oxygen to form water and produce energy.

The energy available to the body from the metabolism of protein is less than that released in the bomb calorimeter. In addition to carbon, hydrogen, and oxygen, proteins contain the element nitrogen. Because the body cannot use nitrogen, it combines with hydrogen to form *urea* (NH_2CONH_2) and is excreted in the urine. This elimination of hydrogen represents a loss of potential energy. For this reason the energy yield from one gram of protein in the body is 4.35 kcal instead of the 5.65 kcal released during its complete oxidation in the bomb calorimeter.

An important consideration in determining the ultimate caloric yield to the body of the various foods is the efficiency of the digestive processes. Efficiency in this sense refers to the completeness or thoroughness of the breakdown of the foods in the digestive tract, as well as their eventual absorption and assimilation as part of the body's various metabolic reactions. Normally about 97% of carbohydrates, 95% of fats, and 92% of proteins are completely digested and absorbed. These average efficiency percentages may vary somewhat depending on the particular foods. This is especially true in the case of protein, where digestive efficiency may vary from a high of 97% with animal protein to a low of 78% for dried legumes. *When the average efficiency of digestion is taken into account, the net kcal value for carbohydrates, fats, and proteins becomes 4.0, 9.0, and 4.0 kcal, respectively.*

By use of these net values, the appropriate caloric content of any portion of food can be determined as long as its composition and weight are known. For example, suppose we wanted to determine the kcal value for one-half cup of creamed chicken. It can be determined from Appendix A that in terms of weight this portion of food is equivalent to 3.5 ounces or about 100 grams. Based on laboratory analysis of portions made from a standard recipe, the nutrient composition of the creamed chicken is approximately 20% protein, 12% fat, and 6% carbohydrate, with the remaining 62% being water. Using these compositional values the kcal value of the creamed chicken can be determined according to the following reasoning: Because of the above proportion of nutrients, each gram of creamed chicken will contain 0.2 g of protein, 0.12 g of fat, and 0.06 g of carbohydrate. The net kcal values indicate that 0.2 g of protein contain 0.8 kcal (0.20×4.00), 0.12 g of fat equal 1.08 kcal (0.12×9.00), and 0.06 g of carbohydrate yield 0.24 kcal (0.06×4.00). The total caloric value of 1 g of creamed chicken would therefore equal 2.12 kcal ($0.80 + 1.08 + 0.24$). Consequently, a 100-g serving would have a caloric value 100 times as large, or 212 kcal. These computations are illustrated in Table 4-1. Although this table shows the method for calculating the kcal value of creamed chicken, the same method could be used to determine the caloric value for a serving of any food. Reducing the size of the portion by half would of course reduce the caloric intake by 50%. Needless to say, if extra fat is added to the preparation of the meal, or if fat-free substitutes are used, the caloric value of the meal will be affected accordingly.

Fortunately, there is seldom a need to compute the kcal value of foods as shown above. These values have already been determined for almost all foods by

Table 4-1. *Method of calculating the caloric value of a food when its composition of nutrients is known.*

Food: creamed chicken

Weight ½ cup = 3.5 oz = 100 g

Composition:	Protein	Fat	Carbohydrates
1. percentage	20%	12%	6%
2. total grams	20	12	6
3. in one gram	0.20 g	0.12 g	0.06 g
Calories per gram:	0.80	1.08	0.24
	(0.20 × 4.00 kcal)	(0.12 × 9.00 kcal)	(0.06 × 4.00 kcal)

Total calories per gram: 0.80 + 1.08 + 0.24 = 2.12 kcal

Total calories per 100 grams: 2.12 × 100 = 212 kcal

the United States Department of Agriculture. What we have done in Appendix A is to present a representative listing of the nutritive value of the more common foods. Included is the weight of an average serving of the food in grams and ounces, the kcal value of the serving, the amount of protein, fat, and carbohydrate present, as well as the quantity of the minerals calcium and iron, and the content of vitamins A and C, thiamin and riboflavin.

For those fortunate to have access to a computer based nutritional analysis system, it is unnecessary to calculate the specific nutrient composition of foods. By specifying the portion size, the computer taps its memory for that particular food item and lists the corresponding nutrient composition. In this way, it is possible to determine the total nutrient intake for any diet and to compare this with the Recommended Dietary Allowances (RDA) specified by the Food and Nutrition Board. This form of nutrient analysis is useful to evaluate nutritional status, as well as to compare individuals and groups in terms of their dietary practices. However, a major drawback with this form of computerized approach for determining nutrient composition is the large amount of time required to enter the "coded" food items into the computer, as well as the uncertainty regarding portion size. At best, the computerized analysis approach is a first approximation of the "true" nutrient intake, ± 10 to 30% even when accurate records are kept by people who consume the typical American diet. In hospital and other institutionalized settings where food intake can be closely supervised, the computerized analysis of nutrient intake may provide a much more valid nutritional evaluation.

If you examine Appendix A carefully you will make a rather striking yet reasonable observation with regard to the energy value of food. Consider for example, five common foods: raw celery, cooked cabbage, cooked asparagus spears, mayonnaise, and salad oil. In order to consume 100 kcal of each of these foods, an individual would need to eat 20 stalks of celery, 4 cups of cabbage, 30 asparagus spears, but only 1 tablespoon of mayonnaise or ⅕ tablespoon of salad oil. The point is that a small serving of some foods can have an equal kcal value as large quantities of other foods. Viewed from a different perspective, one would have to consume over

4000 stalks of celery or 800 cups of cabbage to supply the daily energy needs of a fairly sedentary individual, while the same energy would be supplied by ingesting only ⅖ cup of mayonnaise or about 3 ounces of salad oil. The major difference is that foods with a high fat content exist as relatively concentrated sources of food energy and contain little water. On the other hand, foods low in fat or high in water tend to contain relatively little energy. Keep in mind, however, that 100 kcal from mayonnaise and 100 kcal from celery are exactly the same in terms of energy. There is no difference between calories from an energy standpoint, a calorie being a unit of heat regardless of the food source. Simply stated, a calorie . . . is a calorie . . . is a calorie. It would be incorrect to consider 100 kcal of mayonnaise as being any more fattening than 100 kcal of celery. The number of calories contained in foods are additive: The more you eat the more calories you consume. If the food has a high concentration of calories as in the case of fatty foods, and you consume even a moderate portion, you will of course consume a relatively large number of calories.

Heat Produced by the Body

DIRECT CALORIMETRY

The amount of heat produced by an animal can be measured in a calorimeter similar to that used to determine the caloric content of food. The human calorimeter illustrated in Figure 4-2 consists of an airtight chamber with an oxygen supply in which a person can live and work for an extended period. A known volume of water is circulated through a series of pipes located at the top of the chamber. Because the entire chamber is well insulated, the heat produced and radiated by the individual is absorbed by the circulating water. The change in water temperature reflects the individual's metabolic energy release for a particular time period. To provide adequate ventilation, the subject's exhaled air is drawn from the room

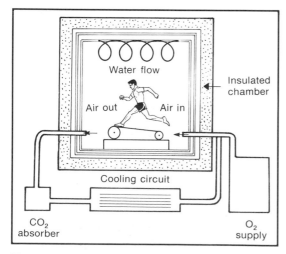

Figure 4-2. *Measuring heat production of the body by direct calorimetry.*

and passed through a series of chemicals that remove the moisture content of the air and absorb carbon dioxide. Oxygen is then added to the air and recirculated through the chamber.

The direct measurement of heat production in humans in a closed chamber is of considerable theoretical importance, yet its use and application are rather limited. The calorimeter is relatively small and quite expensive, accurate measurements of heat production are time-consuming, and its use is generally not applicable for energy determinations during common sport or recreation activities.

INDIRECT CALORIMETRY

All energy-producing reactions in the body depend ultimately on a continual supply of oxygen. By measuring a person's oxygen consumption it is possible to obtain an *indirect* estimate of energy production. Even though the technique of indirect calorimetry is relatively simple and the equipment much less expensive than the direct method previously addressed, it is highly accurate. Researchers have developed two methods of indirect calorimetry termed *closed-circuit* and *open-circuit spirometry.* The open-circuit method is the most widely used technique to measure oxygen consumption, especially during exercise. The subject does not breathe and rebreathe from a prefilled container of oxygen, as in the closed-circuit method, but instead inhales ambient air that has a constant composition. The changes in the percentage of oxygen and carbon dioxide in the exhaled air compared with the ambient air brought into the lungs indirectly reflect the body's constant need for energy to maintain equilibrium of the internal processes. Thus an analysis of two factors, the volume of air breathed and the composition of expired air, provides a relatively simple means to measure the oxygen consumed by the body and indirectly infer the energy expenditure.

Oxygen consumption can easily be converted to a corresponding value for energy production. It has been well established from experiments using the bomb calorimeter that when 1 liter of oxygen is consumed in the burning of a small mixture of carbohydrates, fats, and proteins, approximately 4.82 kcal of heat energy are liberated. This caloric equivalent for oxygen varies only slightly depending on the food mixture. For convenience in calculations, therefore, a value of *5 kcal per liter of oxygen consumed* can be used as an appropriate conversion factor. This amount, 5 kcal, is important to remember for it enables us to determine easily the body's energy production at rest or during steady state exercise simply by measuring the oxygen consumption. The three most common procedures for measuring the rate of oxygen consumption during a variety of physical activities employ a *portable spirometer, Douglas bags* or meteorologic balloons, or *computerized instrumentation.*

Portable Spirometer

German scientists in the early 1940s developed a relatively light and portable system that made it possible to determine indirectly the amount of energy expended during various forms of physical activity. This box-shaped apparatus shown in Figure 4-3 weighs only 8 or 9 pounds and is usually carried on the back during the measurement period. The subject breathes through a two-way valve that allows inspiration of ambient air while the exhaled air passes through a special meter where its volume is measured. Periodically samples of the exhaled air are automatically collected in small rubber bags attached to the meter. Oxygen con-

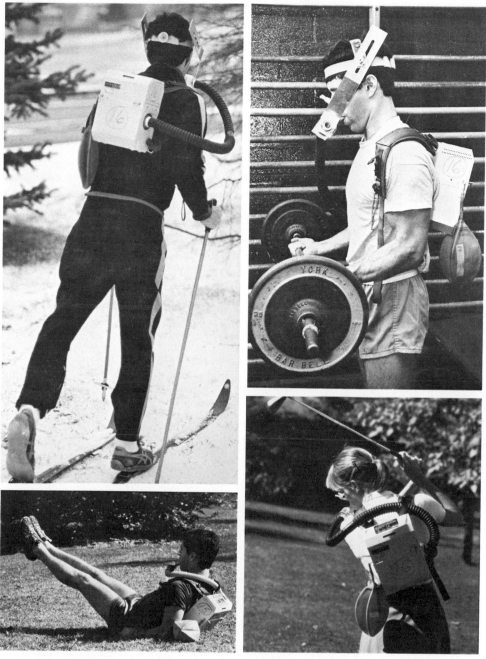

Figure 4-3. *Portable spirometer used to measure oxygen consumption by the open-circuit method during cross country skiing, weight lifting exercise, golf, and calisthenic activities. (Courtesy Exercise Physiology Laboratory, Department of Exercise Science, University of Massachusetts, Amherst.)*

sumption is computed by analyzing the expired air for oxygen and carbon dioxide content. Energy expenditure, expressed in kcal, is then computed from the oxygen consumption. One of the advantages of this particular apparatus is that it allows the subject considerable freedom of movement during the measurement period. The portable spirometer is useful for measuring energy expenditure for activities that do not require intense and sustained physical efforts.

Douglas Bag or Balloon

The subject shown on the left in Figure 4-4 is walking on a motor-driven treadmill. The treadmill provides an excellent way to exercise individuals under controlled conditions because the speed as well as the elevation can be accurately regulated. While exercising, the subject wears a special headgear with a two-way breathing valve. The subject breathes ambient air in through one side of the valve and exhales it from the valve where it is sampled and analyzed for its oxygen and carbon dioxide composition. Energy expenditure is calculated from oxygen consumption just as it was when using the portable spirometer.

As can be seen in the right side of Figure 4-4, oxygen consumption is also being determined for the subject riding the bicycle. This particular bicycle, called

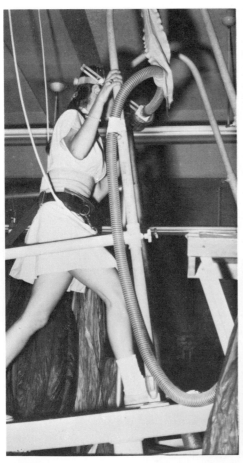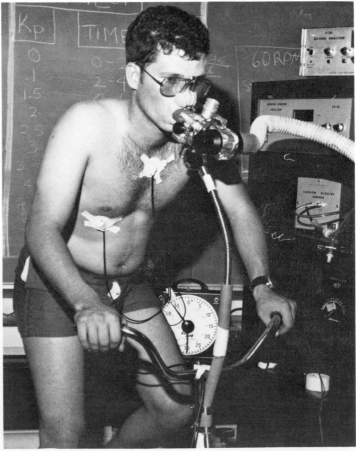

Figure 4-4. *Measurement of oxygen consumption by open-circuit spirometry during treadmill and bicycle ergometer exercise. (Courtesy Exercise Physiology Laboratory, Department of Exercise Science, University of Massachusetts, Amherst.)*

an *ergometer* because it measures the work being done, allows an individual to exercise at a predetermined work level by controlling both the rate of pedaling as well as the resistance to pedaling. The resistance is controlled on this bicycle by increasing or decreasing the tension on a strap surrounding the front flywheel. For other ergometers, resistance is applied by electromechanical means during cycling so that a preset workload can be maintained independently of pedaling rate. These two apparatus, the bicycle ergometer and treadmill, are in common use in physical education and other laboratories where oxygen consumption and energy expenditure during exercise are routinely measured.

Computerized Instrumentation

Recent advances in computer and microprocessor technology enable the sport scientist to efficiently and accurately measure metabolic and cardiovascular response to exercise. A computer is interfaced with at least three instruments: (1) a system to continuously sample the airflow from the subject; (2) a meter to record the volume of air flow, and (3) oxygen and carbon dioxide analyzers to measure the concentration of the gas mixture. The computer is preprogrammed to perform all of the necessary calculations based on the electronic signals it receives from the instrument. A printed or graphic display of the subject's data can occur simultaneously during exercise and recovery. More advanced systems include automated blood pressure, heart rate, and temperature monitors, as well as preset instructions to regulate the speed, duration, and workload of treadmills and bicycle ergometers. The computerized systems currently in use make it possible to rapidly collect, measure, and analyze a vast amount of physiologic information for a wide variety of work and performance tasks.

Basal Metabolic Rate

For each individual there is a minimum level of energy required to sustain the body's vital functions in the waking state. This energy requirement, or *basal metabolic rate* (BMR), is usually determined by measuring oxygen consumption under fairly stringent and standardized laboratory guidelines. No food is eaten for at least 12 hours prior to the measurement so there will be no increase in the energy required for the digestion and absorption of foods in the digestive tract. Abstaining from food in this manner is referred to as the *post-absorptive state*. In addition, no undue muscular exertion should have occurred for at least 12 hours prior to the determination of BMR. During the test, the subject lies in a dimly lit, temperature-controlled room. After lying quietly for 30 to 60 minutes, the subject's oxygen consumption is measured for a 6- to 10-minute period.

The measurement of BMR under strictly controlled laboratory conditions provides a convenient method for studying the relationship between metabolic rate and body size, sex, and age.

INFLUENCE OF BODY SIZE ON RESTING METABOLISM

A general rule is that when individuals of different body size are compared with respect to resting or basal energy metabolism, the value for energy expenditure is usually expressed in terms of surface area and not body weight. The results of numerous experiments have provided data on average values of BMR per unit surface area in men and women of different ages.

The data in Figure 4-5 reveal that the average BMR is *not* equal between the sexes, but is 5 to 10% lower in women than in men at all ages. This difference should not be interpreted to mean that there is an inherent sex difference in the metabolic rate of the body's various tissues. Rather, the lower BMR of women can be attributed to their larger percentage of body fat and smaller muscle mass. In fact, when the BMR is expressed per unit of fat-free or *lean body weight*, the observed sex differences become less apparent. While this observation may be of some theoretical importance, the curves shown in Figure 4-5 still describe the BMR in men and women adequately. From ages 20 to 40, average values for the BMR are 38 kcal per square meter of surface area (m^2) per hour for men, and 35 kcal per m^2 per hour for women. If you desire a more precise estimate of the BMR, you can obtain the actual average value for a given age directly from the curves. By using these values for heat production in conjunction with the appropriate value for surface area, it is easy to compute the approximate resting heat production in kcal per minute, and convert this to the total kcal requirement per day. The nomogram in Figure 4-6 provides a simplified method for computing surface area based on height and weight.

To determine surface area with the nomogram, locate height on Scale I and weight on Scale II. Connect these two points with a straight edge or piece of thread. The intersection at Scale III gives the surface area expressed in square meters (m^2). For example, if height is 6 feet, and weight is 180 pounds, surface area according to Scale III on the nomogram would be 2.04 square meters.

To determine the approximate heat production or kcal requirement of the body during resting conditions, multiply the average kcal per unit surface area per hour by the surface area determined from the nomogram. Then multiply this by 24 to obtain an estimate of the resting energy requirement on a 24-hour basis. For a 22-year-old man whose surface area is 2.04 square meters, the minimum daily

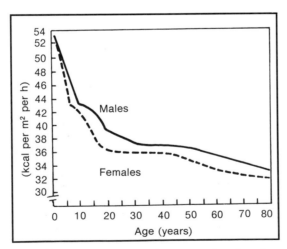

Figure 4-5. *Resting metabolic rate as a function of age and sex. (Data from Altman, P.L., and Dittmer, D.S.: Metabolism, Bethesda, Md., Federation of American Societies for Experimental Biology, 1968.)*

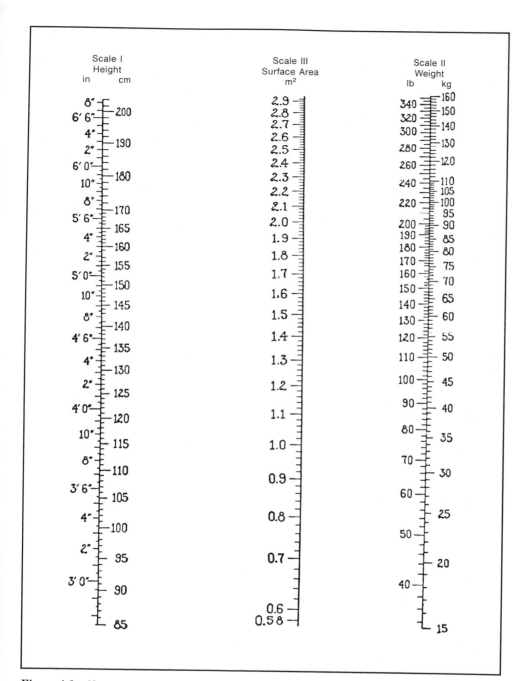

Figure 4-6. *Nomogram to estimate body surface area from height and weight. [Reproduced from "Clinical Spirometry" (as prepared by Boothby and Sandiford of the Mayo Clinic), through the courtesy of Warren E. Collins, Inc., Braintree, Massachusetts.]*

caloric requirement would be 38 kcal/m²/h × 2.04 m² × 24 h, or 1860 kcal per day. In most instances, values calculated in this manner will usually be within 10% of the kcal value per day had the BMR been measured under strict laboratory conditions. Computing the minimum daily energy requirements based on age and surface area gives a much more dependable estimate than simply using the average population value for daily resting energy expenditure, which for men and women ranges from about 900 to 1900 kcal/day.

Another method for determining the daily resting energy expenditure would be to compute the caloric equivalent of the total volume of oxygen consumed for basal functions during a 24-hour period. In the previous section we pointed out that approximately 5 kcal of energy are expended for each liter of oxygen consumed during the combustion of a mixed diet. Because the value for oxygen consumption during resting or basal conditions ranges from about 160 to 290 ml/min (average 0.235 liter/min or 235 ml/min), an average value for energy output per minute at rest would be 1.18 kcal (0.235 × 5 kcal). Because there are 1440 minutes in a day, the daily resting energy expenditure would theoretically equal 1700 kcal (1,440 × 1.18 kcal). This value is only a rough approximation because it does not correct for differences in body size such as surface area, body weight, or lean body weight.

Energy Metabolism during Physical Activity

An understanding of the energy required for maintaining bodily functions in resting conditions provides a frame of reference to evaluate not only the minimum demands for energy, but also the potential to increase the daily metabolic output. According to numerous surveys, about one-third of a person's time is spent in resting activities like those specified in the test of BMR. The remaining 16 to 18 hours are devoted to a wide range of physical activities. Consequently the total amount of energy expended during a day can be considerably greater than the basal requirement, depending of course on the type and duration of physical activity performed.

Researchers have measured the energy expended during such varied physical activities as brushing teeth, cleaning house, mowing the lawn, walking the dog, driving a car, playing Ping-Pong, bowling, dancing, swimming, sawing, and even walking on the moon. The portable spirometer shown in Figure 4-3 has been used extensively for determining the energy requirements of most daily chores and sport activities, while the balloon and computer techniques have provided an accurate means for measuring the oxygen consumed in activities such as cycling, swimming, running, and weight training. Figure 4-7 shows how oxygen consumption was measured during high speed, hydraulic resistive power training and rebound exercise.

In the example of rebound exercise, suppose the time spent exercising was 30 minutes. If the oxygen consumption averaged 1 liter per minute, then in 30 minutes the rebounder would consume 30 liters of oxygen. Because the utilization of 1 liter of oxygen produces about 5 kcal of energy, the researcher can make a reasonably accurate estimate of the energy expended. In this instance the body generated 150 kcal (30 liters × 5 kcal) to power the exercise. All this energy cannot be attributed solely to the requirements of rebounding because the 150 kcal value also

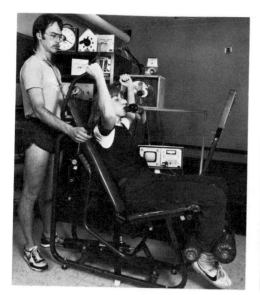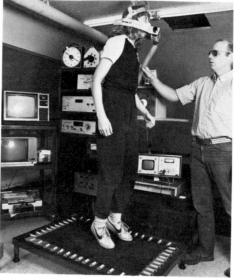

Figure 4-7. *Measurement of oxygen consumption by open-circuit spirometry during high speed hydraulic resistive weight training and rebound exercise on a miniature trampoline. (Courtesy Exercise Physiology Laboratory, Department of Exercise Science, University of Massachusetts, Amherst.)*

includes the normal resting energy requirement during the 30 minutes. By knowing the exerciser's size (weight = 180 pounds; height = 6 feet) surface area can be computed from the nomogram in Figure 4-6. This value for surface area, 2.04 square meters, when multiplied by the average BMR for age (38 kcal/m²/h × 2.04 m²), gives the resting energy production per hour. This amounts to approximately 78 kcal per hour, or 39 kcal in 30-minutes. Based on this computation, the *net energy expenditure* required solely for the exercise can be determined. This is equal to the total energy expenditure of 150 kcal minus that required for resting metabolism which results in a net energy expenditure of approximately 111 kcal.

The energy cost during the weight training exercise would be computed in similar fashion. If the total oxygen consumed in a 30-minute workout was 42 liters for an individual of the same body size as the person performing the rebound exercise, the total or *gross energy expenditure* during the exercise which includes the BMR, would be 210 kcal (42 liters × 5 kcal/liter). By subtracting the appropriate resting value of 39 kcal, the net energy cost for the 30-minute workout would be 171 kcal.

Some investigators have made measurements of the daily rates of energy expenditure for men and women who work in a variety of industrial occupations. They do this by determining the time spent in each activity during the day, and the energy expended for each activity. To calculate the total daily energy expenditure, the time spent in a particular activity is multiplied by the energy cost of the activity. An accurate assessment of the time spent in activities is kept by diary, and energy expenditure is measured with the portable spirometer shown in Figure 4-3. Because it is impractical to carry the spirometer constantly day after day, frequent observations are made for a representative time period. For the miner listed in

technique used to measure oxygen consumption during the floor exercise. Simultaneously, heart rates were monitored by means of radio telemetry. Based on these evaluations, the net caloric expenditure for an entire ballet class averaged only a modest 300 kcal per hour for men and 200 kcal for the women, reflecting a relatively inefficient exercise method for burning calories. A moderate cardiovascular response was also noted as exercise heart rates were generally low, reaching the training sensitive zone only for brief periods during the class. The non-endurance nature of ballet was further substantiated by maximal oxygen uptakes for these elite dancers that were only slightly higher than values for untrained men and women. It can be concluded that standard ballet exercise and training provides a moderate stimulus to enhance aerobic capacity. In terms of its caloric-burning efficiency, it would take a woman approximately eighteen, 1-hour class sessions to burn the calories in a pound of adipose tissues. The same number of calories could be burned in half the time with a program incorporating vigorous running, cycling, or swimming.

Energy Cost of Recreation and Sport Activities

The energy requirements of a group of sport and recreational activities is presented in Appendix B. Table 4-3 lists several examples to illustrate the large variation in energy cost that occurs with participation in various forms of physical activity.

Notice, for example, that golf requires about 6.0 kcal per minute, or 360 kcal per hour for a person who weighs 157 pounds. The same person will expend almost twice this amount of energy, or 708 kcal per hour, while swimming the backstroke. Viewed somewhat differently, 25 minutes of swimming the backstroke

Table 4-3. *Energy cost for a selected group of recreation and sports activities.*

ACTIVITY	KG LBS	50 110	53 117	56 123	59 130	62 137	65 143	68 150	71 157	74 163	77 170	80 176	83 183
Canoeing, leisure		2.2	2.3	2.5	2.6	2.7	2.9	3.0	3.1	3.3	3.4	3.5	3.7
Archery		3.3	3.4	3.6	3.8	4.0	4.2	4.4	4.6	4.8	5.0	5.2	5.4
Golf		4.3	4.5	4.9	5.0	5.3	5.5	5.8	6.0	6.3	6.5	6.8	7.1
Badminton		4.9	5.1	5.4	5.7	6.0	6.3	6.6	6.9	7.2	7.5	7.8	8.1
Swimming, backstroke		8.5	9.0	9.5	10.0	10.5	11.0	11.5	12.0	12.5	13.0	13.5	14.0
Skiing, uphill racing		13.7	14.5	15.3	16.2	17.0	17.8	18.6	19.5	20.3	21.1	21.9	22.7

Source: Data from Appendix B.
Note: Energy expenditure is computed as the number of minutes of participation multiplied by the kcal value in the appropriate body weight column. For example, the kcal cost of one hour of golf for a person weighing 150 pounds is 348 kcal (5.8 kcal × 60 min).

will require about the same number of calories as expended playing golf for 1 hour. If the pace of the swim or golf game is increased, the energy expenditure will also increase proportionally.

As was the case with BMR, body size plays an important role with respect to the energy requirements during exercise. Generally speaking, heavier people expend more energy to perform the same activity than people who weigh less. This is especially true in activities where the body weight must be moved. In fact, energy expenditure during weight bearing exercise increases in direct proportion to body weight. The relationship between body weight and oxygen consumption is so high that energy expenditure during walking or running can be predicted from body weight with almost as much accuracy as from actually measuring the oxygen consumption.

On the other hand, in non-weight-bearing exercise like stationary cycling, there is little or no relationship between body weight and the energy cost of exercise. A practical application of these findings is that walking and other forms of weight-bearing exercise provide a substantial caloric expenditure for heavier people. Notice in Table 4-3 that if a person weighing 183 pounds plays golf or badminton, the total expenditure of energy in kcal is considerably greater than for a lighter person who participates in the same activity. However, when caloric cost is expressed in terms of body weight, that is, kcal per minute per kilogram of body weight (kcal/min·kg), the difference between subjects of different sizes is considerably reduced. When energy expenditure is expressed in this manner, the differences between men and women during exercise are relatively small. Keep in mind, however, that although the average energy requirement in playing a round of golf may be approximately 0.085 kcal/min·kg, regardless of race, sex, or body weight, the *total* energy or calories expended by the heavier player is considerably more than the lighter player. Appendix B presents a more complete list of the energy expended per kilogram of body weight during household, recreational and sports, and occupational and industrial activities. These figures represent average values that can vary considerably depending on skill, pace, and fitness level.

The value listed in the column that corresponds to a particular body weight is the gross caloric cost of the activity for 1 minute, which *includes* the energy cost of rest for the 1-minute period.

HOW TO USE APPENDIX B

Refer to the column that comes closest to your present body weight. Multiply the number in this column by the number of minutes you spend in an activity. For example, suppose an individual weighs 157 pounds and spends 30 minutes playing a casual game of table tennis. To determine the kcal cost of participation, multiply the caloric value of 4.8 kcal obtained in Appendix B by 30 to obtain a total energy expenditure of 144 kcal. If the same individual drives a tractor for 45 minutes the energy expended would be calculated as 2.6 kcal × 45 min or 117 kcal.

Daily Rates of Average Energy Expenditure

A committee of the United States Food and Nutrition Board proposed various norms representing average rates of energy expenditure for men and women living in the United States. These standards apply to males and females who have occupations that could be considered somewhere between sedentary and active, and who participate moderately in recreational activities like weekend swimming, golf, and tennis. As shown in Table 4-4, the average daily energy expenditure is 2700 kcal for men and 2100 kcal for women between the ages of 23 and 50. As can be noted in the bottom part of the table, about 75% of the average man's and woman's day is spent in relatively sedentary activities. This predominance of daily physical *inactivity* has prompted some sociologists to refer to the modern-day American as *Homo sedentarius*, a term that is probably all too appropriate. A survey by the President's Council on Physical Fitness and Sports revealed that for 36% of American men and 51% of American women, walking was the most prevalent form of exercise, regardless of occupation or race. It is probably a fair estimate that only about 50% of adult American men and women engage in physical activities that require an energy expenditure much above the resting level!

Table 4-5 summarizes data on the daily rates of energy expenditure for people with different occupations living in Scotland. Included also are data from Swiss peasants and English army cadets. The number in each group varied from 10 to 30, and the subjects were studied during a 1-week period. Although the average rate of energy expenditure increased for each occupational group as presented from top to bottom in the table, there was considerable individual variation within a particular group. This variability was attributed to differences in time spent outside of work, especially the time devoted to recreational pursuits. Differences in the type of work done within each specific profession were also considered important. One

Table 4-4. *Average daily rates of energy expenditure for men and women living in the United States.*

	AGE, YEARS	WEIGHT, LBS.	HEIGHT, IN.	KCAL
Men	15–18	134	69	3000
	19–22	147	69	3000
	23–50	154	69	2700
	51+	154	69	2400
Women	15–18	119	65	2100
	19–22	128	65	2100
	23–50	128	65	2000
	51+	128	65	1800

AVERAGE TIME SPENT DURING THE DAY FOR MEN AND WOMEN

ACTIVITY	TIME, HOURS
1. Sleeping and lying	8
2. Sitting	6
3. Standing	6
4. Walking	2
5. Recreational: sports or exercises	2

Source: Data from Food and Nutrition Board, National Research Council, *Recommended Dietary Allowances*, 8th rev. ed., National Academy of Sciences, Washington, D.C., 1974. (Also Pub. 1146, 1964.)

Table 4-5. *Daily rates of energy expenditure grouped according to occupation.*

OCCUPATION	ENERGY EXPENDITURE, KCAL/DAY		
	AVERAGE	MINIMUM	MAXIMUM
Men			
Elderly retired	2330	1750	2810
Office workers	2520	1820	3270
Coal mine clerks	2800	2330	3290
Laboratory technicians	2840	2240	3820
Older industrial workers	2840	2180	3710
University students	2930	2270	4410
Building workers	3000	2440	3730
Steel workers	3280	2600	3960
Army cadets	3490	2990	4100
Older peasants (Swiss)	3530	2210	5000
Farmers	3550	2450	4670
Coal miners	3660	2970	4560
Forestry workers	3670	2860	4600
Women			
Older housewives	1990	1490	2410
Middle-aged housewives	2090	1760	2320
Laboratory assistants	2130	1340	2540
Assistants in department store	2250	1820	2850
University students	2290	2090	2500
Factory workers	2320	1970	2980
Bakery workers	2510	1980	3390
Older peasants (Swiss)	2890	2200	3860

Source: Data from J.V.G.A. Durnin and R. Passmore, *Energy, Work and Leisure,* Heinemann Educational Books, London, 1967.

elderly retired man was almost as active as the least energetic of the coal miners and forestry workers. His rate of energy expenditure was therefore much higher than the average for his group.

Classification of Work

All of us at one time or another have done some type of physical work that we would classify as exceedingly "difficult". This might be walking up a flight of stairs, shoveling snow to clear the driveway, running to catch a bus, loading and unloading a truck, digging a trench to fix an underground pipe, skiing through a blizzard, or climbing a steep mountain. There are several factors to consider in rating the difficulty of a particular task. One is the amount of *time* it takes, and the other is the *intensity* of the effort. Both of these factors may vary considerably. For example, two people of the same body size could expend an equal amount of energy to perform the same task. However, one might exert extreme effort over a short period, while the other might exert less effort over a longer period. An example might be climbing several flights of stairs. Suppose the first person ran the stairs at maximum speed, expending 15 kcal of energy. The second person moved more leisurely and took 2 minutes to climb the stairs, yet still expended 15 kcal of energy. The basic difference in achieving the 15 kcal output was the time factor, or more accurately, the intensity of work.

Several systems have been proposed for rating the difficulty of work in terms of intensity. The system we use has classified work into categories designated as light, moderate, heavy, very heavy, and unduly heavy.

The five-level classification system presented in Table 4-6 is based on the energy required by untrained men and women performing different tasks. The amount of energy that corresponds to a particular work level is expressed as kcal per minute and METS, *a MET being defined as a multiple of the resting metabolism.* One MET is equivalent to an average resting energy expenditure or oxygen consumption. Physical work performed at 2 METS requires twice the resting metabolism, 3 METS is three times the resting energy expenditure, and so on. Also listed in the table are caloric equivalents and examples of activities that correspond generally to the different intensities of work effort.

Table 4-6. *Five-level classification of physical work based on intensity of effort.*

WORK CATEGORIES	MEN		WOMEN		ACTIVITIES
	KCAL/MIN	METS	KCAL/MIN	METS	
Light	2.0–4.9	1.6–3.9	1.5–3.4	1.2–2.7	Walking; reading a book; driving a car; shopping; bowling; fishing; golf; pleasure sailing.
Moderate	5.0–7.4	4.0–5.9	3.5–5.4	2.8–4.3	Pleasure cycling; dancing; volleyball; badminton; calisthenics.
Heavy	7.5–9.9	6.0–7.9	5.5–7.4	4.4–5.9	Ice skating; water skiing; competitive tennis; novice mountain climbing; jogging.
Very Heavy	10.0–12.4	8.0–9.9	7.5–9.4	6.0–7.5	Fencing; touch football; scuba diving; basketball game; swim (most strokes).
Unduly Heavy	12.5–>	10.0–>	9.5–>	7.6–>	Handball; squash; cross-country skiing; paddleball; running (fast pace)

II

Body Composition and Weight Control

A N EXCESS ACCUMULATION of body fat is undesirable for a variety of reasons. From a health standpoint, medical problems exist in which obesity or "overfatness" is considered a risk factor, and for which a reduction in excess fat is desirable. These problems include certain types of heart disease, high blood pressure, impaired carbohydrate and fat metabolism, joint, bone, and gallbladder diseases, diabetes, asthma, and various lung disorders. Being too fat is also often accompanied by changes in personality and behavior patterns often manifested as depression, withdrawal, self-pity, irritability, and aggression.

The first step in formulating an intelligent program of weight control is to appraise body size objectively. It is possible to be heavy and even overweight according to height-weight charts, yet possess only a moderate amount of body fat. Many athletes, for example, are quite muscular but are otherwise lean in terms of their overall body composition. For such people a program of dietary modification or exercise for purposes of weight control may be unnecessary. Such an approach would be prudent, however, for others who may be 10 to 15 pounds "overfat." Of even greater importance is the need for effective weight control among the increasingly large segment of the population afflicted with "creeping obesity." During the adult years both body weight and body fat can increase insidiously to the point where the amount of body fat exceeds even the most liberal limits for normalcy. It is at this point that the health-related aspects of obesity become a concern. Unfortunately the correction of adult-acquired obesity through diet or programs of exercise is much more difficult than its early prevention.

The chapters that follow deal with topics relevant to body composition, obesity, and weight control. Chapter 5 discusses the underlying rationale for the evaluation of body composition in terms of body fat and lean body weight. Also included is a simple yet accurate method for assessing the body's total quantity of fat objectively. In Chapter 6 we define overweight in terms of the acceptable limits of body

99

fat for a particular age range for men and women. We discuss the interrelated factors often associated with obesity as well as the efficacy of diet and exercise as a treatment for the overfat condition. In Chapter 7, which deals with weight control, we discuss the question of weight loss and weight gain within the framework of the "energy balance equation." In addition, we present a strategy for quantifying food intake and incorporating exercise and caloric restriction to achieve a desired rate of weight loss. Chapter 8 is concerned with the application of the principles of behavior modification, with emphasis on weight reduction by means of dietary modification and increased energy expenditure through more vigorous physical activity.

Evaluation of Body Composition

I N THE EARLY 1940s Dr. Albert Behnke, a Navy medical doctor and foremost authority on body composition, made detailed measurements of the size, shape, and structure of 25 professional football players, many of whom had achieved All-American status while in college. According to the military standards at that time, a person whose body weight was 15% above the "average weight-for-height," as determined from insurance company statistics, was designated as overweight and rejected by the military. When these overweight standards were applied to the football players who ranged in weight from 170 to 260 pounds, 17 players were classified as too fat and unfit for military service. However, a more careful evaluation of each player's body composition revealed that 11 of the 17 overweight players actually had a relatively low percentage of body fat. The players' excess weight was due primarily to their large muscular development.

These data were among the first to illustrate clearly that the popular height-weight tables provide little information about the *composition* or quality of an individual's body weight. A football player may indeed weigh much more than some "average," "ideal," or "desirable" body weight based on height-weight tables, but more than likely these athletes are not excessively fat or in need of reducing their body size. The extra weight is likely to consist of a considerable amount of muscle mass. Thus the term "overweight" refers only to body weight in excess of some standard, usually the average weight for a specific height, and that's all! Consequently the use of height-weight tables can be quite misleading for the person who wants to know, "How fat am I?"

During the past 50 years many laboratory procedures have been developed to analyze the body in relation to its three major structural components: fat, muscle, and bone. Some of the procedures are time-consuming and require the use of sophisticated, expensive laboratory equipment, while other procedures are fairly simple and inexpensive. In this chapter we will analyze the gross composition of the body and present the rationale underlying the various direct and indirect methods for quantitatively partitioning the body into two basic compartments, *body fat* and *lean body weight*. In addition, we present a simple method for determining the body composition of men and women in terms of percent body fat, pounds of fat, and lean body weight.

Gross Composition of the Human Body

The three major structural components of the human body include muscle, fat, and bone. Because there are marked sex differences in body composition, a convenient basis for evaluation and comparison is to employ the concept proposed by Dr. Behnke of the *reference man* and *reference woman*. Figure 5-1 depicts the gross composition for a reference man and woman in terms of muscle, fat, and

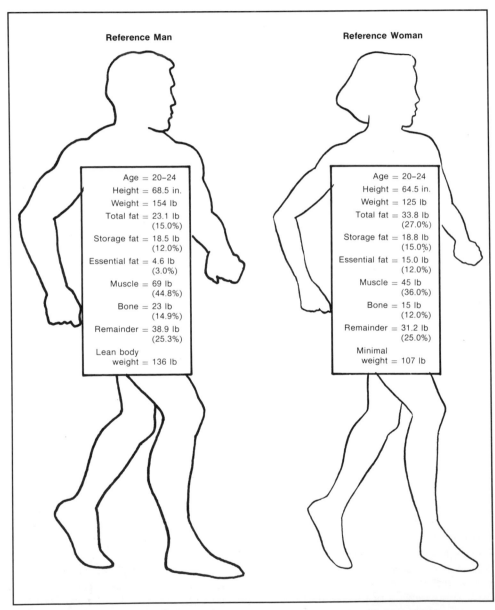

Figure 5-1. *Body composition of a reference man and woman. (McArdle, W.D., Katch, F.I., and Katch, V.L.: Exercise Physiology, Lea & Febiger, 1981.)*

bone. This theoretical model is based upon the average physical dimensions obtained from detailed measurements of thousands of individuals who were subjects in large-scale anthropometric and nutrition assessment surveys.

The reference man is taller by 4 in., heavier by 29 lb; his skeleton weighs more (23 vs. 15 lb); and he has a larger muscle mass (69 vs. 45 lb) and lower total fat content (23.1 vs. 33.8 lb) than the reference female. These sex differences exist even when the amount of fat, muscle, and bone are expressed as a percentage of body weight. This is especially true for body fat which represents 15 and 27% of the total body weight of the average man and woman, respectively. The concept of reference standards does not mean that men and women should strive to achieve the body composition of the reference models, nor that the reference man and woman are in fact "average." The models are useful as a frame of reference to compare different individuals in terms of their body composition.

Essential and Storage Fat

The total amount of body fat exists in two depots or storage sites. The first depot, termed *essential fat*, is the fat stored in the marrow of bones as well as in the heart, lungs, liver, spleen, kidneys, intestines, muscles, and lipid-rich tissues throughout the central nervous system. *This fat is required for normal physiologic functioning.* In the female, essential fat also includes *sex-specific* or *sex-characteristic* fat. It is not at all clear whether this fat depot is expendable or serves as reserve storage. The mammary glands and pelvic region are probably primary storage sites for this fat, although the precise quantitative amounts are unknown. In one recent experiment, the contribution of breast weight to the body's total body fat content was estimated to be no higher than 4% for women who varied in body fat content from 14 to 35%. This must mean that sites other than the breasts contribute a larger proportion of sex-specific fat, perhaps in the lower body region, which includes the pelvis and thighs.

The other major fat depot, the *storage fat*, consists of fat that accumulates in adipose tissue. This nutritional reserve includes the fatty tissues that protect the various internal organs from trauma, as well as the larger subcutaneous fat volume deposited beneath the skin surface. Although the proportional distribution of storage fat in males and females is similar (12% in males, 15% in females), the total quantity of essential fat in females, which includes the sex-specific fat, is four times higher than in males. More than likely, the additional essential fat is biologically important for child-bearing and other hormone-related functions.

MINIMAL STANDARDS FOR LEANNESS

There seems to be a biologically lower limit beyond which a person's body weight cannot be reduced without impairing health status. This lower limit in men is referred to as *lean body weight* and is calculated as body weight minus the weight of storage fat. For the reference man, the lean weight is equivalent to 136 lb; this includes approximately 3% or 4.1 lb essential fat. This amount of fat presumably is a lower limit, and any encroachment into this reserve may impair normal physiologic function or capacity for exercise. Similar low values of body fat have also been obtained for champion male athletes in various sports. The body fat content of world-class, male marathon runners ranges from about 4 to 8%, which is only slightly more than the quantity of essential fat that apparently cannot be reduced. The low fat content and body weight for these exceptional athletes reflect, to some degree, a positive adaptation to the prolonged, severe requirements of distance training. A minimal quantity of body fat permits a more effective transfer of metabolic heat during high intensity exercise, and reduces the quantity of excess weight that the athlete must transport while running. Low values for body fat have also been obtained for other athletes. In our studies of professional football players (1975–1979 New York Jets; 1976–1978 Dallas Cowboys; 1979–1980 Miami Dolphins and New Orleans Saints), values of fatness as low as 1.0% of body weight have been recorded for several defensive backs. This corresponds to the body weight with essentially no storage fat.

Considerable individual differences also are found in the lean body weight of different athletes, with values ranging from a low of 106 pounds in some jockeys to a high of 240 to 250 pounds in All-Pro football defensive linemen and Olympic champion discus throwers and power lifters.

MINIMAL WEIGHT (WOMEN)

In contrast to the lower limit of body weight of males, which includes 3% essential fat in adipose tissue, the lower limit of body weight for the reference female includes 12% essential fat in adipose tissue. This theoretical limit for *minimal weight* for the reference woman is equivalent to 107 pounds. In general, the leanest women in the population do not have body fat levels below about 10 to 12% of body weight. This probably represents the lower limit of fatness for most women in good health. *This concept of minimal weight in females that incorporates about 12% essential fat is equivalent to lean body weight in males that includes 3% essential fat in adipose tissue.*

It should be emphasized that the concept of female minimal weight is based on theoretical considerations, with little actual data other than the fact that in carefully conducted experiments values lower than 10% body fat are rarely reported. Data from female distance runners constitute an exception, where a value of 5.9% body fat was reported for one runner who weighed 52.6 kg.

UNDERWEIGHT AND THIN

The terms underweight and thin are not necessarily synonyomous. In fact, in some cases they describe physical characteristics that differ considerably. For example, in one of our recent studies, the structural characteristics of apparently "thin" females was compared with women who appeared "normal" in size as well as women who appeared obese. The objective of the research was to determine if body frame size (as measured by bone widths) differed among the three groups.

The results were unexpected. While the thin appearing women were indeed relatively low in body fat, 18.2% compared with 25% body fat for the "normal" size women and 32% for the obese group, there were *no differences* in the average structural dimensions between the three groups! What this meant was that for women of approximately the same height, there was no such thing as a predominantly small, medium, or large frame size as defined by four trunk and four extremity bone widths. Thus, appearing thin or skinny does not necessarily mean that skeletal frame size is diminutive or that the body's total fat content is excessively low. Based on our studies, we have classified an underweight adult female as one of three types:

TYPE I. Lean body weight is low, ranging from 35 to 45 kg. These women have similar physical characteristics as preanorexic women and are usually nutritionally deficient. They usually but not always, have a history of underweightness and are not inclined to be physically active.

TYPE II. Lean body weight ranges between 42 to 50 kg. They are physically active but not champion or high performance athletes. Menstrual function and nutritional status are usually normal.

TYPE III. Lean body weight is higher than normal, typically 50 kg. and higher. These women have frequent menstrual irregularities, the most common being amenorrhea. Amenorrhea often coincides with training and reverses when training stops or is reduced. Psychologic stress factors may also be implicated, but are more difficult to clearly define. Nutritional status is normal. These women have good muscle tone and comparatively low levels of subcutaneous fat.

It should be pointed out that basic and clinical research in defining and classifying underweight females is in its infancy; it is not yet possible to precisely state what is abnormal or undesirable regarding underweightness. Further research is required to establish definitive body fat and lean body weight boundaries for the Type I, II, and III underweight female.

Does Low Body Fat Trigger Amenorrhea?

Some researchers have suggested that females with a low percentage of body fat suffer from *amenorrhea* or disruption of the normal menstrual cycle. Harvard researcher, Dr. Rose Frisch, considers the body weight at 17% fat as the critical body weight, and she says reducing below this weight triggers hormonal and metabolic disturbances that can affect the menses. The critical weight hypothesis proposes that the onset and regularity of menstrual function necessitates maintaining body weight above 17% body fat. Although the lean-to-fat ratio does appear to be important, other factors must be considered, however, as there is ample evidence that females who are below 17% body fat have normal menstrual cycles and maintain a high level of physiologic capacity.

A recent report of women in the U.S. Military Academy at West Point demonstrated that participation in a rigorous physical training and exercise program markedly affected previously normal menstrual patterns. Eighty-six percent of the 70 freshmen in 1976 who averaged 19% body fat had normal menstruation before entering West Point, but within 2 months of starting the program 73% reported discontinued menstruation. After 6 months 42% experienced irregularities. After 15 months, 7% had still not resumed their normal periods. This same pattern was observed for the 1977 and 1978 freshman classes. Other recent studies have shown that from one-half to one-third of female athletes have abnormal menstrual functions. It certainly would appear that strenuous physical training per se can affect menstrual patterns, independently of the level of body fat. Conversely, there are currently many outstanding female athletes (long distance runners, gymnasts, body builders) who have normal menses with no disruption of their cycles during intensive training and competition, and who compete at a body fat level in the range of 8 to 13%!

In a recent study from one of our laboratories, 30 female athletes and 30 non-athletes, all below 20% body fat, were compared for menstrual cycle regularity, irregularity, and amenorrhea. Four of the athletes and 3 non-athletes who ranged in body fat from 11 to 15% had regular cycles, while 7 athletes and 2 non-athletes had irregular cycles or were amenorrheic. For the total sample (fat range from 11 to 20%), 14 athletes and 21 non-athletes had regular cycles, respectively. These data corroborate previous findings, and lead us to conclude that the hypothesis of a critical fat level related to the female reproductive cycle needs further research and experimentation. The complex interplay of physical, hormonal, nutritional, psychological, and environmental factors on menstrual function must be considered. In addition, it appears that the exercise-associated disturbances in menstrual function can be reversed with changes in life style without serious consequences. What is not known, however, is the effect sustained amenorrhea may have on the reproductive system. Certainly, detailed studies of reproductive function of athletes in and out of training will provide more definitive answers relative to this important topic.

Female Body Builders

During the late 1970s, body building for females gained widespread popularity throughout the United States as women aggressively pursued this previously male dominated sport. As more women undertook the rigorous demands of training with weights, competition became more intense and the level of achievement increased markedly. Because success in body building is based on a "slim" and lean appearance, complimented by a well-defined musculature, interesting questions were raised with regard to body composition. How lean are such competitors, and does their presumably low level of body fat disrupt normal menstrual function?

The results of a pioneering study of the body composition of 10 competitive female body builders revealed that these athletes were quite lean, averaging 13.3% body fat (range from 8.0 to 18.3%) with an average lean body weight of 46.6 kg. Their body weight averaged 53.8 kg, height 160.8 cm, and age 27.1 years. With the exception of champion gymnasts who also average about 13% body fat, the body builders were shorter in height by 3 to 4%, lower in body weight by 4 to 5%, and possessed 7 to 10% less total weight of body fat compared with other top female athletes. The most striking compositional characteristic of the female body builders was their dramatically large lean-to-fat ratio of 7:1 (weight of the lean mass relative to the weight of the fat mass) in comparison to 4.3:1 for other female athletic groups. Figure 5-2 illustrates the remarkable muscular development of 2 champion female body builders.

As more data become available on other aspects of female body builders, such as strength and fatigue levels and cardiorespiratory and hormonal functions, a more complete picture will emerge regarding the physiologic consequences of both short and long term participation in the sport of body building. It is interesting to note that menstrual function was perfectly normal in 8 of 10 body builders in the previously mentioned study where percent body fat ranged from 8 to 18%.

Common Laboratory Methods to Assess Body Composition

The fat and lean components of the human body have been determined by two general procedures. One procedure measures body composition directly by *chemical analysis*. The second approach assesses body composition indirectly with *hy-*

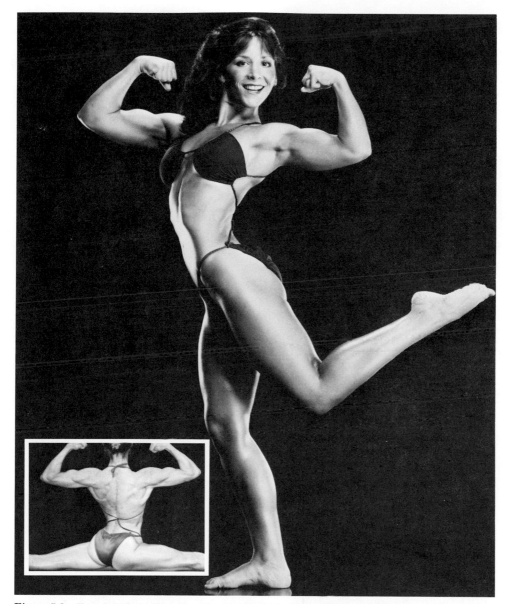

Figure 5-2. *Female body builder. Top, Corrine Machado-Ching. (Courtesy of Muscle and Fitness and Shape Magazines.) Inset, Stephanie Jones. (Courtesy of Stephanie Jones.)*

drostatic weighing or with simple *circumferences* or *fatfold* measurements. While direct methods form the basis for indirect techniques and are useful in animal research and for human cadaver analysis, the use of indirect procedures enables the scientist to assess the body composition of living people accurately.

DIRECT MEASUREMENT
Chemical Analysis

Although there has been considerable research dealing with the direct measurement of body composition in various species of animals, relatively few studies have employed precise chemical techniques to analyze human fat content. Such analyses are time-consuming and tedious, require highly specialized laboratory equipment, and involve many ethical and legal problems in obtaining cadavers for research purposes. For these reasons only a few analyses of human cadavers have been made during the past 100 years. In 1863 detailed dissections were made of a 33-year-old man, a 22-year-old woman, and an 18-year-old boy who died in an accident. In the present century chemical analyses have been made of only 7 cadavers. Of those 7, one subject, a 46-year-old male, 5 feet, 6 inches tall and weight 118 pounds, died of a skull fracture. A 99-pound, 42-year-old woman committed suicide by drowning, while the other 5 male subjects, aged 25, 35, 41, 48, and 60, died of circulatory diseases. Consequently, it is difficult to pinpoint by direct chemical analysis the compositional structure of an "average" subject. This is especially true in terms of body fat which exhibits extreme variability between individuals of the same sex, regardless of height or body weight. Recent studies of cadavers will hopefully provide more detailed information about the chemical composition of the human body.

Data from animals and the limited human cadaver studies also indicate that the weight of the dry, fat-free skeleton remains remarkably constant, even when large variations exist in the percentage of total body fat. Thus the most variable component of the body is its fat. The fact that the skeleton and percentage of water in fat-free tissue remain so invariable in both lean and fat people has enabled researchers to develop accurate mathematical equations to determine the body's fat and lean percentages. This is indeed fortunate, as the direct method for determining the fat content of cadavers, while of considerable theoretical importance, obviously cannot be used with living subjects.

INDIRECT ASSESSMENT

The following section presents two useful indirect procedures to assess body composition. The first procedure describes Archimedes' principle as applied to hydrostatic weighing. With this method percent body fat is computed from *body density,* that is, the ratio of body weight to body volume. The second procedure involves the *prediction* of body fat from circumference or girth measurements. This method is of practical significance because body fat can be predicted both simply and accurately.

Body Volume Determination

About two thousand years ago the Greek mathematician Archimedes discovered a basic principle that is currently applied in the evaluation of body composition. An itinerant scholar of that time described the interesting circumstances surrounding this event:

King Hieron of Syracuse suspected that his pure gold crown had been altered by substitution of silver for gold. The King directed Archimedes to devise a method for testing the crown for its gold content without dismantling it. Archimedes pondered over this problem for many weeks without succeeding until one day he stepped into a bath filled to the top with water and observed the overflow of water. He thought about this for a moment, and then, wild with joy, jumped from the bath and ran naked through the streets of Syracuse shouting "Eureka! Eureka! I have discovered a way to solve the mystery of the King's golden crown." Archimedes reasoned that a substance such as gold must have a volume proportionate to its weight, and the way to measure the volume of an irregular object such as the crown was to submerge it in water and collect the overflow. Archimedes took a lump of gold and silver, each having the same weight as the crown, and submerged each in a container full of water, and to his delight discovered that the crown displaced more water than the lump of gold and less than the lump of silver. What this meant was that the crown was indeed composed of silver *and* gold as the King had suspected.

Essentially, what Archimedes evaluated was the *specific gravity* of the crown (ratio of the weight of the crown to the weight of an equal volume of water) compared to the specific gravities for gold and silver. Archimedes probably also reasoned that an object submerged in water must be buoyed up by a counterforce that equals the weight of the water it displaces. This buoyancy force helps to support an object in water against the downward pull of gravity. Thus the object is said to lose weight in water. Because the object's loss of weight in water equals the weight of the *volume* of water it displaces, we can redefine specific gravity as the ratio of the weight of an object in air divided by its loss of weight in water. Thus,

$$\text{Specific gravity} = \frac{\text{weight of an object in air}}{\text{loss of weight in water or}}$$
$$(\text{weight in air} - \text{weight in water})$$

In practical terms, suppose the crown weighed 5.0 pounds in air and when weighed underwater, as shown in Figure 5-3, weighed 0.29 pounds less or 4.71 pounds. The specific gravity of the crown would then be computed by dividing the weight of the crown (5.0 pounds) by its loss of weight in water (0.29 pounds). This

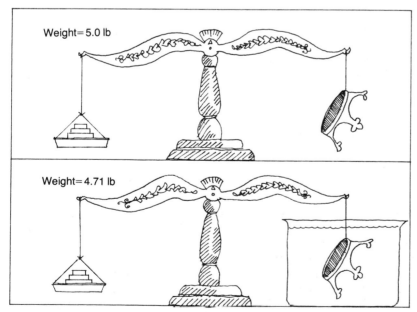

Figure 5-3. *Archimedes' solution for determining the gold content of the king's crown.*

results in a specific gravity of 17.24. Because this ratio is considerably different than the specific gravity of gold (19.3), we too can conclude: "Eureka! Eureka! the crown is a fraud!"

The physical principle Archimedes discovered can be applied directly to the assessment of body composition in humans. This is achieved by determining the volume of the body by water submersion in relation to the total body mass. Because density is mass per unit volume, it becomes a relatively simple matter to compute the body density once the mass and volume are known.

DENSITY OF THE HUMAN BODY   Let us now determine the density of the human body. For illustrative purposes, suppose our subject weighs 50 kg as measured on a conventional scale, and 2 kg when submerged completely underwater. According to Archimedes' principle, the buoyancy or counterforce of the water must equal 48 kg. This loss of weight in water of 48 kg is exactly equal to the weight of the displaced water. Because the density of water at any temperature is known, we can compute the volume of water displaced by this person. In the present example, 48 kg (48,000 g) of water would equal a volume of 48 liters or 48,000 cc (1 g water = 1 cm^3 in volume at 39.2°F). If volume was measured at the cold water temperature of 39.2°F, no density correction would be necessary. In practice, however, researchers use warmer water and apply the appropriate density value for water. The density of the subject, computed as weight ÷ volume, would be 50,000 g (50 kg) ÷ 48,000 g/cm^3 or 1.0417 g/cm^3. This particular value for body density is midway between the value of 0.90 g/cm^3 for fat extracted from adipose tissue and 1.10 g/cm^3 for fat-free tissue. Once body density has been determined, the next step is to determine the amount of fat that corresponds to that value.

COMPUTING PERCENT BODY FAT FROM BODY DENSITY   It is possible to determine the relative percentages of fat in the human body with a simple equation that incorporates density. This equation was derived from the theoretical premise that the densities of fat and fat-free tissues remain relatively constant (density of fat = 0.90 g/cm^3; density of fat-free tissue = 1.10 g/cm^3) even with large variations in total body fat. Thus, the proportions of the fat and lean components can be determined from an algebraic expression that relates these proportions to the density of the whole body. The following equation is used to compute percent body fat by incorporating the determined value of body density.

$$\text{Percent body fat} = \frac{495}{\text{body density}} - 450.$$

The value for body density of 1.0417 g/cm^3 determined for the 50-kg subject in the previous example can now be substituted in the equation for percent body fat as follows:

$$\text{Percent body fat} = \frac{495}{1.0417} - 450 = 25.2 \text{ percent fat.}$$

Thus 25.2% or 12.6 kg of the 50-kg body weight is fat. The remaining 37.4 kg is lean body weight.

The weight of fat is calculated by multiplying body weight by percent fat.

$$\text{Fat weight (kg)} = \frac{\text{body weight (kg)} \times \text{percent fat}}{100}$$

= 50 kg × 0.252
= 12.6 kg.

Lean body weight is calculated by subtracting the weight of fat from body weight.

$$\text{Lean body weight (kg)} = \text{body weight (kg)} - \text{fat weight (kg)}$$

= 50 kg − 12.6 kg
− 37.4 kg.

The determination of body weight and the calculations for body density, percent body fat, and lean body weight are quite simple. The more difficult task is the accurate assessment of body volume and thus body density. By application of the principle discovered by Archimedes, we can do this in two ways: water displacement and underwater or hydrostatic weighing.

Water displacement is essentially the technique used by Archimedes for determining the gold content of the crown. The volume of an object submerged in water can be measured by the corresponding rise in the level of water within a container. Researchers using this technique can measure the rise of water in a thin tube secured to the side of a tank. This finely calibrated tube provides for accurate measurements.

Underwater weighing computes body volume as the difference between body weight measured in air and weight measured during water submersion. In other words, body volume is equal to the loss of weight in water with the appropriate temperature correction for the water's density. Figure 5-4 illustrates the procedure in one of our laboratories for measuring body volume by underwater weighing.

A diver's belt is first secured around the waist to insure that the subject does not float toward the surface during submersion. The subject, who wears a thin nylon swim suit, climbs into the tank and sits in a specially designed chair suspended from the scale and submerged beneath the surface of the water. The subject makes a forced maximal exhalation as the head is lowered underwater. The breath is held for about 5 seconds while the underwater weight is recorded. Ten to 12 repeated weighings are made to insure that a dependable underwater weight score is obtained. Even though the subject has exhaled maximally during the repeated underwater weighings, a small volume of air, the *residual lung volume*, still remains in the lungs. This air volume is measured for each subject just before the underwater weighing and its buoyant effect subtracted in the calculation of body density. The temperature of the water is also recorded and corrected for the density of water at the weighing temperature, as is the hydrostatic effect of water submersion on lung exhalation.

Let us now put theory into practice by showing the sequence of steps used to compute body density, percent fat, pounds of fat, and lean body weight. The sub-

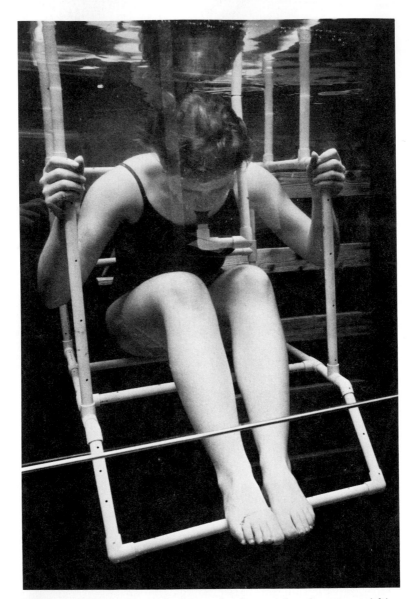

Figure 5-4. *Measuring body volume by the seated underwater weighing method. The subject is submerged in a 5′ × 5′ × 5′ stainless steel tank with plexiglass front. A heater maintains water temperature at 98°F, and a filtration system maintains water purity. A 9 kg, 10 g autopsy scale hangs above the tank to which the lightweight (1.5 kg) tubular chair support is suspended. This subject is breathing through a snorkel. Most younger individuals, however, are able to expel to residual volume without this aid. In our laboratory, we have found no significant differences between residual volume measured during water submersion and residual volume measured prior to underwater weighing in 60 males and 72 females, ages 18 to 30 years. (Photo courtesy of the Department of Exercise Science, University of Massachusetts, Amherst.)*

jects are two professional football players, an offensive guard, and a quarterback. For each player we made the following measurements:

	Offensive guard	Quarterback
Body weight	110 kg	85 kg
Underwater weight	3.5 kg	5.0 kg
Residual lung volume	1.2 liters	1.0 liters
Water temperature correction	0.996	0.996

Because the loss of weight in water is equal to volume, the body volume of the offensive guard is 110 kg − 3.5 kg = 106.5 kg or 106.5 liters; for the quarterback, body volume is 85 kg − 5.0 kg = 80.0 kg or 80 liters. Dividing body volume by the water temperature correction factor of 0.996 increases the volume slightly for both players, from 106.5 liters to 106.9 liters for the offensive guard and from 80.0 liters to 80.3 liters for the quarterback. Because the residual lung volume also contributes to buoyancy, we must now subtract this volume from the body volume. When this is done, the body volume of the offensive guard becomes 105.7 liters (106.9 liters − 1.2 liters); for the quarterback, body volume is 79.3 liters (80.3 liters − 1.0 liters). Body density is then computed as weight ÷ volume. For the offensive guard, body density is 110 kg ÷ 105.7 liters = 1.0407 kg/liters or 1.0407 g/cm³. For the quarterback, body density is 85.0 ÷ 79.3 = 1.0719 g/cm³.

$$\text{Body density} = \frac{\text{weight in air}}{\dfrac{\text{weight in air} - \text{weight in water}}{\text{water temperature correction}} - \begin{array}{c}\text{residual}\\\text{lung volume}\end{array}}$$

Offensive guard

$$\text{Body density} = \frac{110 \text{ kg}}{\dfrac{110 \text{ kg} - 3.5 \text{ kg}}{0.996} - 1.2 \text{ liters}}$$

$$= 1.0407 \text{ g/cc.}$$

Quarterback

$$\text{Body density} = \frac{85 \text{ kg}}{\dfrac{85 \text{ kg} - 5.0 \text{ kg}}{0.996} - 1.0 \text{ liters}}$$

$$= 1.0719 \text{ g/cc.}$$

Percent body fat is calculated as follows:

$$\text{Percent fat} = \frac{495}{\text{density}} - 450$$

Offensive guard

$$\text{Percent fat} = \frac{495}{1.0407} - 450$$

$$= 25.6 \text{ percent.}$$

Quarterback

$$\text{Percent fat} = \frac{495}{1.0719} - 450$$

$$= 11.8 \text{ percent.}$$

The total weight of body fat is calculated as follows:

$$\text{Weight of fat} = \frac{\text{body weight} \times \text{percent fat}}{100}$$

Offensive guard

Weight of fat = 110 kg × 0.256
= 28.2 kg.

Quarterback

Weight of fat = 85 kg × 0.118
= 10.0 kg.

Lean body weight is calculated as follows:

Lean body weight (LBW) = body weight − weight of fat

Offensive guard

LBW = 110 kg − 28.2 kg
= 81.8 kg.

Quarterback

LBW = 85 kg = 10.0 kg
= 75.0 kg.

This analysis of body composition clearly illustrates that the offensive guard possesses more than twice the percentage of body fat than the quarterback (25.6 versus 11.8%) and almost 3 times as much total fat (28.2 kg versus 10.0 kg). On the other hand, lean body weight, which provides a good indication of muscle mass, is also larger for the guard than for the quarterback. Although the offensive guard is 25 kg heavier than the quarterback, similar differences in body composition can also be demonstrated for people of the *same* body weight, especially between physically active and sedentary people. Results such as these demonstrate clearly that the crucial aspect of body composition evaluation is to determine the fat and lean components of the body, and *not* to rely solely on body weight as an index of "acceptability" regarding body size and shape.

Prediction of Body Fat from Circumference Measurements

Hydrostatic weighing is one of the most accurate indirect methods currently available to assess the body's fat content. However, proper measurement with this technique requires equipment and facilities not normally available in a doctor's office, hospital, physical education department, or physical conditioning center. Thus alternative but simple procedures to predict body fatness have been developed. One of these procedures is to measure the girth or circumferences at selected sites on the body. It is easy to take circumferences with a cloth measuring tape and you can achieve accuracy with a minimum of practice. For added precision, record measurements in centimeters.

In taking the measurement, apply the tape lightly to the skin surface so it is taut but not tight. If you pull the tape too tightly, it will compress the underlying soft tissue and make the value smaller than it actually is. Take duplicate measurements at each site and use the average value as the circumference score.

USEFULNESS OF CIRCUMFERENCE SCORES

In recent experiments we have determined the best combination of circumference measures for predicting body fatness in a sample of young adult and older men and women. The younger group ranged in age from 17 to 26 years; the age range of the older subjects was 27 to 50 years. The criterion values for body density and percent body fat were determined in the laboratory by hydrostatic weighing or water displacement methods. The data were analyzed to determine the combination of circumference measures that came closest to predicting actual body fatness as determined by the more sophisticated laboratory techniques. A combination of three circumferences resulted in an accurate prediction of fatness for all subjects. *These predicted values for body fat were within 2.5 to 4.0% of values determined in the laboratory.* The practical significance of this finding was obvious; percent body fat could be predicted easily from a few simple circumference measurements.

The anatomic landmarks used in taking the various circumference measurements for the young and older women and men are described below and illustrated in Figure 5-5.

Young women	Older women	Young men	Older men
1. Abdomen	1. Abdomen	1. Right upper arm	1. Buttocks
2. Right thigh	2. Right thigh	2. Abdomen	2. Abdomen
3. Right forearm	3. Right calf	3. Right forearm	3. Right forearm

Abdomen—one inch above the umbilicus

Buttocks—maximum protrusion with the heels together

Right thigh—upper thigh just below the buttocks

Right upper arm—arm straight, palm up and extended in front of the body (measure at the midpoint between the shoulder and elbow)

Right forearm—maximum circumference with the arm extended in front of the body with palm up

Right calf—widest circumference midway between the ankle and knee

CALCULATION OF PERCENT BODY FAT

Percent body fat can be calculated directly by use of the three constants *A*, *B*, and *C*, presented in Table 5-1 for young women, Table 5-2 for older women, Table 5-3 for young men, and Table 5-4 for older men. The values corresponding to each constant are substituted in the formula at the bottom of the appropriate table. Percent body fat is obtained after performing the two additions and two subtrac-

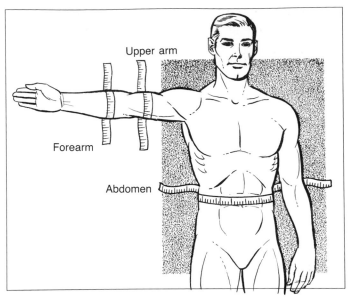

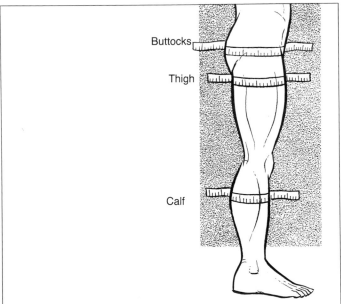

Figure 5-5. *Measurement of circumferences with a tape.*

tions in the formula. It should be emphasized that the equations to predict percent body fat from circumferences may not be valid when applied to athletic young men and women who regularly engage in strenuous physical training, or for large or small individuals who could be visually classified as thin or obese.

The following five-step example illustrates how percent fat, weight of fat, and lean body weight were calculated for a 24-year-old woman who weighed 125 pounds.

TABLE 5-1. *Conversion constants to predict percent body fat for* **young women.**
(Tables 5-1 to 5-4 from McArdle, W.D., Katch, F.I. and Katch, V.L.: Exercise Physiology,
Lea & Febiger, 1981.)

ABDOMEN			THIGH			FOREARM		
IN.	CM	CONSTANT A	IN.	CM	CONSTANT B	IN.	CM	CONSTANT C
20.00	50.80	26.74	14.00	35.56	29.13	6.00	15.24	25.86
20.25	51.43	27.07	14.25	36.19	29.65	6.25	15.87	26.94
20.50	52.07	27.41	14.50	36.83	30.17	6.50	16.51	28.02
20.75	52.70	27.74	14.75	37.46	30.69	6.75	17.14	29.10
21.00	53.34	28.07	15.00	38.10	31.21	7.00	17.78	30.17
21.25	53.97	28.41	15.25	38.73	31.73	7.25	18.41	31.25
21.50	54.61	28.74	15.50	39.37	32.25	7.50	19.05	32.33
21.75	55.24	29.08	15.75	40.00	32.77	7.75	19.68	33.41
22.00	55.88	29.41	16.00	40.64	33.29	8.00	20.32	34.48
22.25	56.51	29.74	16.25	41.27	33.81	8.25	20.95	35.56
22.50	57.15	30.08	16.50	41.91	34.33	8.50	21.59	36.64
22.75	57.78	30.41	16.75	42.54	34.85	8.75	22.22	37.72
23.00	58.42	30.75	17.00	43.18	35.37	9.00	22.86	38.79
23.25	59.05	31.08	17.25	43.81	35.89	9.25	23.49	39.87
23.50	59.69	31.42	17.50	44.45	36.41	9.50	24.13	40.95
23.75	60.32	31.75	17.75	45.08	36.93	9.75	24.76	42.03
24.00	60.96	32.08	18.00	45.72	37.45	10.00	25.40	43.10
24.25	61.59	32.42	18.25	46.35	37.97	10.25	26.03	44.18
24.50	62.23	32.75	18.50	46.99	38.49	10.50	26.67	45.26
24.75	62.86	33.09	18.75	47.62	39.01	10.75	27.30	46.34
25.00	63.50	33.42	19.00	48.26	39.53	11.00	27.94	47.41
25.25	64.13	33.76	19.25	48.89	40.05	11.25	28.57	48.49
25.50	64.77	34.09	19.50	49.53	40.57	11.50	29.21	49.57
25.75	65.40	34.42	19.75	50.16	41.09	11.75	29.84	50.65
26.00	66.04	34.76	20.00	50.80	41.61	12.00	30.48	51.73
26.25	66.67	35.09	20.25	51.43	42.13	12.25	31.11	52.80
26.50	67.31	35.43	20.50	52.07	42.65	12.50	31.75	53.88
26.75	67.94	35.76	20.75	52.70	43.17	12.75	32.38	54.96
27.00	68.58	36.10	21.00	53.34	43.69	13.00	33.02	56.04
27.25	69.21	36.43	21.25	53.97	44.21	13.25	33.65	57.11
27.50	69.85	36.76	21.50	54.61	44.73	13.50	34.29	58.19
27.75	70.48	37.10	21.75	55.24	45.25	13.75	34.92	59.27
28.00	71.12	37.43	22.00	55.88	45.77	14.00	35.56	60.35
28.25	71.75	37.77	22.25	56.51	46.29	14.25	36.19	61.42
28.50	72.39	38.10	22.50	57.15	46.81	14.50	36.83	62.50
28.75	73.02	38.43	22.75	57.78	47.33	14.75	37.46	63.58
29.00	73.66	38.77	23.00	58.42	47.85	15.00	38.10	64.66
29.25	74.29	39.10	23.25	59.05	48.37	15.25	38.73	65.73
29.50	74.93	39.44	23.50	59.69	48.89	15.50	39.37	66.81
29.75	75.56	39.77	23.75	60.32	49.41	15.75	40.00	67.89
30.00	76.20	40.11	24.00	60.96	49.93	16.00	40.64	68.97
30.25	76.83	40.44	24.25	61.59	50.45	16.25	41.27	70.04
30.50	77.47	40.77	24.50	62.23	50.97	16.50	41.91	71.12
30.75	78.10	41.11	24.75	62.86	51.49	16.75	42.54	72.20
31.00	78.74	41.44	25.00	63.50	52.01	17.00	43.18	73.28
31.25	79.37	41.78	25.25	64.13	52.53	17.25	43.81	74.36
31.50	80.01	42.11	25.50	64.77	53.05	17.50	44.45	75.43
31.75	80.64	42.45	25.75	65.40	53.57	17.75	45.08	76.51
32.00	81.28	42.78	26.00	66.04	54.09	18.00	45.72	77.59
32.25	81.91	43.11	26.25	66.67	54.61	18.25	46.35	78.67
32.50	82.55	43.45	26.50	67.31	55.13	18.50	46.99	79.74
32.75	83.18	43.78	26.75	67.94	55.65	18.75	47.62	80.82
33.00	83.82	44.12	27.00	68.58	56.17	19.00	48.26	81.90
33.25	84.45	44.45	27.25	69.21	56.69	19.25	48.89	82.98
33.50	85.09	44.78	27.50	69.85	57.21	19.50	49.53	84.05
33.75	85.72	45.12	27.75	70.48	57.73	19.75	50.16	85.13
34.00	86.36	45.45	28.00	71.12	58.26	20.00	50.80	86.21

TABLE 5-1. *continued*

ABDOMEN			THIGH			FOREARM		
IN.	CM	CONSTANT A	IN.	CM	CONSTANT B	IN.	CM	CONSTANT C
34.25	86.99	45.79	28.25	71.75	58.78	20.25	51.44	87.29
34.50	87.63	46.12	28.50	72.39	59.30	20.50	52.07	88.34
34.75	88.26	46.46	38.75	73.02	59.82	20.75	52.71	92.42
35.00	88.90	46.79	29.00	73.66	60.34	21.00	53.34	93.50
35.25	89.53	47.12	29.25	74.29	60.86			
35.50	90.17	47.46	29.50	74.93	61.38			
35.75	90.80	47.79	29.75	75.56	61.90			
36.00	91.44	48.13	30.00	76.20	62.42			
36.25	92.07	48.46	30.25	76.83	62.94			
36.50	92.71	48.80	30.50	77.47	63.46			
36.75	93.34	49.13	30.75	78.10	63.98			
37.00	93.98	49.46	31.00	78.74	64.50			
37.25	94.61	49.80	31.25	79.37	65.02			
37.50	95.25	50.13	31.50	80.01	65.54			
37.75	95.88	50.47	31.75	80.64	66.06			
38.00	96.52	50.80	32.00	81.28	66.58			
38.25	97.15	51.13	32.25	81.91	67.10			
38.50	97.79	51.47	32.50	82.55	67.62			
38.75	98.42	51.80	32.75	83.18	68.14			
39.00	99.06	52.14	33.00	83.82	68.66			
39.25	99.69	52.47	33.25	84.45	69.18			
39.50	100.33	52.81	33.50	85.09	69.70			
39.75	100.96	53.14	33.75	85.72	70.22			
40.00	101.60	53.47	34.00	86.36	70.74			

Note: Percent fat = Constant A + Constant B − Constant C − 19.6. For athletic people, the age correction is 22.6.

TABLE 5-2. *Conversion constants to predict percent body fat for **older women***

ABDOMEN			THIGH			CALF		
IN.	CM	CONSTANT A	IN.	CM	CONSTANT B	IN.	CM	CONSTANT C
25.00	63.50	29.69	14.00	35.56	17.31	10.00	25.40	14.46
25.25	64.13	29.98	14.25	36.19	17.62	10.25	26.03	14.82
25.50	64.77	30.28	14.50	36.83	17.93	10.50	26.67	15.18
25.75	65.40	30.58	14.75	37.46	18.24	10.75	27.30	15.54
26.00	66.04	30.87	15.00	38.10	18.55	11.00	27.94	15.91
26.25	66.67	31.17	15.25	38.73	18.86	11.25	28.57	16.27
26.50	67.31	31.47	15.50	39.37	19.17	11.50	29.21	16.63
26.75	67.94	31.76	15.75	40.00	19.47	11.75	29.84	16.99
27.00	68.58	32.06	16.00	40.64	19.78	12.00	30.48	17.35
27.25	69.21	32.36	16.25	41.27	20.09	12.25	31.11	17.71
27.50	69.85	32.65	16.50	41.91	20.40	12.50	31.75	18.08
27.75	70.48	32.95	16.75	42.54	20.71	12.75	32.38	18.44
28.00	71.12	33.25	17.00	43.18	21.02	13.00	33.02	18.80
28.25	71.75	33.55	17.25	43.81	21.33	13.25	33.65	19.16
28.50	72.39	33.84	17.50	44.45	21.64	13.50	34.29	19.52
28.75	73.02	34.14	17.75	45.08	21.95	13.75	34.92	19.88
29.00	73.66	34.44	18.00	45.72	22.26	14.00	35.56	20.24
29.25	74.29	34.73	18.25	46.35	22.57	14.25	36.19	20.61
29.50	74.93	35.03	18.50	46.99	22.87	14.50	36.83	20.97
29.75	75.56	35.33	18.75	47.62	23.18	14.75	37.46	21.33
30.00	76.20	35.62	19.00	48.26	23.49	15.00	38.10	21.69
30.25	76.83	35.92	19.25	48.89	23.80	15.25	38.73	22.05
30.50	77.47	36.22	19.50	49.53	24.11	15.50	39.37	22.41
30.75	78.10	36.51	19.75	50.16	24.42	15.75	40.00	22.77

TABLE 5-2. *continued*

ABDOMEN			THIGH			CALF		
IN.	CM	CONSTANT A	IN.	CM	CONSTANT B	IN.	CM	CONSTANT C
31.00	78.74	36.81	20.00	50.80	24.73	16.00	40.64	23.14
31.25	79.37	37.11	20.25	51.43	25.04	16.25	41.27	23.50
31.50	80.01	37.40	20.50	52.07	25.35	16.50	41.91	23.86
31.75	80.64	37.70	20.75	52.70	25.66	16.75	42.54	24.22
32.00	81.28	38.00	21.00	53.34	25.97	17.00	43.18	24.58
32.25	81.91	38.30	21.25	53.97	26.28	17.25	43.81	24.94
32.50	82.55	38.59	21.50	54.61	26.58	17.50	44.45	25.31
32.75	83.18	38.89	21.75	55.24	26.89	17.75	45.08	25.67
33.00	83.82	39.19	22.00	55.88	27.20	18.00	45.72	26.03
33.25	84.45	39.48	22.25	56.51	27.51	18.25	46.35	26.39
33.50	85.09	39.78	22.50	57.15	27.82	18.50	46.99	26.75
33.75	85.72	40.08	22.75	57.78	28.13	18.75	47.62	27.11
34.00	86.36	40.37	23.00	58.42	28.44	19.00	48.26	27.47
34.25	86.99	40.67	23.25	59.05	28.75	19.25	48.89	27.84
34.50	87.63	40.97	23.50	59.69	29.06	19.50	49.53	28.20
34.75	88.26	41.26	23.75	60.32	29.37	19.75	50.16	28.56
35.00	88.90	41.56	24.00	60.96	29.68	20.00	50.80	28.92
35.25	89.53	41.86	24.25	61.59	29.98	20.25	51.43	29.28
35.50	90.17	42.15	24.50	62.23	30.29	20.50	52.07	29.64
35.75	90.80	42.45	24.75	62.86	30.60	20.75	52.70	30.00
36.00	91.44	42.75	25.00	63.50	30.91	21.00	53.34	30.37
36.25	92.07	43.05	25.25	64.13	31.22	21.25	53.97	30.73
36.50	92.71	43.34	25.50	64.77	31.53	21.50	54.61	31.09
36.75	93.35	43.64	25.75	65.40	31.84	21.75	55.24	31.45
37.00	93.98	43.94	26.00	66.04	32.15	22.00	55.88	31.81
37.25	94.62	44.23	26.25	66.67	32.46	22.25	56.51	32.17
37.50	95.25	44.53	26.50	67.31	32.77	22.50	57.15	32.54
37.75	95.89	44.83	26.75	67.94	33.08	22.75	57.78	32.90
38.00	96.52	45.12	27.00	68.58	33.38	23.00	58.42	33.26
38.25	97.16	45.42	27.25	69.21	33.69	23.25	59.05	33.62
38.50	97.79	45.72	27.50	69.85	34.00	23.50	59.69	33.98
38.75	98.43	46.01	27.75	70.48	34.31	23.75	60.32	34.34
39.00	99.06	46.31	28.00	71.12	34.62	24.00	60.96	34.70
39.25	99.70	46.61	28.25	71.75	34.93	24.25	61.59	35.07
39.50	100.33	46.90	28.50	72.39	35.24	24.50	62.23	35.43
39.75	100.97	47.20	28.75	73.02	35.55	24.75	62.86	35.79
40.00	101.60	47.50	29.00	73.66	35.86	25.00	63.50	36.15
40.25	101.24	47.79	29.25	74.29	36.17			
40.50	102.87	48.09	29.50	74.93	36.48			
40.75	103.51	48.39	29.75	75.56	36.79			
41.00	104.14	48.69	30.00	76.20	37.09			
41.25	104.78	48.98	30.25	76.83	37.40			
41.50	105.41	49.28	30.50	77.47	37.71			
41.75	106.05	49.58	30.75	78.10	38.02			
42.00	106.68	49.87	31.00	78.74	38.33			
42.25	107.32	50.17	31.25	79.37	38.64			
42.50	107.95	50.47	31.50	80.01	38.95			
42.75	108.59	50.76	31.75	80.64	39.26			
43.00	109.22	51.06	32.00	81.28	39.57			
43.25	109.86	51.36	32.25	81.91	39.88			
43.50	110.49	51.65	32.50	82.55	40.19			
43.75	111.13	51.95	32.75	83.18	40.49			
44.00	111.76	52.25	33.00	83.82	40.80			
44.25	112.40	52.54	33.25	84.45	41.11			
44.50	113.03	52.84	33.50	85.09	41.42			
44.75	113.67	53.14	33.75	85.72	41.73			
45.00	114.30	53.44	34.00	86.36	42.04			

Note: Percent fat = Constant A + Constant B − Constant C − 18.4. For athletic people, the age correction is 21.4.

TABLE 5-3. *Conversion constants to predict percent body fat for* **young men**

UPPER ARM			ABDOMEN			FOREARM		
IN	CM	CONSTANT A	IN	CM	CONSTANT B	IN	CM	CONSTANT C
7.00	17.78	25.91	21.00	53.34	27.56	7.00	17.78	38.01
7.25	18.41	26.83	21.25	53.97	27.88	7.25	18.41	39.37
7.50	19.05	27.76	21.50	54.61	28.21	7.50	19.05	40.72
7.75	19.68	28.68	21.75	55.24	28.54	7.75	19.68	42.08
8.00	20.32	29.61	22.00	55.88	28.87	8.00	20.32	43.44
8.25	20.95	30.53	22.25	56.51	29.20	8.25	20.95	44.80
8.50	21.59	31.46	22.50	57.15	29.52	8.50	21.59	46.15
8.75	22.22	32.38	22.75	57.78	29.85	8.75	22.22	47.51
9.00	22.86	33.31	23.00	58.42	30.18	9.00	22.86	48.87
9.25	23.49	34.24	23.25	59.05	30.51	9.25	23.49	50.23
9.50	24.13	35.16	23.50	59.69	30.84	9.50	24.13	51.58
9.75	24.76	36.09	23.75	60.32	31.16	9.75	24.76	52.94
10.00	25.40	37.01	24.00	60.96	31.49	10.00	25.40	54.30
10.25	26.03	37.94	24.25	61.59	31.82	10.25	26.03	55.65
10.50	26.67	38.86	24.50	62.23	32.15	10.50	26.67	57.01
10.75	27.30	39.79	24.75	62.86	32.48	10.75	27.30	58.37
11.00	27.94	40.71	25.00	63.50	32.80	11.00	27.94	59.73
11.25	28.57	41.64	25.25	64.13	33.13	11.25	28.57	61.08
11.50	29.21	42.56	25.50	64.77	33.46	11.50	29.21	62.44
11.75	29.84	43.49	25.75	65.40	33.79	11.75	29.84	63.80
12.00	30.48	44.41	26.00	66.04	34.12	12.00	30.48	65.16
12.25	31.11	45.34	26.25	66.67	34.44	12.25	31.11	66.51
12.50	31.75	46.26	26.50	67.31	34.77	12.50	31.75	67.87
12.75	32.38	47.19	26.75	67.94	35.10	12.75	32.38	69.23
13.00	33.02	48.11	27.00	68.58	35.43	13.00	33.02	70.59
13.25	33.65	49.04	27.25	69.21	35.76	13.25	33.65	71.94
13.50	34.29	49.96	27.50	69.85	36.09	13.50	34.29	73.30
13.75	34.92	50.89	27.75	70.48	36.41	13.75	34.92	74.66
14.00	35.56	51.82	28.00	71.12	36.74	14.00	35.56	76.02
14.25	36.19	52.74	28.25	71.75	37.07	14.25	36.19	77.37
14.50	36.83	53.67	28.50	72.39	37.40	14.50	36.83	78.73
14.75	37.46	54.59	28.75	73.02	37.73	14.75	37.46	80.09
15.00	38.10	55.52	29.00	73.66	38.05	15.00	38.10	81.45
15.25	38.73	56.44	29.25	74.29	38.38	15.25	38.73	82.80
15.50	39.37	57.37	29.50	74.93	38.71	15.50	39.37	84.16
15.75	40.00	58.29	29.75	75.56	39.04	15.75	40.00	85.52
16.00	40.64	59.22	30.00	76.20	39.37	16.00	40.64	86.88
16.25	41.27	60.14	30.25	76.83	39.69	16.25	41.27	88.23
16.50	41.91	61.07	30.50	77.47	40.02	16.50	41.91	89.59
16.75	42.54	61.99	30.75	78.10	40.35	16.75	42.54	90.95
17.00	43.18	62.92	31.00	78.74	40.68	17.00	43.18	92.31
17.25	43.81	63.84	31.25	79.37	41.01	17.25	43.81	93.66
17.50	44.45	64.77	31.50	80.01	41.33	17.50	44.45	95.02
17.75	45.08	65.69	31.75	80.64	41.66	17.75	45.08	96.38
18.00	45.72	66.62	32.00	81.28	41.99	18.00	45.72	97.74
18.25	46.35	67.54	32.25	81.91	42.32	18.25	46.35	99.09
18.50	46.99	68.47	32.50	82.55	42.65	18.50	46.99	100.45
18.75	47.62	69.40	32.75	83.18	42.97	18.75	47.62	101.81
19.00	48.26	70.32	33.00	83.82	43.30	19.00	48.26	103.17
19.25	48.89	71.25	33.25	84.45	43.63	19.25	48.89	104.52
19.50	49.53	72.17	33.50	85.09	43.96	19.50	49.53	105.88
19.75	50.16	73.10	33.75	85.72	44.29	19.75	50.16	107.24
20.00	50.80	74.02	34.00	86.36	44.61	20.00	50.80	108.60
20.25	51.43	74.95	34.25	86.99	44.94	20.25	51.43	109.95
20.50	52.07	75.87	34.50	87.63	45.27	20.50	52.07	111.31
20.75	52.70	76.80	34.75	88.26	45.60	20.75	52.70	112.67
21.00	53.34	77.72	35.00	88.90	45.93	21.00	53.34	114.02
21.25	53.97	78.65	35.25	89.53	46.25	21.25	53.97	115.38
21.50	54.61	79.57	35.50	90.17	46.58	21.50	54.61	116.74
21.75	55.24	80.50	35.75	90.80	46.91	21.75	55.24	118.10

TABLE 5.3. *continued*

UPPER ARM			ABDOMEN			FOREARM		
IN.	CM	CONSTANT A	IN.	CM	CONSTANT B	IN.	CM	CONSTANT C
22.00	55.88	81.42	36.00	91.44	47.24	22.00	55.88	119.45
22.25	56.52	82.34	36.25	92.07	47.57	22.25	56.52	120.80
22.50	57.15	83.26	36.50	92.71	47.89	22.50	57.15	122.15
22.75	57.79	84.18	36.75	93.34	48.22	22.75	57.79	123.50
23.00	58.42	85.10	37.00	93.98	48.55	23.00	58.42	124.85
			37.25	94.61	48.88			
			37.50	95.25	49.21			
			37.75	95.88	49.54			
			38.00	96.52	49.86			
			38.25	97.15	50.19			
			38.50	97.79	50.52			
			38.75	98.42	50.85			
			39.00	99.06	51.18			
			39.25	99.69	51.50			
			39.50	100.33	51.83			
			39.75	100.96	52.16			
			40.00	101.60	52.49			
			40.25	102.23	52.82			
			40.50	102.87	53.14			
			40.75	103.50	53.47			
			41.00	104.14	53.80			
			41.25	104.77	54.13			
			41.50	105.41	54.46			
			41.75	106.04	54.78			
			42.00	106.68	55.11			

Note: Percent fat = Constant A + Constant B − Constant C − 10.2. For athletic people, the age correction is 14.2.

TABLE 5-4. *Conversion constants to predict percent body fat for **older men***

BUTTOCKS			ABDOMEN			FOREARM		
IN.	CM	CONSTANT A	IN.	CM	CONSTANT B	IN.	CM	CONSTANT C
28.00	71.12	29.34	25.50	64.77	22.84	7.00	17.78	21.01
28.25	71.75	29.60	25.75	65.40	23.06	7.25	18.41	21.76
28.50	72.39	29.87	26.00	66.04	23.29	7.50	19.05	22.52
28.75	73.02	30.13	26.25	66.67	23.51	7.75	19.68	23.26
29.00	73.66	30.39	26.50	67.31	23.73	8.00	20.32	24.02
29.25	74.29	30.65	26.75	67.94	23.96	8.25	20.95	24.76
29.50	74.93	30.92	27.00	68.58	24.18	8.50	21.59	25.52
29.75	75.56	31.18	27.25	69.21	24.40	8.75	22.22	26.26
30.00	76.20	31.44	27.50	69.85	24.63	9.00	22.86	27.02
30.25	76.83	31.70	27.75	70.48	24.85	9.25	23.49	27.76
30.50	77.47	31.96	28.00	71.12	25.08	9.50	24.13	28.52
30.75	78.10	32.22	28.25	71.75	25.29	9.75	24.76	29.26
31.00	78.74	32.49	28.50	72.39	25.52	10.00	25.40	30.02
31.25	79.37	32.75	28.75	73.02	25.75	10.25	26.03	30.76
31.50	80.01	33.01	29.00	73.66	25.97	10.50	26.67	31.52
31.75	80.64	33.27	29.25	74.29	26.19	10.75	27.30	32.27
32.00	81.28	33.54	29.50	74.93	26.42	11.00	27.94	33.02
32.25	81.91	33.80	29.75	75.56	26.64	11.25	28.57	33.77
32.50	82.55	34.06	30.00	76.20	26.87	11.50	29.21	34.52
32.75	83.18	34.32	30.25	76.83	27.09	11.75	29.84	35.27
33.00	83.82	34.58	30.50	77.47	27.32	12.00	30.48	36.02
33.25	84.45	34.84	30.75	78.10	27.54	12.25	31.11	36.77
33.50	85.09	35.11	31.00	78.74	27.70	12.50	31.75	37.53
33.75	85.72	35.37	31.25	79.37	27.98	12.75	32.38	38.27
34.00	86.36	35.63	31.50	80.01	28.21	13.00	33.02	39.03
34.25	86.99	35.89	31.75	80.64	28.43	13.25	33.65	39.77
34.50	87.63	36.16	32.00	81.28	28.66	13.50	34.29	40.53
34.75	88.26	36.42	32.25	81.91	28.88	13.75	34.92	41.27

TABLE 5-4. *continued*

BUTTOCKS			ABDOMEN			FOREARM		
IN.	CM	CONSTANT A	IN.	CM	CONSTANT B	IN.	CM	CONSTANT C
35.00	88.90	36.68	32.50	82.55	29.11	14.00	35.56	42.03
35.25	89.53	36.94	32.75	83.18	29.33	14.25	36.19	42.77
35.50	90.17	37.20	33.00	83.82	29.55	14.50	36.83	43.53
35.75	90.80	37.46	33.25	84.45	29.78	14.75	37.46	44.27
36.00	91.44	37.73	33.50	85.09	30.00	15.00	38.10	45.03
36.25	92.07	37.99	33.75	85.72	30.22	15.25	38.73	45.77
36.50	92.71	38.25	34.00	86.36	30.45	15.50	39.37	46.53
36.75	93.34	38.51	34.25	86.99	30.67	15.75	40.00	47.28
37.00	93.98	38.78	34.50	87.63	30.89	16.00	40.64	48.03
37.25	94.61	39.04	34.75	88.26	31.12	16.25	41.27	48.78
37.50	95.25	39.30	35.00	88.90	31.35	16.50	41.91	49.53
37.75	95.88	39.56	35.25	89.53	31.57	16.75	42.54	50.28
38.00	96.52	39.82	35.50	90.17	31.79	17.00	43.18	51.03
38.25	97.15	40.08	35.75	90.80	32.02	17.25	43.81	51.78
38.50	97.79	40.35	36.00	91.44	32.24	17.50	44.45	52.54
38.75	98.42	40.61	36.25	92.07	32.46	17.75	45.08	53.28
39.00	99.06	40.87	36.50	92.71	32.69	18.00	45.72	54.04
39.25	99.69	41.13	36.75	93.34	32.91	18.25	46.35	54.78
39.50	100.33	41.39	37.00	93.98	33.14			
39.75	100.96	41.66	37.25	94.61	33.36			
40.00	101.60	41.92	37.50	95.25	33.58			
40.25	102.23	42.18	37.75	95.88	33.81			
40.50	102.87	42.44	38.00	96.52	34.03			
40.75	103.50	42.70	38.25	97.15	34.26			
41.00	104.14	42.97	38.50	97.79	34.48			
42.25	104.77	43.23	38.75	98.42	34.70			
41.50	105.41	43.49	39.00	99.06	34.93			
41.75	106.04	43.75	39.25	99.69	35.15			
42.00	106.68	44.02	39.50	100.33	35.38			
42.25	107.31	44.28	39.75	100.96	35.59			
42.50	107.95	44.54	40.00	101.60	35.82			
42.75	108.58	44.80	40.25	102.23	36.05			
43.00	109.22	45.06	40.50	102.87	36.27			
43.25	109.85	45.32	40.75	103.50	36.49			
43.50	110.49	45.59	41.00	104.14	36.72			
43.75	111.12	45.85	41.25	104.77	36.94			
44.00	111.76	46.12	41.50	105.41	37.17			
44.25	112.39	46.37	41.75	106.04	37.39			
44.50	113.03	46.64	42.00	106.68	37.62			
44.75	113.66	46.89	42.25	107.31	37.87			
45.00	114.30	47.16	42.50	107.95	38.06			
42.25	114.93	47.42	42.75	108.58	38.28			
45.50	115.57	47.68	43.00	109.22	38.51			
45.75	116.20	47.94	43.25	109.85	38.73			
46.00	116.84	48.21	43.50	110.49	38.96			
46.25	117.47	48.47	43.75	111.12	39.18			
46.50	118.11	48.73	44.00	111.76	39.41			
46.75	118.74	48.99	44.25	112.39	39.63			
47.00	119.38	49.26	44.50	113.03	39.85			
47.25	120.01	49.52	44.75	113.66	40.08			
47.50	120.65	49.78	45.00	114.30	40.30			
47.75	121.28	50.04						
48.00	121.92	50.30						
48.25	122.55	50.56						
48.50	123.19	50.83						
48.75	123.82	51.09						
49.00	124.46	51.35						

Note: Percent fat = Constant A + Constant B − Constant C − 15.0. For athletic people, the age correction is 19.0.

1. The abdomen, right thigh, and right forearm circumference were taken with a cloth tape, and accuracy was to the nearest one-eighth inch. Convert inches to centimeters by multiplying by 2.54 (1 in. = 2.54 cm).
   Abdomen = 28.0 in. (71.1 cm)
   Right thigh = 20.0 in. (50.8 cm)
   Right forearm = 8.0 in. (20.3 cm).

2. The three constants A, B, and C, corresponding to the three circumference measures, were determined from Table 5-1.
   Constant A, corresponding to 28.0 in. = 37.4
   Constant B, corresponding to 20.0 in. = 41.6
   Constant C, corresponding to 8.0 in. = 34.5

3. Percent body fat was computed by substituting the appropriate constants in the formula shown at the bottom of Table 5-1.
   $$
   \begin{aligned}
   \text{Percent fat} &= \text{constant } A + \text{constant } B - \text{constant } C - 19.6 \\
   &= \quad 37.4 + 41.6 \quad - \quad 34.5 \quad - 19.6 \\
   &= \quad\quad 79.0 \quad\quad - \quad 34.5 \quad - 19.6 \\
   &= \quad 44.5 - 19.6 \\
   &= \quad 24.9 \text{ percent}
   \end{aligned}
   $$

4. Weight of fat $= \dfrac{\text{percent fat}}{100 \times \text{body weight}}$

   $$
   \begin{aligned}
   \text{Weight of fat} &= 24.9/100 \times 125 \text{ lb} \\
   &= 0.249 \quad \times 125 \text{ lb} \\
   &= 31.1 \text{ lb.}
   \end{aligned}
   $$

5. Lean body weight = body weight − weight of fat
   $$
   \begin{aligned}
   \text{Lean body weight} &= 125 \text{ pounds} - 31.1 \text{ pounds} \\
   &= 93.9 \text{ pounds.}
   \end{aligned}
   $$

Measurement of Subcutaneous Fat by the Fatfold Technique

Approximately one-half of the body's total fat content is located in the tissues beneath the skin. The feasibility of measuring this *subcutaneous fat* was suggested by anthropologists at the end of World War I. By 1930 researchers developed a special pincer-type caliper that enabled them to measure this fat at representative sites on the body with relative accuracy. The caliper works on the same principle as the micrometer used to measure the distance between two points. The procedure for measuring fatfold thickness is to grasp firmly with the thumb and forefinger a fold of skin and subcutaneous fat away from the underlying muscular tissue following the natural contour of the fatfold. The pincer arms of the caliper exert constant tension at their point of contact with the skin. The thickness of the double layer of skin and subcutaneous tissues can then be read directly from the caliper dial. The procedure for taking the fatfold measurements, as well as the precise location of the skinfold sites, must be standardized if results are to be reliable and used for comparative purposes.

There are two ways to use fatfolds. The first is to add the scores from the various measurements and use this value as an indication of the relative degree of fatness among subjects. The sites most commonly measured are at the back of the right, upper arm (referred to as triceps), the fatfold measured just below the tip of the right scapula (subscapula), the vertical fold measured just above the hipbone (supra-iliac), the vertical fold measured 1 inch to the right of the umbilicus (abdomen), and the vertical fold measured at the midline of the thigh, two-thirds the distance from the knee cap to the hip. The sum of fatfolds can be used to reflect changes in fatness before and after a physical conditioning or weight reduction program.

A second way to use fatfolds is in conjunction with the mathematical equations that have been developed to predict body density or percent body fat. These equations are often quite useful in ranking or ordering individuals within a group in terms of relative fatness. The equations are *population specific*, in that they accurately predict fatness in samples of subjects similar to those on which the equations were derived.

While the fatfold technique has been widely used in the fields of physical education, nutrition, and medicine, it presents a major drawback in that the person taking the measurements must have considerable expertise with the proper techniques to obtain consistent and accurate fatfold values. When fatfolds are measured for research purposes, for example, the investigator has usually had experience taking several thousand measurements and is quite consistent in duplicating values for the same subject made on the same day, on consecutive days, or even weeks apart. In such cases the fatfold technique can provide a useful means for body composition evaluation.

New Indirect Procedures for Assessment of Body Composition

During the past 5 years, several new procedures have been developed that enable the researcher to gain valuable information about body composition. The first technique makes use of ultrasonic technology to measure fat and muscle thickness at selected body sites. A second technique converts the fat thickness at three sites from an upper arm x-ray to an accurate estimate of percentage body fat, while a third procedure, called computerized axial tomography (CT) scanning, creates images of fat distribution within the body.

Ultrasound

A lightweight, portable ultrasound meter is used to measure the distance between the skin and fat-muscle layer, and fat-muscle layer and bone. The ultrasound meter operates by emitting high frequency sound waves that penetrate the skin surface. The sound waves pass through adipose tissue until the muscle layer is reached; here the sound waves are then reflected from the fat-muscle interface to produce an echo that returns to the ultrasound unit. The time for sound wave transmission through the tissues and back to the receiver is converted to a distance score and displayed on a light emitting diode (LED) scale.

In one of our laboratories, we are evaluating the pattern of fat gain and loss on the trunk and extremities in athletes and in obese and normal weight non-athletes before and after sports and exercise training. Figure 5-6 displays the details of the ultrasound meter for recording fat and muscle thickness in a female distance runner. This use of ultrasound for "mapping" muscle and fat thickness at various sites on the body should prove to be a valuable technique for assessment of body composition.

X-Ray

Figure 5-7 illustrates a new procedure developed in one of our laboratories for determining an individual's body fat content. A standard x-ray picture is taken of the right upper arm. The thickness of the fat layers at point A, B, and C are measured accurately with either a caliper or electronic measuring instrument interfaced with a sonic digitizer and computer graphics system. Muscle and bone (medullary and cortex) thickness can also be measured. Total radiation (10 millirems) is low; it is approximately one-half that of a chest x-ray film or about one-tenth the background radiation accumulated in 1 year living at sea level.

The effectiveness of the x-ray film measurements of arm fat in relation to total percentage of body fat was evaluated in 50 young (18 to 30 years) and 50 older (30 to 40 years) men and women. A high degree of association was obtained between percent body fat determined by hydrostatic weighing and fat thickness from the x-ray picture (correlation of $r = .90$). This remarkable relationship, in conjunction with a person's height and weight, permits the conversion of the fat thickness shown on x-ray film to total body fat. For a given individual, the conversion to percent body fat is accurate to within plus or minus 2% of body fat determined by the hydrostatic weighing method. Similar results were obtained in another sample of 190 men and women of different ages and fitness capacities.

The results from these initial series of experiments have established the validity of the arm x-ray method for determining percent body fat in men and women of different ages who vary in body size and fitness status. The applications will include cross-sectional and longitudinal studies of body composition and aging, effects of resistive training on muscular hypertrophy, as well as clinical evaluation of nutritional status. The x-ray method appears to have a promising future in body composition research.

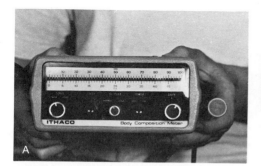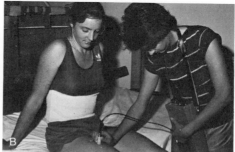

Figure 5-6. *Ultrasound measurement. A. Portable body composition meter that includes a display scale on the meter to provide a direct readout of distance between skin-to-fat, fat-to-muscle, and muscle-to-bone. B. Measurement of upper leg fat and muscle thickness. (Photos courtesy of the Department of Exercise Science, University of Massachusetts, Amherst.)*

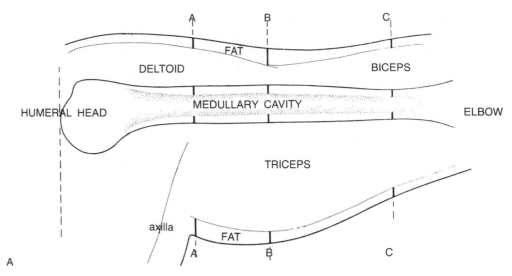

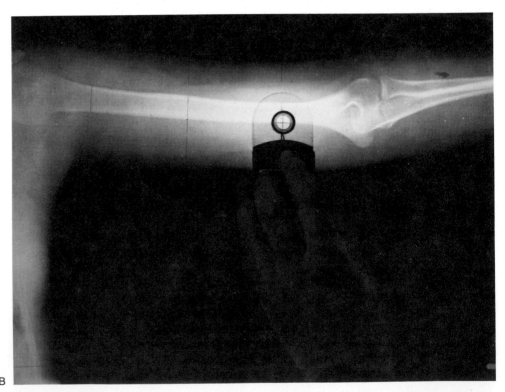

Figure 5-7. *A. Schematic drawing of an arm x-ray of a 24-year-old female. The six fat widths are represented by the vertical lines drawn perpendicular to the long axis of the humerus at points A, B, and C. B. There is a demarcation on the x-ray between fat, muscle, and bone that permits an accurate assessment of radiographic widths. Total body fat determined from this x-ray was 23.6%; by underwater weighing, body fat was 23.3%. The technician is using a digitizer to calculate fat width on the x-ray. The information from the digitizer is processed by a computer to a printer and graphics plotter. (Photos courtesy of the Department of Exercise Science, University of Massachusetts, Amherst.)*

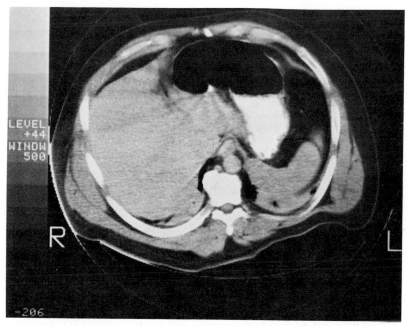

Figure 5-8. *CT abdominal scan of a patient with observable differences in subcutaneous and intra-abdominal fat.*

Computed Tomography (CT)

The CT scanning procedure produces radiographic images at any section of the body. In the first studies to use CT for body composition evaluation, researchers were able to accurately differentiate fat accumulation in the abdominal area. By use of appropriate computer software, the scan provides pictorial and quantitative information for total tissue area, total fat area, and intra-abdominal fat area. Figure 5-8 shows a CT abdominal scan for a patient with differing amounts of subcutaneous and intra-abdominal fat. The technological advances of CT open up whole new areas for body composition research. CT will make it possible to evaluate directly changes in sex-specific essential and storage fat depots consequent to dietary and exercise regimens. Basic research with CT will also delve into the origins and development of obesity and underweightness, hopefully to provide a clearer understanding of the reasons for these disease conditions.

DETERMINE YOUR BODY COMPOSITION

The five-step procedure outlined in the previous example to determine your body composition (percent fat, weight of fat, and lean body weight) is as follows:

1. With a tape, measure the three circumferences that correspond to your sex and age group. Record all values in centimeters or to the nearest one-eighth inch.

Measurement Site	cm	in.
1. _____	___	___
2. _____	___	___
3. _____	___	___

2. Determine the three constants *A*, *B*, and *C* that correspond to the appropriate circumference in Step 1. Use Tables 5-2, 5-3, 5-4, or 5-5 to determine the constants depending on your age and gender.

	cm	Constant
Measurement 1	_____	A = _____
Measurement 2	_____	B = _____
Measurement 3	_____	C = _____

3. Substitute the value for each constant in the equation below. Enter the age constant at the end of the equation depending on your sex and age group; young men = 10.2; older men = 15.0; young women = 19.6; older women = 18.4.

   If you participate in a regular program of *vigorous physical activity* a minimum of 240 minutes a week, use the following age-correction factors that incorporate this significantly higher than normal level of physical activity: young men, 14.2; older men, 19.0; young women, 22.6; older women, 21.4.

$$\text{Percent fat} = \underset{A}{\text{Constant}} + \underset{B}{\text{Constant}} - \underset{C}{\text{Constant}} - \frac{}{\text{Age Constant}}$$

$$=$$
$$=$$
$$=$$

Percent fat =

4. Weight of fat = percent fat (step 3)/100 × body weight (lb).

$$\text{Weight of fat} = \frac{}{\text{percent of fat}} \times \frac{}{\text{body weight}}$$

$$=$$
$$=$$

5. Compute lean body weight by subtracting the weight of fat from body weight.

$$\text{Lean body weight} = \frac{}{\text{body weight, lb}} - \frac{}{\text{weight of fat, lb}}$$

AVERAGE VALUES FOR BODY COMPOSITION

Values for body fat for a sample of men and women throughout the United States are presented in Table 5-5. In comparing your values for body fat with these results, keep in mind that these data represent *average* values. We have also included values that are plus and minus one standard deviation in the table to give some indication of the amount of variation or spread from the average. The column headed "68% variation limits" indicates the range of values for percent body fat, which include ±1 standard deviation or about 68 of every 100 people measured. As an example, the average value for percent body fat for young men from the New York sample is 15.0%, and the 68% variation limits are from 8.9 to 21.1% body fat. Interpreting this statistically, it could be expected that for 68 of every 100 people measured, values for percent fat would range between 8.9 to 21.1%. Of the remaining 32 young men, 16 would possess more than 21% body fat, while for the other 16 people, body fat would be less than 8.9%. Certainly a value within the 68% variation limits for body fat could be considered "normal." In the next chapter we will discuss what is considered abnormal or excessive fatness.

Although considerable data are available concerning the average body composition of many groups of men and women of different ages and fitness levels, there has been no systematic evaluation of the body composition of representative samples from the general population that would warrant setting up precise norms or desirable values of body composition. At this time the best we can do is to present the average values from various studies of different age groups.

Table 5-5. *Average values of percent body fat for younger and older women and men from selected studies.*

STUDY	AGE RANGE	HEIGHT cm	WEIGHT kg	PERCENT FAT[a]	68% VARIATION LIMITS
Younger Women					
North Carolina, 1962	17–25	165.0	55.5	22.9	17.5–28.5
New York, 1962	16–30	167.5	59.0	28.7	24.6–32.9
California, 1968	19–23	165.9	58.4	21.9	17.0–26.9
California, 1970	17–29	164.9	58.6	25.5	21.0–30.1
Air Force, 1972	17–22	164.1	55.8	28.7	22.3–35.3
New York, 1973	17–26	160.4	59.0	26.2	23.4–33.3
North Carolina, 1975		166.1	57.5	24.6	—
Texas, 1978	18–26	165.0	57.4	25.5	21.1–30.0
Massachusetts, 1983	17–30	165.3	57.6	21.9	16.7–27.1
Older Women					
Minnesota, 1953	31–45	163.3	60.7	28.9	25.1–32.8
	43–68	160.0	60.9	34.2	28.0–40.5
New York, 1963	30–40	164.9	59.6	28.6	22.1–35.3
	40–50	163.1	56.4	34.4	29.5–39.5
North Carolina, 1975	33–50	—	—	29.7	23.1–36.5
Massachusetts, 1983	31–50	165.2	58.9	25.1	19.2–31.0
Younger Men					
Minnesota, 1951	17–26	177.8	69.1	11.8	5.9–11.8
Colorado, 1956	17–25	172.4	68.3	13.5	8.3–18.8
Indiana, 1966	18–23	180.1	75.5	12.6	8.7–16.5
California, 1968	16–31	175.7	74.1	15.2	6.3–24.2
New York, 1973	17–26	176.4	71.4	15.0	8.9–21.1
Texas, 1977	18–24	179.9	74.6	13.4	7.4–19.4
Massachusetts, 1983	17–30	178.2	76.3	12.9	7.8–18.0
Older Men					
Indiana, 1966	24–38	179.0	76.6	17.8	11.3–24.3
	40–48	177.0	80.5	22.3	16.3–28.3
North Carolina, 1976	27–50	—	—	23.7	17.9–30.1
Texas, 1977	27–59	180.0	85.3	27.1	23.7–30.5
Massachusetts, 1983	31–50	177.0	77.3	19.8	13.2–26.4

[a]Percent body fat was computed from body density measured by hydrostatic weighing, where percent fat = 495/density − 450.

A general conclusion based on these data is that with increasing age the percentage of body fat tends to increase in both men and women. This average change does not necessarily mean the trend should be interpreted as being desirable or "normal." This increase in fat could be due in part to the fact that the aging skeleton becomes demineralized and porous. Such a process reduces body density because of the decrease in bone density. Another reason for the relative increase in body fat with age is the reduction in the level of daily physical activity. The adaptation of a more sedentary life style could increase the deposition of storage fat and reduce the quantity of muscle mass. This would occur even if the daily caloric consumption remained unchanged. The exact interaction of the aging process per se and the numerous ramifications of the sociology and psychology of aging on fitness and body composition in industralized societies have not as yet been adequately evaluated.

DESIRABLE BODY WEIGHT

Although large quantities of body fat are undesirable for good health and fitness, precise statements cannot be made as to an optimum level of body fat or body weight for a particular individual. More than likely, this optimum varies from person to person and is greatly influenced by a variety of genetic factors. Certainly, we are hard pressed to find objective evidence to indicate that a 5-or 10-pound increase in body weight is, in and of itself, a health risk. Based on data from active young adults and competitive athletes, however, it does appear that it would be desirable to maintain body fat at about 15% of body weight or *less* for men, and 25% or *less* for women. This "optimal" or *desirable body weight* can be computed (based on a desired body fat level) as follows:

$$\frac{\text{Desirable body}}{\text{weight}} = \frac{\text{Lean body weight}}{1.00 - \% \text{ fat desired}}$$

Suppose a 200-lb man who is 20% body fat wishes to know the weight he should attain so that this new lower body weight would contain 10% body fat. The computations would be:

$$\text{Fat weight} = 200 \text{ lb} \times .20 = 40 \text{ lb}$$
$$\text{Lean body weight} = 200 \text{ lb} - 40 \text{ lb} = 160 \text{ lb}$$

$$\text{Desirable body weight} = \frac{160 \text{ lb}}{1.00 - .10}$$

$$= \frac{160 \text{ lb}}{.90}$$

$$= 177.8 \text{ lb}$$

$$\boxed{\text{Desirable fat loss} = \text{Present body weight} - \text{Desirable body weight}}$$

$$= 200 \text{ lb} - 177.8 \text{ lb}$$
$$= 22.2 \text{ lb}$$

If this man lost 22.2 lb of body fat, his new body weight of 177.8 lb would have a fat content equal to 10% of body weight. For practical purposes, it is prudent to recommend a *desirable weight range*, rather than an absolute value for the desirable weight. In this example, an appropriate weight range would be 175 to 180 lb. We believe that the notion of an upper and lower limit around the desired weight is the best procedure to use when prescribing optimal levels of body composition.

More detailed information about the ultrasound and x-ray procedures can be found in the following articles:

1. Katch, F.I. Individual differences of ultrasound assessment of subcutaneous fat: effects of body position. *Human Biology.* December, 1984.

2. Katch, F.I., and A.R. Behnke. Arm x-ray assessment of percent body fat in men and women. *Medicine and Science in Sports and Exercise* 16, No. 3. 1984.

3. Katch, F.I. and V.L. Katch. The body composition profile. Techniques of measurement and applications. *Clinics in Sports Medicine.* Vol. 3. No. 1. January, 1984. W.B. Saunders Co. Philadelphia, p. 31–63.

6

Obesity

AMERICANS CONSUME more fat per capita than any other nation in the world. They also consume more than 90% of the foods high in saturated fats and processed sugars. The end result of this national preoccupation with food and effortless living is that an estimated 60 to 70 million adults and 10 to 12 million teenagers are "too fat" by a total of 2.3 billion pounds. In calories, this excess fat represents an energy equivalent of 5.7 trillion kcal, or the potential energy in 1.3 billion gallons of gasoline! This is sufficient energy to power 900,000 automobiles a year or provide the annual residential electrical requirements of Boston, Chicago, San Francisco, and Washington, D.C.

Until recently, it was commonly believed that the major cause of progressive weight gain (and resulting obesity) was simply a problem of overeating. However, if gluttony and overindulgence were the only factors associated with accumulation of excess fat, the easiest way to reduce body fat would simply be to decrease food intake. As we all know, it's much more complicated. If there were a simple method to help cure the overfat condition, obesity would surely be eliminated as a major health concern. There are obviously other factors that include genetic, environmental, psychological, and social influences. Recent research suggests that individual differences in specific factors such as eating patterns, body image, resting metabolic rate, basal body temperature, hypothalamic control, and levels of cellular adenosine triphosphatase and other enzymes, and brown fat may predispose a person to excessive fat gain. It is also becoming increasingly clear that the lack of adequate energy expenditure in daily physical activity is an important predisposing factor to obesity.

We can state with certainty that excess fat is the end result of an imbalance between the number of calories consumed and the number of calories expended to sustain daily activities. It also seems clear to us that treatment procedures devised so far, be they dietary, surgical, drug, or behavioral, either alone or in combination, have not been particularly successful in controlling obesity on a long-term basis. Although research has provided some information about the possible causes of the imbalance between calorie intake and energy output, as yet no unifying theory has emerged to explain exactly why some people become too fat, while others remain relatively thin despite an apparently large caloric intake.

This chapter deals with the development of obesity and examines the following topics: (1) the definition of obesity; (2) medical and health aspects of obesity; (3) methods of determining the size and number of fat cells and their comparison in normal and obese subjects before and after weight gain and reduction; (4) development of adipose cellularity in animals and humans; and (5) the influence of diet and exercise in modifying fat cell size and number.

What Is Obesity?

PERCENT BODY FAT AS A CRITERION

Obesity can be defined as an excessive enlargement of the body's total quantity of fat. The line of demarcation between normal levels of body fat and obesity is somewhat arbitrary. In the previous chapter we suggested that the normal range of body fat in adult men and women encompasses at least plus and minus one unit of variation from the average population value for body fat. This variation unit is approximately 5% body fat for men and women between the ages 17 to 50 years. Within this statistical boundary, overfatness would correspond to any value for percent body fat that exceeds the average value for fatness for a particular age and sex, plus 5%. Thus in young men whose body weight averages 15% fat, the borderline for obesity is 20% body fat. For older men average fatness is approximately 25%. Consequently, overfatness for this group would be a body fat content in excess of 30%. For young women aged 17 to 27, obesity would correspond to a body fat content above 31%, while for older women aged 27 to 50, borderline obesity would be about 37% body fat. It should be emphasized that although the average population value for percent body fat increases with age, *this does NOT imply that men and women should be expected to get fatter as they grow older.* To the contrary, the criterion for overfatness should be that established for younger men and women—*above 20% for men and above 30% for women.*

It should also be pointed out that there is a gradation of obesity that progresses from the upper limit of normal—20% for men and 30% for women—to as high as 50 to 70% of body weight in those massively obese. Common terms for the gradation of obesity include pleasantly plump for those just above the cut off, to moderately obese, excessively obese, and massively obese. The latter category includes people who weigh in the range of 375 to about 600 pounds, and whose fat content is above 55% of body weight, and often 60 to 65% or higher. In this situation body fat exceeds the lean body weight and obesity may be a life threatening condition.

> Standards for Overfatness
> Men —above 20%
> Women—above 30%

FAT CELL SIZE AND NUMBER AS CRITERIA

In addition to the total percent of body fat, scientists have also proposed the *size* and *number* of fat cells as a means to identify and study what is normal and abnormal with regard to body fatness. The body increases its quantity of adipose tissue in two ways. The first is by enlarging or filling existing fat cells with more fat. We refer to this as *fat cell hypertrophy*. The second way is by increasing the total number of fat cells, or *fat cell hyperplasia*.

MEDICAL AND HEALTH ASPECTS OF OBESITY

It is well established in the medical literature that chronic disease is more prevalent in obese than individuals of normal body fat. While it is not clear the degree to which obesity causes specific medical problems, the plight of the obese person in terms of increased medical and health complications include the following: (1) hypertension and increased risk of stroke, (2) renal disease, (3) gallbladder disease, (4) diabetes mellitus, (5) pulmonary diseases, (6) problems with anesthesia during surgery, (7) osteoarthritis and gout, (8) breast and endometrial cancer, (9) abnormal plasma lipid and lipoprotein concentrations, (10) impairment of cardiac function due to an increase in the heart's mechanical work, (11) menstrual irregularities and toxemia of pregnancy, (12) psychologic trauma, (13) flat feet and intertriginous dermatitis (infection in skin folds), (14) organ compression by adipose tissue, and (15) impaired heat tolerance.

It should be pointed out that obesity *per se* may not in itself be detrimental to overall health. Unfortunately, the obese condition is usually intimately related to a number of other indicators that directly affects the risk of medical complications. For example, obesity by itself does not reveal the extent of coronary heart disease or of its development. Rather, obesity is linked strongly with such factors as hypertension and diabetes, both of which are significant coronary heart disease risk factors. Clearly, obesity is associated with multiple atherogenic traits, and excessive fat accumulation after age 30 contributes to the increased risk of heart disease.

Methods of Determining Fat Cell Size and Number

Researchers have used a variety of techniques to study adipose cellularity in humans and animals. The most accurate method was developed in the 1960s in the laboratory of Dr. Jules Hirsch at Rockefeller University, New York City. The technique involves sucking small fragments of subcutaneous tissue, usually from the buttocks and abdomen, into a syringe through a needle inserted directly into a fat depot. The adipose tissue is then treated chemically so that the fat cells can be separated and counted.

Once the number of cells is determined for a known weight of fat tissue, the average quantity of fat per cell is determined by dividing the quantity of fat in the sample by the total number of cells present in the sample. If total body fat is known, a reasonable estimate can be made of the total number of fat cells in the body. Let us assume that a subject weighs 70 kg and is 18% fat as determined by the underwater weighing method outlined in Chapter 5. The weight of fat for this person is computed as body weight × percent body fat and equals 12.6 kg of fat. By dividing this value for the weight of fat by the average content of fat per cell, the total number of fat cells in the body can be determined.

$$\text{Total number of cells} = \frac{\text{Weight of body fat}}{\text{Fat content per cell}}$$

In this example, if the average fat cell contains 0.53 micrograms (μg) of fat, then there are 23.8 billion fat cells contained in the 12.6 kg adipose tissue depot.

In one of our laboratories, the needle biopsy procedure coupled with photomicrographic techniques are used to extract and measure the average size of fat cells in the buttocks, abdomen, and upper back area. After the fat sample is extracted, it is treated chemically and then photographed for later projection on a large screen. Figure 6-1 shows the biopsy procedure from the buttocks region and a photomicrograph of the fat cells that are counted and measured for diameter and volume with a light emitting pen that interfaces with a computer. For the middle-aged professor whose total fat content prior to a successful marathon run was 14.4 kg (184 lbs or 83.4 kg body weight, 17.2% body fat) with 0.68 μg of lipid per cell, the total number of fat cells was estimated to be 21.2 billion (14.4 kg $\div$ 0.68 μg).

Fat Cell Size and Number in Normal and Obese Adult Subjects

There have been several comparative studies of adipose cellularity in obese and nonobese human subjects. These studies show quite conclusively that the accumulation of excess calories as fat in the obese is brought about either by the storage of larger quantities of fat in existing adipose cells (hypertrophy), by the actual formation of new fat cells (hyperplasia), or by a combination of both hypertrophy and hyperplasia.

Figure 6-2 graphically compares the body weight, total fat content, cell size, and cell number in a group of 20 subjects clinically classified as obese and in 5 nonobese subjects.

The body weight of the obese subjects averaged more than twice that of the nonobese, while their total fat content was nearly triple that of the leaner group. The weight of body fat in the obese ranged from 92 pounds to 227 pounds, while the average weight of fat for the nonobese was about 40 pounds. Further analysis of fat composition indicated that the average amount of fat within each fat cell was about 35% greater in the obese than in the nonobese. In addition, the total *number* of fat cells in the obese subjects was approximately three times greater than the number of fat cells in the nonobese: 75 billion fat cells compared to 27 billion fat cells. This vividly illustrates that the major structural difference in adipose tissue mass between obese and nonobese people is in cell number.

We can illustrate the role of fat cell number in obesity further by relating total fat content to both cell size and cell number. The data in the left side of Figure 6-3 demonstrate the strong positive relationship between total weight of fat in the obese and the total number of fat cells. The obese person with the lowest fat content had the fewest number of fat cells, while the fattest subject had considerably more fat cells than the less fat subjects. On the other hand, the data displayed in the right panel of Figure 6-3 clearly show that there was little or no relationship between the total body fat of obese people and the average size of fat cells. This information suggests that there may be some biologic upper limit to how large fat

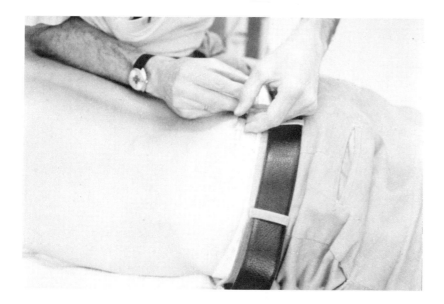

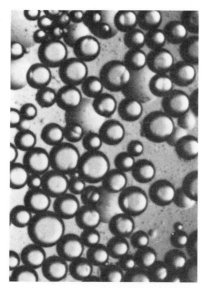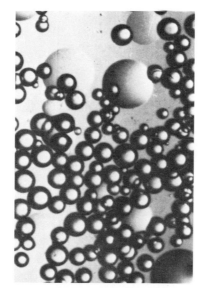

Figure 6-1. *Upper panel. Needle biopsy procedure for extraction of fat cells in the buttocks region. Bottom panels. Photomicrograph of fat cells biopsied from the buttocks of the middle-aged, physically active professor. The large spherical structures in the background are lipid droplets. During a period of relative inactivity prior to 6 months of marathon training (5 days/week, 10 to 16 miles/day), the average diameter of the buttocks fat cells was 8.6% larger than following the training regimen. The average volume of fat in each cell decreased by 18.2% compared to pretraining values. (Courtesy of Debra Spiak and Muscle Biochemistry Laboratory, Department of Exercise Science, University of Massachusetts, Amherst.)*

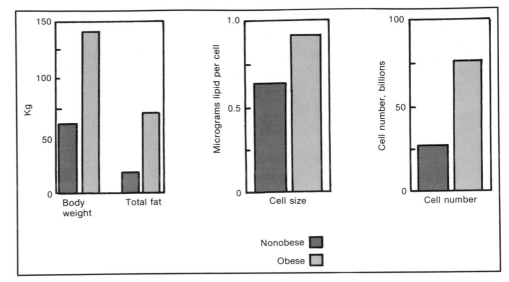

Figure 6-2. *Comparison of body weight, total body fat, cell size, and cell number in obese and non-obese subjects. (Reprinted and modified from J. Hirsch and J. Knittle, "Cellularity of Obese and Non-obese Human Adipose Tissue," Federation Proceedings, 29:1518–1519, 1970.)*

cells can become. After this size is reached, cell number probably becomes the key factor in determining the extent of obesity. Even if the size of fat cells could double, their size would not account for the tremendous difference in the amount of fat in obese and nonobese people. Therefore the excessive quantity of adipose tissue in obesity must occur by fat cell hyperplasia. As a frame of reference, an average nonobese person has about 25 to 30 billion fat cells. For the moderately

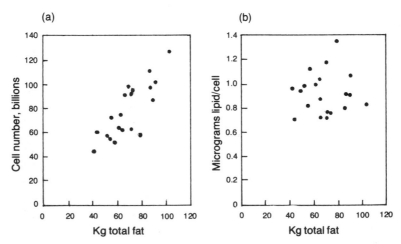

Figure 6-3. *Left panel: Adipose cell number related to the body's total weight of fat; right panel: Adipose cell size related to the body's total weight of fat. (Reprinted from J. Hirsch and J. Knittle, "Cellularity of Obese and Non-obese Human Adipose Tissue," Federation Proceedings, 29:1518–1519, 1970.)*

obese the number of fat cells is about 60 to 100 billion, while for the massively obese, the number of fat cells may be as high as 200 billion.

Table 6-1 presents recent data on fat cell (adipocyte) size and number, total body fat, and percentage body fat in men and women by 5-year age intervals from 20 to 50 years. The interesting observation in this sample of 217 subjects was the lack of sex differences among the variables, except the 20 to 24 year age group where the women had significantly larger adipocytes and more total body fat than the men. On a percentage basis, women had the greatest amount of body fat in every age group except at 45 to 50 years of age. Longitudinal data, where the same subjects are remeasured over time, will confirm whether or not adipocyte number can increase (as it appears to do in these cross-sectional data) as people get older. If this is true, then the notion that cell number becomes fixed early in life will require reexamination.

Fat Cell Size and Number after Weight Reduction

Weight reduction in obese adults and children is accompanied by a decrease in the size of fat cells but *no change* in the number of cells. If a weight reduction program achieves normal body weight and fatness, then the individual fat cells will shrink and actually become smaller in size than the fat cells of people who have never been obese. The results of one study of weight reduction in obese adults are depicted in Figure 6-4.

Table 6-1. *Comparison of adipocyte size and number, and body composition in men and women by 5-year age groups.*

AGE GROUP	SEX	ADIPOCYTE SIZE MICROGRAMS LIPID/CELL	ADIPOCYTE NUMBER BILLIONS	TOTAL BODY FAT, kg	% BODY FAT[a]
20–24	M	.37[b]	28.83	9.4[b]	13.0[b]
	F	.47	33.48	15.1	25.0
25–29	M	.37	34.62	13.0	17.5[b]
	F	.41	38.37	14.2	24.7
30–34	M	.42	34.85	13.4	17.8[b]
	F	.47	32.87	15.7	26.4
35–39	M	.41	42.08	16.6	21.8[b]
	F	.44	40.28	17.3	27.9
40–44	M	.39	45.57	18.9	22.7[b]
	F	.46	43.34	19.7	31.5
45–50	M	.51	50.07	22.0[b]	26.3
	F	.49	39.33	17.1	29.0

[a] Determined by underwater weighing.
[b] Differences between the sexes statistically significant.
Source: Chumlea, W.C. and others. Adipocytes and adiposity in adults. *American Journal of Clinical Nutrition, 34*:1798–1803, 1981.

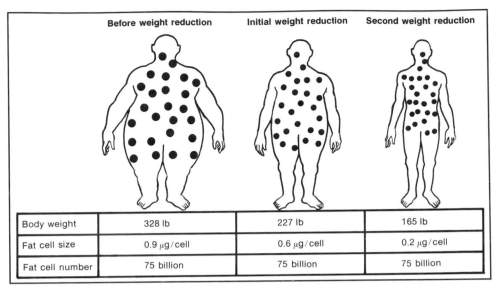

	Before weight reduction	Initial weight reduction	Second weight reduction
Body weight	328 lb	227 lb	165 lb
Fat cell size	0.9 μg/cell	0.6 μg/cell	0.2 μg/cell
Fat cell number	75 billion	75 billion	75 billion

Figure 6-4. *Changes in adipose cellularity with weight reduction in obese subjects. (Data from J. Hirsch, "Adipose Cellularity in Relation to Human Obesity," in G.H. Stollerman, ed., Advances in Internal Medicine, vol. 17. Copyright © 1971 by Year Book Medical Publishers, Inc. Used by permission.)*

In this study 19 obese subjects who initially weighed 328 pounds reduced body weight by 101 pounds, weighing 227 pounds at the end of the first part of the experiment. Prior to weight reduction the average number of fat cells was approximately 75 billion. This number remained essentially unchanged after weight reduction. The average size of the fat cells, on the other hand, was reduced 33%, from 0.9 to 0.6 μg of fat per cell. When they lost 62 more pounds, the subjects attained a normal body weight. Cell number again remained unchanged, while cell size continued to shrink to about one-third the size of the fat cells of normal, nonobese subjects. Other experiments have confirmed these findings in adults and young children. *The major anatomical or structural change after weight reduction is a shrinkage in fat cell size with little or no change in cell number.*

These findings suggest that the formerly obese person who reduces body weight and even body fat to near average levels is still not "cured" of his or her obesity, at least in terms of the number of fat cells present. Clinical evidence reveals that such formerly obese patients have an extremely difficult time maintaining their new body size. It is tempting to suggest that this large number of relatively small fat cells in the reduced obese is somehow related to the appetite control center in the brain. When this appetite center is stimulated, the person craves food, overeats, and regains the lost weight. Some nutritionists have referred to the repetitive "yo-yo-like" cycle of weight loss and weight gain among the obese as the "plight of the starving fat cells."

Research indicates that using various dietary manipulations to help adult obese persons to reduce is not likely to alter their large number of fat cells, even if the dietary intervention is successful over a long period. This is a somewhat pessimistic outlook for the obese person who hopes to stay permanently reduced.

Fat Cell Size and Number after Weight Gain

An interesting series of studies dealing with the experimental development of obesity in humans was carried out by researchers at the College of Medicine, University of Vermont. Over a period of 40 weeks, adult male volunteers with an initial average body fat content of 15% deliberately tripled their caloric intake to about 7000 kcal per day. The subject shown in Figure 6-5 increased 25% in body

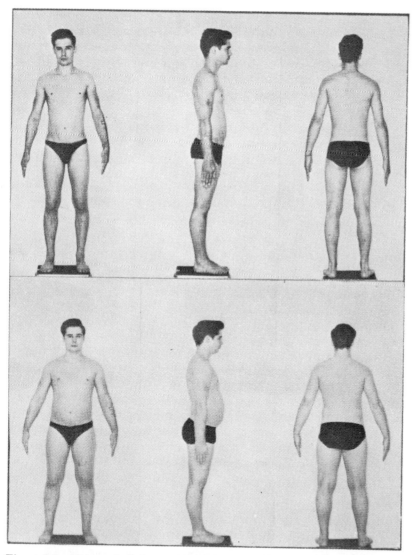

Figure 6-5. *Changes in body weight and percent body fat by deliberate overeating (top: 14.6% body fat; bottom: 28.2% body fat). A 25% increase in body weight was accompanied by a 100% increase in body fat. (Courtesy of Dr. E. A. Sims, School of Medicine, University of Vermont.)*

weight, from 110 to 138 pounds. Body fat for this subject doubled from 14.6 to 28.2% of body weight. Consequently, of the 28 pounds gained during the period of overeating, 23 were caused by increased deposition of body fat.

In a similar experiment with a group of nonobese subjects with no previous personal or family history of obesity, body weight increased an average of 36 pounds from voluntary overeating. When the size and number of fat cells were compared before and after the four-month experimental period, the average size of the fat cells had increased substantially, with no corresponding change in cell number. When the subjects were once again reduced to their normal weight by restricting caloric intake, body fat was reduced and the fat cells returned to their original size. These results indicate that the acquisition of excess fat produced in adults by overeating is caused by filling existing adipose cells with more fat rather than by increasing or proliferating new fat cells. However, there is also recent evidence to indicate that in mature-onset moderate to massive obesity, where the already fat adult becomes even fatter, *new* fat cells may be developed in addition to the expansion in size of the already existing cells.

Development of Adipose Cellularity

The development of adipose tissue during growth has been studied by several laboratories and can be categorized in terms of animal research and human research.

ANIMAL STUDIES

Studies of fat cell development in different species of animals reveals two basic ways in which fat depots develop. The guinea pig, for example, expands its adipose tissue mass from 6 weeks to 1 year primarily by hyperplasia. The hamster and rat, on the other hand, increase adipose tissue mainly by fat cell hypertrophy, although hyperplasia also occurs. The most extensive studies of adipose cellularity have been conducted with rats, as these mammals have a relatively short life span and various diets and exercise regimes can be studied quite easily during the growth cycle. In establishing these growth curves, the experimenter determines adipose cellularity periodically from three main fat depots in the rat. What usually occurs is that the number and size of fat cells increases during weeks 6 through 16. Thereafter, as animals continue to gain in body weight and body fat, there is a corresponding increase only in the size of the fat cells. Thus, the additional increase in body fat occurs by filling existing cells rather than by developing new fat cells.

HUMAN STUDIES

In contrast to the many longitudinal studies of animals during their growth periods, scientists have made very few investigations of the time course of adipose tissue development in humans. In one human experiment, fat cell size and number were determined for 34 infants and children ranging in age from a few days to age 13. Figure 6-6 plots some of these data that illustrate the relationship between fat

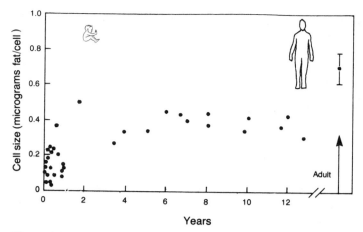

Figure 6-6. *Changes in fat cell size from birth to adulthood. (Reprinted and modified from J. Hirsch and J. Knittle, "Cellularity of Obese and Non-obese Human Adipose Tissue," Federation Proceedings, 29:1518–1519, 1970.)*

cell size and age. The value for average cell size in normal adults is shown at the right of the figure.

These data suggest that the size of fat cells in newborn infants and children up to the age of 1 year is about one-fourth the size of adult fat cells. It is also evident from Figure 6-6 that fat cells triple in size during the first 6 years with little further increase in size to age 13. Data on adipose cell size during adolescence are scarce. We can assume, however, that cell size increases further during this growth period because in adulthood it is significantly larger than it was at age 13. Figure 6-7 illustrates data on fat cell number from birth to age 13.

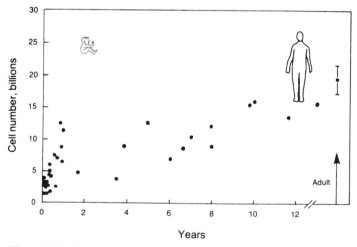

Figure 6-7. *Changes in fat cell number from birth to adulthood. (Reprinted and modified from J. Hirsch and J. Knittle, "Cellularity of Obese and Non-obese Human Adipose Tissue," Federation Proceedings, 29:1517, 1520, 1970.)*

During the *first year of life* cell number increases fairly rapidly, for the total number of fat cells is about three times greater at 1 year than at birth. Scientists believe that most of the fat cells existing prior to birth are formed during the *last 3 months of pregnancy.* After the first year of life cell number increases more gradually up to the age of about 10. As was the case with cell size, the number of cells formed after age 13 continues to increase during *the growth spurt in adolescence* until adulthood; thereafter, there is little further increase in cell number. Thus there appear to be three critical periods when the number of fat cells increases significantly. The first is during the last trimester of pregnancy, the second is during the first year of life, and the third occurs during the adolescent growth spurt. It is during adulthood that the total number of fat cells probably cannot be altered to any significant degree; the only exception appears to be in the moderately or massively obese adult where further cell proliferation can occur. However, there are still no substantial data to indicate clearly if the final number of adult fat cells can be modified through some form of intervention at an earlier period of life. It is impossible to state with certainty whether the rate of fat cell development in humans can be reversed or at least slowed down. The fundamental question remains, "Can fat cell number be altered before adulthood, or is overfatness predetermined primarily by genetic code?"

Modification of Adipose Cellularity

Although the precise causes for fat cell development are poorly understood, it does appear that certain practices can affect body fat. In humans, for example, nutritional practices of the mother during pregnancy may modify the body composition of the developing fetus. A weight gain by the mother in excess of 40 lb was associated with a significantly larger skinfold thickness of the offspring than that in a woman who followed a recommended weight gain during pregnancy. Bottle feeding and the early introduction of solid food may also be associated with the development of obesity. Conversely, breast feeding, allowing the infant to set the limits to food consumption, and a delayed introduction to solid food may prevent overfeeding, the development of poor eating habits, and subsequent obesity.

Research in animals suggests that alterations in fat cell size and number can be achieved in two ways: (1) modification of early nutrition, and (2) exercise.

NUTRITIONAL INFLUENCES

Studies have demonstrated that *early nutritional practices* can influence the development of body fatness and adipose cellularity at a later time period in the animal's life. In one well-controlled study large numbers of rats were redistributed at birth, giving some mothers large litters of 22 animals and others smaller litters of 4 animals. After weaning at 21 days both groups were given unlimited access to food. At weaning and at each subsequent 5-week period to 20 weeks of age, both groups of rats differed significantly in body weight. Thus, the early (calorically deprived) nutritional deprivation produced by rearing animals in large litters for the first 21 days of life resulted in the permanent stunting of their growth, even though both groups of animals had free access to food after weaning.

In both groups the weight of one of the fat depots increased from weaning to 20 weeks of age. The most dramatic differences in fat weight occurred, however, in animals reared in small litters, especially at weeks 15 and 20. These relative differences were larger than the differences observed in body weight for the same period. Figure 6-8 shows that in terms of cell size and number, the nutritionally deprived animals from large litters had fewer and smaller fat cells at all age intervals than animals reared in small litters.

At 5 and 10 weeks of age, the height of the rectangles is greater than the base, indicating that the proliferation of fat cells made a greater contribution to adipose mass than cell size. For the 15- and 20-week periods, the shape of the bar approaches a square, indicating that cell size plays an increasingly important role in the development of adipose tissue. An interesting comparison is seen in the two shaded areas of the bar that represent animals raised in large and small litters. The total area of the bar represents the fat depot of the overnourished animals raised in small litters, the darker area denotes the data from animals raised in large litters, and the lighter area illustrates the difference in depot size between the two groups.

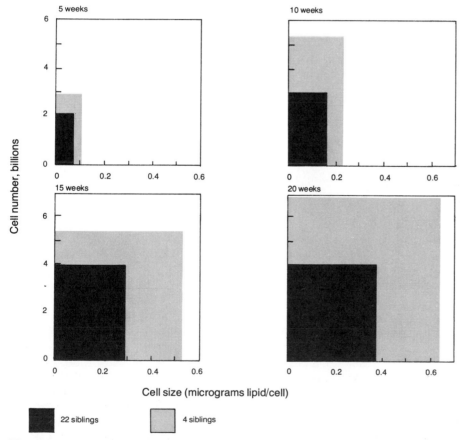

Figure 6-8. *Changes in cell size and number in animals raised in small and large litters. (Adapted from J. Knittle and J. Hirsch, "Effect of Early Nutrition on the Development of Rat Epididymal Fat Pads: Cellularity and Metabolism," Journal of Clinical Investigation, 47:2095, 1968.)*

The underfed group reached a definite plateau in the number of fat cells by 15 weeks of age. In contrast, cell number continued to increase in the overfed, small-litter animals. In both groups cell size increased progressively during the 20-week experiment. These data certainly suggest there may be a critical time during the early growth period when permanent modifications in adipose tissue occur.

We would like to point out that it is difficult to extrapolate experimental results from rats to humans. However, some striking similarities appear in human and rat adipose tissue development. It appears that the excessive quantity of body fat of obese humans is associated primarily with a large increase in the number of fat cells, and to a lesser extent by increased size of individual fat cells. When obese adults lose a considerable amount of weight, the number of fat cells remains unchanged and they reduce total body fat almost exclusively by reducing fat cell size. Similar findings concerning fat cell number have been observed in studies with adult rats. When adult rats are calorically deprived by acute starvation or more prolonged semistarvation, the decrease in body weight is only temporary and is rapidly reinstated upon refeeding. The weight loss in such food-restricted animals is due to a decrease in fat cell size with no corresponding change in cell number. When the animals again have normal access to food, the fat cells refill and attain the size they had prior to food deprivation. Except in cases of already obese animals, overfeeding of *adult* animals produces an increase in total body fat, but as with humans, this increase is generally brought about by "stuffing" of cells with fat rather than by increases in cell number. Thus in both humans and rats dietary manipulation does not appear to affect adipose cell number in adulthood, and any changes in the total quantity of body fat are brought about primarily by cellular enlargement. Furthermore, when the fat content of adult humans is reduced, cell size shrinks accordingly, only to expand again when the body's content of fat is restored.

More recent studies have also shown that the early nutritional patterns in rats (controlled by weaning in small and large litters), can have a sustained effect on the total fat mass and total number of cells, but not necessarily the size of the cells. If the influence of early nutrition in the rat are paralleled by similar effects in man, then overfeeding during childhood may increase the tendency to adult obesity. Thus, it seems prudent to encourage the parents of young children to avoid overfeeding their youngsters, as this may temper their proclivity to obesity as adults. This is especially true prior to 2 years of age.

EXERCISE INFLUENCES

Only a few experiments have evaluated the contribution of exercise to modifying adipose tissue cell size and number. Figure 6-9 summarizes the results of one such experiment on the effects of physical activity and food restriction on the growth of rats. In this study an exercise group with free access to food was subjected to a 14- to 16-week program of swimming early in the animals' growth period. The animals swam in plastic barrels 6 days a week. Initially the exercise sessions lasted 15 minutes; they lengthened gradually until the animals were swimming for 360 minutes at the end of 4 weeks. They continued to swim for 360 minutes until the end of the experimental period. They were then sacrificed and analyzed for fat content and adipose cellularity. During the experiment two adult groups of rats remained sedentary; one group had free access to food and water,

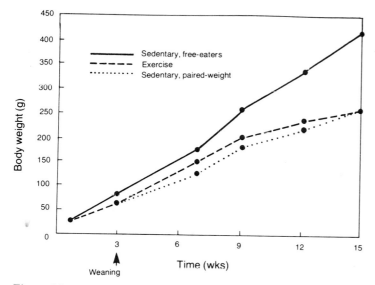

Figure 6-9. *Effects of exercise and of food restriction on body weight of rats. (From L. Oscai et al., "Effects of Exercise and of Food Restriction on Adipose Tissue Cellularity," Journal of Lipid Research, 13.590, 1972.)*

while the other group was restricted in food intake to maintain their body weight at the same level as the exercise group.

The results were convincing; animals given unlimited food but forced to exercise for 15 weeks gained weight more slowly and had a lower final body weight then sedentary, freely eating rats. Because both groups consumed *the same* number of calories each day, the lower rate of weight gain in the exercisers could be attributed to the increased caloric requirements of the exercise. It was also shown that the total fat content of the nonexercise group was about four times higher than the fat content of the freely eating exercise group. The exercise intervention program during the growth period resulted in a significant reduction in total body fat due to a decrease in both cell size *and* number.

The total fat content of the sedentary, food-restricted group was lower than that of the sedentary animals who could eat ad libitum. Reducing food intake resulted in a reduction in cell size and cell number. When the body fat of the food restricted and exercised animals was compared, the exercisers had fewer fat cells and less fat per cell, even though the final body weights of both groups were approximately equal. The results demonstrated that exercise performed *early* during the growth period depressed the growth of new fat cells. In a follow-up experiment, the fat-retarding effects of exercise or diet early in an animal's life were studied to determine whether either would reduce fat accumulation in adulthood.

Three groups of animals were used: an exercise group, a sedentary group with free access to food and water, and a sedentary group with restricted food intake. Exercise and food restriction were terminated after 28 weeks. Several animals from each group were then sacrificed and the groups compared for growth, body fat, and adipose cell size and number. The remaining animals were subjected to 34

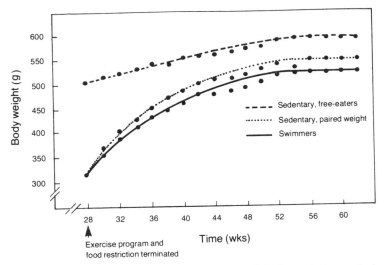

Figure 6-10. *Effects of 28 weeks of exercise and food restriction on body weight in rats followed by no exercise with unlimited access to foods. (Data from L. Oscai et al., "Exercise or Food Restriction: Effect on Adipose Tissue Cellularity," American Journal of Physiology, 227:902, 1974.)*

weeks of sedentary living without exercise and were allowed unlimited food and water. The animals were then sacrificed and the groups compared for body weight cell size, and cell number. The data in Figure 6-10 show that the exercised animals had lower body weights at 28 weeks of age than the other groups.

During the next 34 weeks of inactivity, the previously exercised animals continued to maintain a lower body weight than the sedentary animals. Thus, the 28-week exercise program performed earlier in life caused a reduction in body weight that was still evident at the end of the experiment. Comparing cell size and number at the end of the training period revealed that the exercised group had *fewer* and *smaller* fat cells than either sedentary group of animals. These results were in agreement with the previous experiment. The exercise group had a lower final body weight and reduced total body fat content than their sedentary counterparts, as well as significantly *fewer* fat cells in later life than animals in the other groups. Twenty-six weeks of exercise, begun early in life and then terminated, retarded the expansion and proliferation of fat cells during the growth period to adulthood, even though the exercise period was followed by 34 weeks of inactivity.

If these findings can be applied to humans, it is possible that the introduction of a diet and/or exercise program during the early stages of growth may aid in controlling the proliferation of new fat cells and the filling up of previously dormant ones. Programs of exercise and weight control begun later in life and maintained thereafter can be effective in lowering the body's total quantity of fat. As far as we know, however, it is only cell size and *not* cell number than can be reduced. If exercise or dietary intervention is discontinued, then the existing adipose tissue mass is likely to increase again by expansion of the cellular volume. *Early prevention of obesity through exercise and diet, rather than correction of obesity once it is present, may be the most effective method to curb the grossly "overfat" condition so common in teenagers and adults.*

There is widespread belief that by exercising one area of the body, more fat will be lost from that area in comparison to other body parts. It is also believed that disuse of a muscle group causes a disproportionate accumulation of local subcutaneous fat and, conversely, an increase in a muscle's activity facilitates a relatively large fat mobilization from the specific storage sites. While the notion of "spot-reduction" through selective exercise such as leg raises, sit ups, side bends, or twists is especially attractive from an aesthetic stand point (and monitarily to those who peddle special creams, shakers and rollers), the scientific evidence does not support such practices.

The following experiment was conducted to critically evaluate the spot reducing hypothesis. Thirteen college men at the University of Massachusetts, Amherst, performed 5,004 sit-ups during a 27-day progressive sit-up exercise program. Sit-ups were performed with hands clasped behind the head and legs bent at a 90° angle at the knee. Cadence was maintained with a metronome. Table 6-2 outlines the regimen used to progressively increase the number of sit-ups. Detailed measurements of body composition were made before and following the experimental period. Total body fat was measured by the water immersion method outlined in Chapter 5, as were selected fatfolds and girths. In addition, fat biopsies were taken from the abdominal, buttocks, and subscapular (base of shoulder blade) regions and the number of fat cells determined by the photomicrographic, computer-digitizing method discussed in a previous section.

If spot reducing worked due to the sit-up exercise, then the amount of fat in the abdominal fat cells should have reduced to a greater extent than the storage fat in the fat cells of the other areas. However, this did not occur. The reduction in cell diameter was the *same* for the three sites. While the amount of change in cell diameter was about 5% (equivalent to a 15 to 17% change in volume), there were no alterations in gross measures of body composition (body density, fatfolds, or girths) for the experimental subjects or control subjects that did not exercise. Thus, under the conditions of this experiment, the notion of spot reducing was

Table 6-2. *Progressive sit-up training program.*[a]

DAYS	BOUTS	TIME PER BOUT, sec	SIT-UPS COMPLETED PER BOUT	TOTAL SIT-UPS
1–6	10 increase to 20	10	7	630
7–12	10 increase to 20	15	10	900
13–18	10 increase to 20	20	14	1260
19–24	10 increase to 20	25	15	1350
25–27	10 increase to 14	30	24	864
				5004

[a] A 10-sec rest interval remained constant between bouts on all training days.

From: Katch, F.I., Clarkson, P.M., Kroll, W., McBride, T., and A. Wilcox. Preferential effects of abdominal exercise training on regional adipose cell size. *Research Quarterly for Exercise and Sport.* 1984.

considered to be unattainable. Similar findings have been observed in comparisons of the circumferences and subcutaneous fat stores of the right and left forearms of elite tennis players. While the dominant or playing arm was significantly larger than the non-dominant arm, this was due entirely to a modest muscular hypertrophy as there was no difference between the arms in terms of quantity of subcutaneous forearm fat. It seems clear that the mobilization of fat during selective exercise is not restricted to the underlying fatty area of the body part being exercised. Mobilization of fatty acids occurs from the fat depots throughout the body and the areas of greatest fat storage probably supply the greatest amount of energy.

7

Weight Control

I T IS TRULY REMARKABLE that the body weight of most adults fluctuates only
slightly during the year, even though the annual intake of food averages between 1600 to 1900 pounds; this includes 280 eggs, 15.6 pounds of breakfast
cereal, 184 pounds of meat, 200 pounds of fruit, 250 pounds of vegetables, 68
pounds of bread, and 429 soft drinks, 2 gallons of wine, 24 gallons of beer, and 2
gallons of liquor! This relative stability in body weight is rather impressive when
you consider that a slight but prolonged increase in food intake can cause a substantial increase in body weight. Eating just an extra handful of peanuts each day
would increase body weight by about 10 pounds in 1 year. However, the fact that
the body weight of most adults does not usually increase by this amount illustrates
the body's exquisite regulatory control in balancing caloric intake with daily energy expenditure. *It is only when the number of calories ingested as food exceeds
the daily energy requirements that the excess calories are stored as fat in adipose
tissue.* To prevent an increase in body weight and body fat because of a caloric
imbalance, an effective program of weight control must establish a balance between energy input and energy output.

Balancing Energy Input with Energy Output

The many popular books that advocate exotic diets or exercise plans to help
reduce body weight have one thing in common: They all claim their plans are so
easy and effortless to follow that results can be guaranteed! If this were the case,
and a simple procedure could maintain the "perfect" body size permanently, then
the estimated 60 to 70 million American adults and at least 10 million American
teenagers who are overfat could be cured easily. Even when a particular diet plan
gains widespread popularity as a result of an advertising blitz that "documents"
examples of actual weight loss, these schemes often place a dieter's total health in
jeopardy. Many professional organizations have voiced strong opposition to various dietary practices, in particular the *low-carbohydrate, high-fat,* and *high-
protein* diets. The American Medical Association Council on Food and Nutrition
severely criticized the popular Atkins high-fat diet as "bizarre" by stating it was

without scientific merit, and lacked prior experimentation concerning the validity of the claims made. Advocates of this diet emphasize carbohydrate restriction while ignoring the total caloric content of the diet. It is argued that with minimal carbohydrate for energy the body must metabolize its fat stores. This supposedly generates sufficient ketones bodies (by-products of incomplete fat breakdown) to cause urinary loss of these unused calories to account for significant weight loss despite an allegedly high caloric intake. It is argued that this caloric loss will be so great that the dieter can eat all he or she wishes, as long as carbohydrates are restricted. At best, the calories lost by a urinary excretion of ketones would equal only 100 to 150 calories a day. This would account for only a small weight loss of approximately 1 pound a month—not very appealing when the major proportion of the daily calorie intake amounts to a fat intake that may be as high as 60 to 70% of the food consumed. Also, any initial weight loss on this diet may be due largely to dehydration brought about by sodium loss and extra solute load on the kidneys which increases the excretion of urinary water. Such water loss is of no lasting significance in a program designed to reduce body fat. Low carbohydrate diets have the potential for causing the body to lose significant amounts of lean tissue. This is certainly an *undesirable* side effect for a diet designed to bring about fat loss.

High-fat, low-carbohydrate diets are also potentially hazardous in a number of ways. The diet can raise serum uric acid levels, lower potassium levels, which facilitates undesirable cardiac arrhythmias, cause acidosis, aggravate kidney problems due to the extra solute burden placed on the renal system, elevate blood lipids thus increasing a primary heart disease risk factor, deplete glycogen reserves and contribute to a fatigued state, and cause a relative dehydration. The diet is definitely contraindicated during pregnancy as adequate carbohydrate metabolism is essential for proper fetal development.

A *starvation diet* or *therapeutic fast* may be recommended in cases of severe obesity where body fat exceeds 40 to 50% of body weight. Such diets are usually prescribed for up to 3 months, but only as a "last resort" prior to undertaking more extreme medical approaches which include various surgical treatments. The starvation approach to weight loss is predicated on the hope that abstinence from food will break established dietary habits and this, in turn, may improve the long term prospects for successful weight loss. This form of dieting must be closely supervised, usually in a hospital setting.

Other dietary plans, specifically the various modifications of a high-protein diet, can be potentially harmful. The high-protein diet has been extrolled as the "last chance diet" for the obese as well as those who are less overweight. It is argued that protein diets cause suppression of appetite through the body's excessive reliance on fat mobilization. This effect has yet to be supported with careful research. It is also argued that the elevated calorie-burning SDA effect of dietary protein as well as its relatively low coefficient of digestability ultimately reduce the net calories available from this food compared to a well-balanced meal of equal caloric value. This calorigenic effect of protein ingestion is believed to be due largely to digestive processes as well as the extra energy required by the liver to assimilate amino acids. Although this point may have some validity, many other factors must be considered in formulating a sound program for weight loss—not to mention the potentially harmful strain on kidney and liver function, and accompanying dehydration, electrolyte imbalance, and lean tissue loss resulting from diets excessively high in protein. When the protein is in liquid form, the "miracle liquid" is made palatable with artificial flavoring, and often includes a blend of ground-up animal hooves and horns, and pigskin mixed in a broth with enzymes and tenderizers to "predigest" it. In 1979, according to the Federal Drug Administration, this particular brand of protein elixir and others like it were associated with 58 deaths. Sixteen of the victims were obese women who lost an average of 83 pounds within 2 to 8 months. None had a previous history of heart disease; they all died suddenly while on the diet or shortly thereafter. Formal complaints were received from 165 people who reported a variety of side effects that included hair loss, nausea, headaches, constipation, neural disorders, bad breath, faintness, muscle weakness, decreased libido, and gastrointestinal disorders. Table 7-1 summarizes the principles and main advantages and disadvantages of some of the popular dietary approaches to weight loss.

While most diets produce a weight loss during the first several weeks, most of the weight lost is body water. Unless a person can maintain a reduced caloric intake for a considerable time, the weight will eventually be regained. The net result is a return to original body size, often at the expense of feelings of hunger and other psychological stresses while the diet plan is actually followed. Anyone who has seriously tried to maintain a diet knows the difficulties encountered. While it is certainly possible to lose 15, 20, or even 30 or more pounds through diet, few people have enough self-control to stick with a diet plan long enough to change body size successfully and permanently.

A review of the scientific literature dealing with weight loss in obese subjects reveals that people who are initially successful in modifying their body composition are usually unsuccessful in permanently maintaining their desired body size and shape. This has been pointed out in numerous studies dealing with follow-up measurements of patients who have participated in weight reduction programs where caloric intake was carefully regulated and monitored. In one survey of the effectiveness of obesity clinics in weight control management during a 10 year period, it was observed that the dropout rate varied from 20 to 80%. Of those who remained in a program, no more than 25% lost as much as 20 pounds and only 5% lost 40 pounds or more. Such statistics are rather discouraging and indicate that the long-term maintenance of a particular low-calorie diet is extremely difficult; it is especially difficult in the relaxed atmosphere of a person's home, where access to food is relatively easy. Similarly, increasing energy expenditure through physical activity, while not unpleasant in itself, does require a personal commitment in terms of time and life style that many people are not willing to make. *Reducing body size through diet and exercise is only half the battle; staying reduced requires a serious commitment to a new life style.*

WHEN IS IT TIME TO REDUCE?

In the previous chapter on evaluating body composition we described a simple tape measure technique for determining the body's fat content. By referring to the suggested guidelines for optimal fatness in Chapter 6, you can make a good estimate of whether or not you are overfat for your age and sex. Consider the example of a 23-year-old female who weighs 175 pounds.

The three circumference measurements used to compute fatness from Table 5-1 are mid-abdomen = 36 inches, right thigh = 26.5 inches, and right forearm = 10.0 inches. By using the appropriate constants and substituting into the formula, percent body fat is computed as 40.6% of total body weight. This amounts to a total

Table 7-1. *Some popular weight loss methods.*

TYPE OF METHOD	PRINCIPLE	ADVANTAGES	DISADVANTAGES	COMMENTS
Surgical procedures	Alteration of the gastrointestinal tract changes capacity or amount of absorptive surface	Caloric restriction is less necessary	Risks of surgery and post-surgical complications include death	Radical procedures include stapling of the stomach and removal of a section of the small intestine (a jejunoilieal bypass)
Fasting	No energy input assures negative energy balance	Weight loss is rapid (which may be a disadvantage) Exposure to temptation is reduced	Ketogenic A large portion of weight lost is from lean body mass Nutrients are lacking	Medical supervision is mandatory and hospitalization is recommended
Protein-sparing modified fast	Same as fasting except protein intake helps preserve lean body mass	Same as above	Ketogenic Nutrients are lacking Some unconfirmed deaths have been reported, possibly from potassium depletion	Medical supervision is mandatory Popular presentation was made in Linn's *The Last Chance Diet*
One-food-centered diets	Low-caloric intake favors negative energy balance	Being easy to follow has initial psychological appeal	Being too restrictive means nutrients are probably lacking Repetitious nature may cause boredom	No food or food combination is known to "burn off" fat Examples include the grapefruit diet and the egg diet
Low-carbohydrate high-fat diets	Increased ketone excretion removes energy-containing substances from the body Fat intake is often voluntarily decreased; a low caloric diet results	Inclusion of rich foods may have psychological appeal Initial rapid loss of water may be an incentive	Ketogenic High-fat intake is contraindicated for heart and diabetes patients Nutrients are often lacking	Popular versions have been offered by Taller and Atkins; some have been called the "Mayo," "Drinking Man's," and "Air Force" diets
Low-carbohydrate/ high-protein diets	Low-caloric intake favors negative energy balance		Expense and repetitious nature may make it difficult to sustain	If meat is emphasized, the diet becomes one that is high in fat The Pennington diet is an example
High-carbohydrate/ low-fat diets	Low-caloric intake favors negative energy balance	Wise food selections can make the diet nutritionally sound	Initial water retention may be discouraging	

quantity of body fat of 71.1 pounds (175 pounds × 0.406), and 103.9 pounds of lean body weight (175 pounds body weight − 71.1 pounds fat). Knowing these values of body composition, you could ask, "How do these body composition measures compare to the average woman for this age range?" Referring to Table 5-5 compare the obtained value for percent body fat and that of an average woman. The last two columns in this table show the average values for percent body fat as well as the acceptable limits for body fat. A value of 40.6% body fat is well above the average and even exceeds one variation unit that includes the normal range. When compared to the 1983 Massachusetts data, the value for fat is 18.7% units higher than the 21.9% average fat value for the Massachusetts women, and 6.3% units higher than the upper range of the 1967 data for young women in Colorado. Thus this hypothetical 23-year-old woman possesses considerably more fat than the average woman reported in these studies.

Recall also that the average value plus or minus one variation unit gives a range for body fat that includes about 68 out of every 100 persons tested. The value of one variation unit is 5% body fat; thus two variation units above average would correspond to the average percent of fat plus an additional 10%. If you use the 1967 values of fatness for New York women, then 37% would represent the body fat value two variation units above the average. The observed value of 40.6% body fat is still above this limit; this woman is fatter than about 95 out of every 100 women measured. Admittedly, the diagnosis is not too cheerful, especially when her degree of fatness is related to what is known about fat cell size and fat cell number. Compared to the average young woman who possesses about 25 to 30 billion fat cells, this woman could have anywhere from 60 to 260 billion fat cells. To complicate matters further, the average size of her fat cells is also much larger than that of the fat cells of normal people. The important question to ask in this situation is, "What can be done to reduce to normal body size?"

THE ENERGY BALANCE EQUATION

Before someone develops a plan for establishing normal body composition, the rationale underlying the *energy balance equation* must be considered. The equation states that *body weight will remain constant when caloric intake equals caloric expenditure*. Any imbalance in energy output or energy input will result in a change in body weight. Figure 7-1 shows the ideal situation in which energy input (calories in food) *exactly balances* energy output (calories expended in daily physical activities). As long as this equilibrium is maintained within narrow limits, there will be relatively little fluctuation in body weight. The middle part of the figure depicts what happens all too frequently when energy input *exceeds* energy output. Under such conditions the number of calories consumed in excess of daily requirements is stored as fat in the adipose tissue depots. As we will discuss shortly, *3500 "extra" kcal on either the input or output side of the equation equal approximately 1 pound of stored fat*. The body has a way of keeping track of the extra calories consumed above the requirement level. It simply does not forget about the extra slice of cheese, cola or additional helping of pizza or strawberry ice cream with chocolate jimmies on top. The bottom of the figure illustrates what occurs when energy intake is *less than* energy output. In this case, the body obtains the required calories from its energy stores and weight and fat become reduced.

There are three ways to "unbalance" the energy balance equation and cause a reduction in body weight: (1) reduce caloric intake *below* daily energy requirements, (2) maintain regular food intake and *increase* caloric output through additional physical activity *above* daily energy requirements, and (3) combine methods (1) and (2) by *decreasing* daily food intake and *increasing* daily energy expenditure.

To understand how sensitive the energy balance equation is in regulating overall energy balance, consider the situation in which calorie intake exceeds calorie

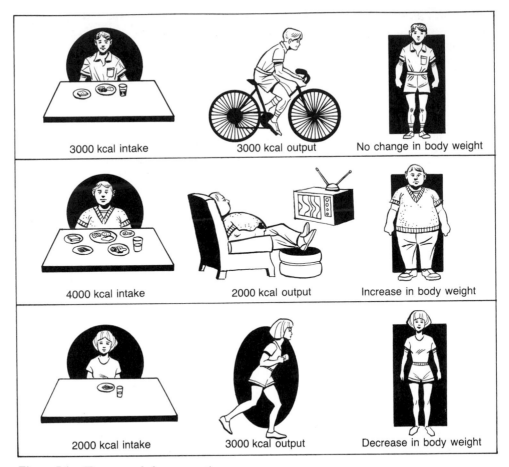

Figure 7-1. *The energy balance equation.*

output by only a hundred kcal per day. This could be achieved by eating only one extra banana each day. On an annual basis, the surplus number of kcal consumed would be 365 days × 100 kcal or 36,500 kcal. Because 1 pound of body fat contains about 3500 kcal, the small daily increase in calories consumed would result in a gain of 10.4 pounds of fat in a year. If the same eating habits were maintained and energy output remained unchanged, then theoretically there would be a gain in fat weight of 52 pounds in 5 years! On the other hand, reducing food intake by only 100 kcal a day *and* increasing energy expenditure by 100 kcal by jogging a mile each day would reduce total body fat by 21 pounds in 1 year. There's simply no way of getting around the fact that when the total extra calories consumed add up to 3500, approximately 1 extra pound of fat is gained. This cannot be undone by magic potions, trick diets, or special formula foods.

We believe one of the major reasons that weight control is so difficult is because most Americans are not willing to display the discipline or initiative to curb their appetites and get their bodies moving. We are all mesmerized to varying degrees by modern technologies that provide convenience rather than rely on the body's own power for movement and exercise. In the next chapter, we will discuss practical ways to help 20th century man and woman fight the battle of the energy balance equation to avoid defeat by 21st century technologies.

157

Weight Control

Personal Assessment of Eating Behavior

We usually eat for two reasons. First, we consume food because we are truly hungry. This hunger enables us to maintain a food intake to supply the energy to power the body's vital processes and sustain life. Second, we eat food to satisfy our appetites, which in America are usually "programmed" to be stimulated three times each day. Even after finishing the most delicious and satisfying meal, few of us could not be coaxed into eating "just a bit more," even if we felt full. Such overeating, although quite common, apparently occurs more in obese than in lean people. It appears that human eating behavior is intimately tied to environmental cues as well as to internal biochemical cues that signal a real need for caloric intake. The external "food cues" include the sight of food, its packaging, display, and advertising, the time and physical environment in which the food is eaten, and the taste, smell, and size of the portions.

Several experiments have demonstrated how external factors can influence eating behavior. In one study, normal and obese subjects were deceived into believing they were participating in an elaborate psychologic experiment. In actuality the experimenters wished to determine whether or not the visual presence of food affects eating behavior. After missing lunch, normal and obese subjects were tested in their responses to meaningless psychophysical stimuli. They were then left in a room to complete a questionnaire supposedly concerned with the experiment. In the room subjects found either 1 or 3 roast beef sandwiches and soda. Subjects were told to eat as much as they wanted and to help themselves to more food from the refrigerator. When 3 sandwiches were left in the room, the obese subjects consumed an average of 2.3 sandwiches compared with 1.9 sandwiches eaten by the normal-sized subjects; when only 1 sandwich was in view, the obese subjects ate fewer sandwiches (1.5) then the nonobese subjects (2.0).

Another experiment concerned the effects of taste on eating behavior. Before the experiment, obese subjects normally consumed 3500 kcal per day while nonobese subjects consumed 2200 kcal per day. Then for 3 weeks subjects in both groups were offered a bland liquid diet; the nonobese subjects continued to consume 2200 kcal of this liquid meal each day, whereas the obese subjects decreased their daily caloric intake to only 500 kcal. These results demonstrated that obese subjects were influenced considerably more by the *taste of food* then by its caloric content. Results of this type illustrate how external environmental cues can significantly affect eating behavior, especially in the obese.

Daily events quite unrelated to food itself can also trigger the urge to eat. Depression, frustration, boredom, "uptight" or anxious feelings, guilt, sadness, or anger can all be linked to periods of excessive food intake. The importance of food cues in dieting is that the prospective dieter must learn to make an accurate appraisal of his or her eating behavior in terms of the quantity, frequency, and circumstances of eating. A first step in such a self-analysis is to become keenly aware of daily caloric intake. Once this is accomplished, "undesirable" food cues must be eliminated, and a new set of desirable eating responses must replace previously learned behaviors. In the following chapter we will discuss such a process, which is referred to as *eating behavior modification.*

In addition to caloric restriction through diet coupled with attempts to modify eating behavior, we believe that the final component of a successful program of weight control is the adoption of a physically active life style. This does not mean that the dieter simply plays a token game of tennis twice a year, goes for a swim on weekends during the summer, or walks to the store when the car is being repaired. *Modifying personal exercise habits entails a serious commitment to changing the daily routine to include regular periods of relatively vigorous physical activity.*

HOW TO DETERMINE CALORIC INTAKE FROM FOODS

There is a relatively simple yet accurate method to determine the average total number of calories consumed each day. The dieter should keep a *daily log* of food intake for 7 consecutive days. Many experiments have shown that people who calculate caloric intake from accurate records of their daily food consumption are usually within 10% of the actual number of calories consumed. For example, suppose the caloric value of your daily food intake were directly measured in the bomb calorimeter and averaged 2130 kcal. If you kept a 7-day dietary history and estimated your daily caloric intake, the daily value would vary by about 10% from the actual value or from 1920 to 2350 kcal. As long as you maintained a careful record, the degree of accuracy for daily caloric determinations would be within acceptable limits.

Before beginning to record daily caloric intake for the 7-day period, you must become familiar with "honest" calorie counting. To do this you must first acquire four items for measuring food: a plastic ruler, a standard measuring cup, measuring spoons, and a small, inexpensive balance or weighing scale. You can purchase these items at most hardware stores. Second, familiarize yourself with the caloric value of foods. Consult Appendix A for this purpose that includes a listing for alcoholic beverages as well as the nutritive value of specialty and "fast-food" items sold at 12 popular take-out restaurants. You should obtain an inexpensive calorie-counting guide as a supplement. This is available at newsstands and bookstores and gives the average caloric values for most foods. Guides that list foods according to brand names are also helpful.

Measure or weigh each of the food items in your diet that are listed below. This is the only reliable way to get an accurate estimate of the size of a food portion. If you elect to use Appendix A to estimate kcal value, you need only to weigh each food item. If you use a supplementary calorie-counting guide, you may have to use the measuring cup, spoons, and ruler.

Food Categories

Meat and fish: Measure the portion of meat or fish by thickness, length, and width, or record weight on the scale.

Vegetables, mashed potatoes, rice, cereals, salads: Measure the portion in a measuring cup or record weight on the scale.

Cream or sugar added to coffee or tea: Measure the portion with the measuring spoons before adding to the drink or record weight on the scale.

Fluids and bottled drinks: Check the labels for volume or empty the container into the measuring cup. If you weigh the fluid, be sure to subtract the weight of the cup or glass. Sugar-free soft drinks usually have kcal values listed on their labels.

Cookies, cakes, pies: For cookies, measure the diameter and thickness with a ruler, or weigh on the scale. Evaluate frosting or sauces separately.

Fruits: Cut them in half before eating and measure the diameters, or weigh on the scale. For fruits that must be peeled or have rinds or cores, be sure the weight of the nonedible portion is subtracted from the total weight of the food. Do this for items such as oranges, apples, and bananas.

Jam, salad dressing, catsup, mayonnaise: Measure the condiment with the measuring spoon or weigh the portion on the scale.

If you eat a food item not listed in Appendix A or in the calorie guide, try to make an intelligent guess as to the ingredients and amount eaten. Sometimes this is impossible, however, and the only alternative is to use a somewhat arbitrary average value. If you are completely baffled, use 400 kcal for small portions, 600 kcal for medium to large portions, and 800 kcal for "giant" portions. It is better to overestimate the number of kcal consumed than to underestimate or to make no estimation at all. If you go to a restaurant for dinner, or to a friend's house where it may be inappropriate to take the measurements, then omit this day from the counting procedure and resume record-keeping the following day. Be sure to include a Friday, Saturday, and Sunday sequence as part of the 7-day record. Research has shown that caloric intake is significantly higher on the weekend than on weekdays. Because the purpose of keeping records for 7 days is to obtain an accurate appraisal of the average daily caloric intake, recordkeeping during the weekend is extremely important. Be sure to record everything you eat. If you are not completely "honest" you are wasting your time. Most people find it easier to keep accurate records if they record food items while preparing a meal or immediately afterwards when eating snack items. Table 7-2 presents an example of a daily dietary intake form for the 7-day period. The caloric value for each food item consumed during the day was estimated from Appendix A.

COMPUTE DAILY CALORIC INTAKE FOR 7 DAYS

You should keep meticulous records of food intake for 7 consecutive days. At first it is normal to become preoccupied with the food you eat, so much so that you may unconsciously begin to diet by omitting foods you would usually eat. Be aware of this temptation and try not to limit normal food intake during the evaluation period. It is important at this point to obtain an accurate estimate of daily caloric intake. Many people like to believe they eat less than they actually do. An overfat person rarely takes delight in knowing that he or she consumes 5000 or 8000 calories per day. Initially, most people who need to restrict food intake will underestimate their true kcal intake, perhaps from fear of confirming what they already know. We have had experience with overfat people who actually believed they were consuming only 500 to 600 kcal each day. These people never seemed to lose weight and some even gained weight during a 16-week physical conditioning course. We kept a 7-day dietary record for one middle-aged woman who stated she was adhering strictly to a low-calorie diet; however, we determined that her total daily calorie intake was approximately 6 times higher than she had originally "guesstimated."

Table 7-2. *Form used to record the caloric equivalent of food consumed on a daily basis.*

FOOD ITEM	AMOUNT	KCAL VALUE
Breakfast		
eggs, boiled	2	160
orange juice	6 oz	110
corn flakes	1 cup	100
skim milk	8 oz	90
Snack		
none		
Lunch		
tuna fish, white	2 oz	113
white bread	2 pieces	140
mayonnaise	1 tbsp	100
skim milk	8 oz	90
plums	4	100
Snack		
ice cream, Rocky Road, sugar cone	2¼	204
Dinner		
McDonald's "Big Mac"	2	1114
French fries	small	215
banana split, 3 scoops vanilla, topping, whipped cream	average	550
Snack		
McDonald's strawberry milkshake	8 oz	315
	Total	3401

Once the number of calories consumed for 7 days is determined, it is possible to compute the number of kcal consumed for a typical day by dividing the total by 7. For a quick but less reliable appraisal of caloric and nutrient intake, a 3-day recall could be used but is not recommended. Record keeping such as this accomplishes two things; (1) it provides the dieter with an objective list of the foods actually consumed (rather than a guess as to what had been eaten), and (2) it triggers an important aspect of the dietary process that must occur before any measure of success can really be achieved—self realization or awareness of current food habits and preferences. Most people who keep meticulous records are often "shocked" at not only how much they actually eat, but the wide range of foods they consume. For many people, the act of eating food has truly become an unconscious act, so much so that they have difficulty remembering what they ate, let alone the quantity of food consumed, the frequency of consumption, or the situations that trigger the urge to eat.

Unbalancing the Energy Balance Equation

The preceding means for estimating caloric intake provides useful information with regard to the energy balance equation. By knowing the average daily caloric input and whether or not body weight is increasing, decreasing, or remaining stable, it is relatively easy to determine if caloric intake is equal to, less than, or exceeds the average daily expenditure of energy. If body weight remains relatively stable from week to week, caloric input exactly matches the caloric requirements of daily living. Part of this food energy is needed to maintain the resting requirements and the remainder is used for physical activity. On the other hand, if the intake of calories *exceeds* that expended for rest plus other daily energy needs, then a positive caloric imbalance will result and body weight will *increase*. *It is simply not possible to consume more calories than are expended without increasing body weight*. If, however, the equilibrium is disturbed in favor of *less* input than output, body weight will *decrease*.

In a previous section we pointed out that 1 pound of adipose tissue contains approximately 3500 kcal of energy. It follows that consuming an additional 3500 kcal above that required to sustain the daily energy requirements will result in a weight gain equal to about 1 pound of body fat. Conversely, to decrease the body's fat content by 1 pound, it would be necessary to create a caloric deficit of 3500 kcal. If the goal is to reduce 2 pounds of fat, then the caloric deficit must be about 7000 kcal. For a 3-pound fat loss, the deficit would be 10,500 kcal; to lose 4 pounds, the necessary deficit would be 14,000 kcal, and so on.

Unbalancing the energy balance equation is the most important step in a weight control program, and it puts theory into practice by creating a *disequilibrium* of the equation. Energy input must become *less* than energy output, or energy output must become *greater* than energy input. In either instance, weight reduction will occur.

DIETING TO TIP THE ENERGY BALANCE EQUATION

This approach to weight loss creates an imbalance in the energy balance equation by reducing energy intake, usually by about 500 to 1000 kcal a day below the daily energy expenditure. Let us assume that a hypothetical 23-year-old obese woman who consumes 2833 kcal per day and maintains body weight at 175 pounds wishes to lose 5 pounds. If her daily level of physical activity remains unchanged, her energy output of 2833 kcal would remain the same. Suppose the woman decreases her daily food intake to create a caloric deficit of 1000 kcal. Caloric restriction of greater than 1000 kcal per day is poorly tolerated over prolonged periods, and this form of semi-starvation greatly increases the chances for poor nourishment. Instead of consuming 2833 kcal each day, she reduces daily caloric intake to 1833 kcal. In 7 days, the caloric deficit would equal 7000 kcal (1000 kcal/day × 7 days). This would be accompanied by a corresponding loss of approximately 2 pounds of body fat. Actually, more than 2 pounds would be lost during the first week because the carbohydrate stores that contain fewer calories per pound than fat, and considerably more water, would be metabolized first. To reduce fat content by another 3 pounds the reduced daily caloric intake of 1833 kcal would have to be maintained for another 10.5 days. By adhering to the 1833 kcal diet, she would reduce body fat at the rate of 1 pound of fat every 3.5 days, provided that caloric output remained at 2833 kcal. If the dieter continued to maintain this energy deficit for a prolonged period, she would lose 10 pounds of fat after 35 days, 20 pounds after 70 days, and 30 pounds within 100 days. While the mathematics of weight loss through caloric restriction may seem rather straightforward, uncomplicated, and encouraging, several basic assumptions could, if violated, reduce the effectiveness of weight loss through diet or even cause the energy balance equation to become unbalanced in the opposite direction.

The *first assumption* is that energy expenditure remains relatively unchanged throughout the period of caloric restriction. This is somewhat difficult to control, however, as there can be considerable variation in someone's daily and weekly energy output. For some people, caloric restriction and its resulting depletion of the body's carbohydrate stores may cause lethargy and actually *decrease* the level of energy expenditure. In addition, as body weight is reduced the energy cost of moving the body is reduced proportionately. Again, the energy output side of the equation may become smaller. The *second assumption* is that a dieter can maintain reduced caloric intake until the desired body size is achieved. These two assumptions could probably be met quite adequately if humans functioned without individual variation. Because physiologic functioning is in continuous interaction with the internal and external environment and subject to its many and varied fluctuations, we cannot expect "perfect" results with regard to weight loss with a low-calorie diet. If weight loss was indeed proportional to caloric restriction, a progressive decrease in body weight would depend directly on the extent of the caloric deprivation. However, changes take place during caloric restriction that can affect the rate at which weight loss occurs. One such change is in the resting metabolic rate.

SETPOINT THEORY: A CASE AGAINST DIETING

When reviewing the scientific literature on the success of weight loss through dieting, one is forced to conclude that, on a long-term basis, dieting just does not work. Surely, one can crash off large amounts of body weight in a relatively short time period by simply not eating. However, this success is short-lived and eventually the urge to eat wins out and weight is regained. The reason for this failure lies in "setpoints" that differ from what the dieter would like to have. The proponents of a *setpoint theory* argue that the body has an internal control mechanism, a setpoint, probably located deep within the brain's *hypothalamus*, that drives the body to maintain a particular level of *body fat.* In a practical sense, this would be the body weight you would tend to achieve when you are not counting calories. The problem is that we all have different setpoints, and various factors such as the drugs amphetamine and nicotine, as well as exercise, lower the particular setting—while dieting has no effect. Each time we manage to reduce our fat level below our "natural" setpoint the body makes internal adjustments to resist this change and conserve body fat. One well-documented occurrence is the dramatic reduction in resting metabolic rate. In fact, the decrease in resting metabolism is often greater than the decrease attributable to the weight loss. For example, severe caloric restriction depresses resting metabolism by as much as 45%! This calorie-sparing effect may even become more apparent with repeated bouts of dieting so the depression of resting metabolism is enhanced with each subsequent attempt to reduce caloric intake. This greatly conserves energy and causes the diet to become progressively less effective. As a result, a plateau in weight loss is reached and further decreases in weight are considerably less than predicted from the mathematics of the restricted food intake. When the rewards of one's efforts are no longer apparent, the dieter usually quits and reverts to the previous eating behaviors. Figure 7-2 displays the results from one study of 6 obese men in which body weight, resting oxygen consumption (minimal energy requirements), and caloric intake were carefully monitored for 31 consecutive days. The subjects consumed 3500 kcal per day for the first 7 days of the experiment. For the remaining 24 days the daily caloric intake was reduced markedly to 450 kcal.

During the prediet period, body weight and resting oxygen consumption remained stable. For this group, 3500 kcal a day was just adequate to equal the daily energy expenditure. However, when the subjects switched to the low-calorie semistarvation diet, both body weight and resting metabolism declined. Interestingly, the percentage decline in resting energy expenditure was greater than the decrease in body weight. The dashed line represents the expected weight loss for this 450-kcal diet. The decline in resting energy metabolism actually conserved energy and caused the diet to be less effective. More than half the 22.6-pound total weight loss occurred within the first 8 days of the 24-day diet, with the remain-

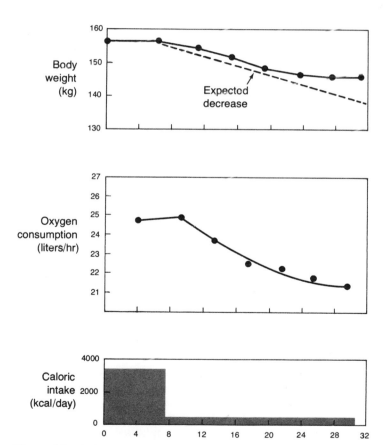

Figure 7-2. *Effects of two levels of caloric intake on changes in body weight and resting oxygen consumption. (Adapted from G. Bray, "Effect of Caloric Restriction on Energy Expenditure in Obese Subjects," Lancet, 2:397–398, 1969.)*

ing weight loss occurring during the final *16* days. This slowing up of the theoretical weight loss curve often leaves the dieter frustrated and discouraged. Dieters are anxious for weight loss to occur rapidly and according to an expected schedule.

Classic starvation studies in the 1940s to help the military plan the repatriation of war prisoners showed that even when an extreme diet ends and food intake is increased above the daily energy output, the dieter usually remains preoccupied with food. In fact, binge eating and psychologic distress continued until the original weight and fat level were attained. The fact that the body itself demands a certain amount of adipose tissue, as proposed by the setpoint theory, was further substantiated by a series of experiments in 1960 in which sedentary prisoners gained weight by increasing their food intake. As body weight and fat increased, concurrently the resting metabolic rate decreased so it took an astounding 7000 kcal per day for weight gain to continue!

What then can safely effect the setpoint and lower it toward a more desirable level? One factor put forth by the setpoint theorists is *sustained, vigorous exercise.* Americans now eat about 10% fewer calories than they did 15 years ago, yet they weigh an average of 4 or 5 pounds more. Certainly, if dieting were effective this reduction in caloric intake should bring the national body weight to a lower, not higher level. Notwithstanding the renewed interest in exercise, the American population has become increasingly sedentary, *not* increasingly gluttonous. Most fat people eat normal quantities of food and sometimes even less than thin people eat. The main difference between fat and lean people is the level of daily physical activity—lean people move around much more and consequently expend more calories than their obese counterparts. For overweight men and women who exercise regularly, food intake tends to drop initially, despite the increase in caloric output, and body fat decreases. Eventually, as an active lifestyle is maintained, caloric intake balances the daily energy requirements so body weight is stabilized at a *lower* level.

HOW TO SELECT A DIET PLAN

The most difficult aspect of dieting is to decide on exactly what foods to include as part of the daily menu. There are literally hundreds of diet plans to choose from. There are water diets, drinking man's diets, fruit diets, egg diets, meat diets, fast food diets, ice cream diets, and vegetable diets, not to mention the potentially dangerous varieties of the high-fat, low-carbohydrate and protein diets. Some authors have even preached that it's not total calories that contribute to weight loss, but the order in which foods are eaten! One popular diet book states that eating a grapefruit every morning counteracts the effects of consuming foods high in calories, and another that drinking extra water dilutes the number of calories in the foods ingested. Of course, such claims are erroneous and misleading, but for those desperate to shed excess weight, such plans establish or reinforce negative eating behaviors. A vicious cycle of failures is repeated. Someone who wants to reduce a given amount of weight tries a particular diet plan that, for whatever reason, is not accompanied by the expected weight loss. The dieter, who may have lost a few pounds, is easily discouraged and quickly regains the lost weight. After a pep talk or some counseling by friends, another attempt is made, this time with a diet "guaranteed" to work! The cycle continues, usually with the same results—the dieter has not changed appreciably in appearance and is still overfat.

As a general rule, it is unwise to follow some prescribed or packaged exotic diet plan in a book or magazine. Instead, *dieters should eat well-balanced meals but in smaller quantities*. A calorie counting approach to weight loss should provide a well-balanced diet containing all the essential nutrients. The general recommendation is that low-calorie diets be composed of approximately 12% protein, 20 to 30% fat (with reduced saturated fats), and the remainder consisting predominantly of unrefined, fiber-rich, complex carbohydrates. The dietary fiber may add to a feeling of fullness and speed the transit of food through the digestive tract so that fewer calories are absorbed. *Calories do count;* the trick is to keep within the specified daily limits as determined by the amount and rate of fat loss desired. Recall from the previous section that the daily energy requirement is determined by two factors: (1) the minimal resting energy requirements, and (2) energy expenditure accounted for by daily physical activities. As long as the diet is nutritionally sound, it really isn't of concern *what* is eaten, but rather *how many calories* are consumed. If a true caloric deficit exists and calorie input is less than calorie output, weight loss *must* occur quite independently of the diet's composition. When caloric intake is below the daily energy requirement, the initial decrease in body weight occurs primarily from water loss and a corresponding depletion of the body's carbohydrate reserves. With further weight loss, a larger proportion of body fat is metabolized to supply the caloric deficit created by restricting food intake or increasing physical activity.

There is simply no compelling evidence to support the contention that the popular "fad" diets have any advantage over a calorically-restricted, well-balanced diet. Weight loss occurs with reduced caloric intake regardless of the diet's composition of carbohydrate, protein, and fat. When obese patients consumed either a high-fat or high-carbohydrate 800 kcal diet, weight loss on each diet was nearly identical, as was the percentage of fat tissue lost during a 10-day period. These findings illustrate an important principle of dieting and weight control; *there is no magic metabolic mixture to assure a more effective weight loss than a well-balanced, low-calorie diet,* even though a low-calorie diet high in fat content may seem more filling and perhaps produce less hunger. A physician with particular expertise in nutrition and the energetics of weight control should be consulted in planning a dietary modification that deviates from the recommended low-calorie but well-balanced meal plan.

USING THE COMPUTERIZED MEAL PLAN AND EXERCISE APPROACH

The computerized meal and exercise plan discussed in Chapter 2 and illustrated in Appendix C is an alternative method to combine dietary control with exercise. The weight loss curve provides a picture of the progress likely to be made if one follows the nutrition *and* exercise prescription. As will be pointed out in Chapter 8, it is crucial to modify both eating and exercise behaviors if positive and permanent changes are to occur in body size and shape. The weight loss curve on the computer printout is not a straight line, but rather is curvilinear to account for *changes* that occur in metabolism and body composition as one progresses through the program of exercise and reduced food consumption.

In addition to speed and reasonable accuracy, there are three major advantages of utilizing a computer in the dietary and exercise prescription.

1. Because the meal plans are based on the dietary exchange method, foods of one's preference can easily be substituted within a given meal to offer tremendous variety in planning the daily menus. Such flexibility still maintains the integrity of the nutritional adequacy of the meals, and assures a constancy to the recommended level of caloric intake.

2. The major difference between the computer meal plan for dieting and the myriad of typical "diets" is that with the former, there is direct participation in the creation of well-balanced meals without having to follow a preset selection of foods chosen by someone else, often some self-appointed "expert." People who become actively involved in planning their daily meals are much more likely to remain with the program than if nutritional choices are unavailable. If a person selects to eat a particular food, then he or she probably will; having to eat disliked foods as part of a particular diet regimen is negative reinforcement and usually leads to failure (reject the diet) before achieving a particular goal (15 pound weight loss). The same is true for the exercise. If the plan calls for jogging, and jogging is despised with a passion, what are the chances of sticking with it? Slim of course. We all know men and women who refuse to exercise regularly because they've been led to believe that long-distance running is the only beneficial exercise. With a choice of activities, as well as an appropriate starting level, however, the chances are excellent for rapid progress. To this end the computer stands ready with its variety of *choices.*

3. The computerized exercise prescription allows a person to interchange between activities and still expend about the same number of calories. For example, if it rains one day and jogging is not preferred, then the computer allows alternative activities like swimming, cycling or racquetball to be performed at about the same caloric expenditure. The example in Appendix C shows the equivalency in gross caloric output between walking, swimming, cycling, and nine sport activities. Without a computer, such calculations would literally require hundreds of hours, particularly because the exercise output is matched to the dietary plan, and both are individualized to the needs of the particular person desiring a particular weight loss.

EXERCISE TO TIP THE ENERGY BALANCE EQUATION

Exercise can play an important role in helping to unbalance the energy balance equation and produce a caloric deficit. Too frequently, however, the importance of exercise in weight control has been played down. One reason is the common belief that participation in additional exercise *always* causes an increase in appetite and food intake. Also, it is often believed that the amount of energy expended during physical activity is so *small* that a dieter would have to spend an inordinate amount of time exercising before achieving a substantial caloric deficit. In the following section we will explore the basis for these two misconceptions.

Misconception One. Exercise Effects on Appetite. It appears that physical activity is necessary for the normal functioning of the brain's feeding control mechanisms. A fine balance between energy expenditure and food intake is not maintained in sedentary people. For them, the daily caloric intake generally exceeds energy requirement. This lack of precision in regulating food intake at the low end of the physical activity spectrum may account for the "creeping obesity" commonly observed in highly mechanized and technically advanced societies. On the other hand, for individuals who exercise on a regular basis, appetite control is in a "reactive zone" where it is simpler to match food intake with the daily level of energy expenditure. In considering the effects of exercise on appetite and food consumption, we must make a distinction between the type and duration of the exercise. There is no question that lumberjacks, farm laborers, and certain athletes who regularly perform hard, physical labor, often consume about twice the daily calories (4000 to 7000 kcal) than do more sedentary people (2000 to 3000 kcal).

In a study of 32 Scandinavian woodcutters who spent 4 days in national competition splitting and cutting lumber, the daily kcal intake ranged from 4120 to 7210 kcal, with an average intake of 5460 kcal. Other studies of Swedish lumbermen also revealed similar high daily caloric intakes. In one study the average caloric ingestion was 5700 kcal per day, while another study reported a 6200-kcal daily food consumption. This latter value is similar to 6425 kcal consumed each day by loggers in the Pacific Northwest and slightly lower than the value of 8083 kcal estimated for lumberjacks working in the forests of Maine. Because these workers are usually quite lean, such high caloric intakes are necessarily required to balance the extremely high caloric expenditure during lumberjacking and logging.

The same situation exists for many athletes who devote considerable time to strenuous physical training. Table 7-3 lists the estimated daily caloric intake of various international-caliber athletes. It should be emphasized that athletes of this status devote as much as 8 hours a day to training. Notice that endurance athletes like marathon runners, cross-country skiers, and cyclists consume about 6000 kcal each day. Yet some of these athletes are the leanest in the world! Obviously, this extreme caloric intake is required just to meet the energy requirements of their training.

When an evaluation of dietary intake is made for people who train for relatively short periods of time, the appetite-stimulating effect of exercise is *not* readily apparent. This was demonstrated for college women in an experiment that evaluated daily calorie intake before and after a season of competitive swimming and tennis. The physical conditioning programs for the two groups of women differed both in duration and intensity. Swimming workouts were conducted each day for 2 hours from January to May. Daily swimming distance ranged from between 2000 and 4000 meters during January and March to 1000 to 2000 meters in April and May. The tennis players practiced daily for 1 hour. The workouts consisted of 10 minutes of rope-skipping, 45 minutes of organized practice and games, followed by a half-mile jog. Rope-skipping and jogging were discontinued after January. Average daily caloric intake was assessed for each woman before and after the 5-month training and competitive season by use of the 7-day dietary inventory discussed previously.

Inspection of Table 7-4 shows that the average caloric intake of the swimmers remained about 15% higher than that of the tennis players. Within each group, however, there were only small increases in caloric intake during the season compared with values before and after the experiment. This was also true for proportions of proteins, fats, and carbohydrates consumed. During the 5-month evaluation there was no change in body weight, percent body fat, and lean body weight for both groups of athletes. Average body weight remained constant at 132 pounds for the swimmers and 129 pounds for the tennis players.

Table 7-3. *Estimated daily caloric intake for athletes in various sport activities.*

SPORT	AVERAGE BODY WEIGHT KILOGRAMS	ESTIMATED DAILY KCAL INTAKE
Cross-country skiing	67.5	6105
Bicycle racing	68.0	5995
Canoe racing	75.0	5995
Marathon racing	68.0	5940
Soccer	74.0	5885
Field hockey (men)	75.0	5720
Handball (European)	75.0	5610
Basketball	75.0	5610
Ice hockey	68.0	5390
Gymnastics (men)	67.0	5000
Sailing	74.0	5170
Fencing	73.0	5000
Sprinting (track)	69.0	4675
Boxing (middle and welter weight)	63.5	4675
Diving	61.0	4620
Pole vault	73.0	4620

Reprinted with permission of Macmillan Publishing Co., Inc., from Encyclopedia of Sport Sciences and Medicine by the American College of Sports Medicine. Copyright © 1971 by Macmillan Publishing Co., Inc.

Many other studies provide supporting evidence that vigorous exercise of moderate duration does not markedly increase appetite and food intake. In one study, obese young men participated in a three-phase, 18-week physical conditioning program. For the first 8 weeks (phase 1), subjects exercised 1 hour each day by running, swimming, performing calisthenics, and playing handball. For the next 5 weeks (phase 2) the daily exercise was terminated and subjects resumed their sedentary life styles. Then the daily exercise program was resumed for another

Table 7-4. *Average kcal intakes of swimmers and tennis players before and after a five-month training and competitive season.*

GROUP	CALORIES BEFORE	CALORIES AFTER	PROTEINS BEFORE	PROTEINS AFTER	FATS BEFORE	FATS AFTER	CARBOHYDRATES BEFORE	CARBOHYDRATES AFTER
Swimmers	2091	2065	80.8	71.8	92.3	90.0	247.9	240.6
Tennis players	1811	1797	78.1	74.2	78.9	78.8	192.6	195.2

Values for proteins, fats, and carbohydrates are expressed in grams.
Source: F.I. Katch et al.: Effects of physical training on the body composition and diet of females, *Research Quarterly, 40:*99–104, 1969.

5 weeks (phase 3). Daily caloric intake was assessed before and during the experiment. Before the program of physical activity, daily caloric intake averaged 2003 kcal. During the first 8 weeks of exercise caloric intake increased only slightly to 2148 kcal. During the next 5-week period of sedentary living, daily caloric intake increased only slightly. These data are in agreement with the pattern of caloric intake of the swimmers and tennis players reported in Table 7-4.

In summary, vigorous exercise of relatively short duration does not necessarily stimulate appetite and cause increased food intake. While there were no changes in body composition for the female swimmers and tennis players who were already within the normal range, exercise produced significant reductions in body weight and body fat for the obese men. Compared to their initial values before the exercise program, there was a 12.3% decrease in body weight, a 17% decrease in total pounds of fat, a 5.2% increase in lean body weight, and an 80% reduction in the sum of eight skinfold measures. These modifications in body size can be attributed to the calorigenic effects of the exercise per se, since caloric intake remained essentially *unchanged.*

Misconception Two. Exercise Effects on Energy Expenditure. The second misconception concerns the number of calories that can be expended through regular exercise. Some authors argue that a person must perform an inordinate amount of exercise just to lose 1 pound of body fat. Usually cited is the fact that one must chop wood for 10 hours, golf for 20 hours, perform mild calisthenic exercises for 22 hours, or play Ping-Pong for 28 hours or volleyball for 32 hours or run 35 miles just to reduce body fat by 1 pound. Understandably, such a commitment is overwhelming and discouraging to the overweight person who plans to lose up to 20 or 30 pounds or more. From a different perspective, however, if golf was played only 2 hours (about 350 kcal per day), 2 days per week (700 kcal), it would take about 5 weeks or 10 golfing days to lose 1 pound of fat (3500 kcal). Assuming you could play golf year round, playing golf 2 days a week would result in a 10-pound loss of fat during the year, provided the food intake remained fairly constant. While most of us would probably not play golf this frequently (nor are we likely to play golf for 20 consecutive hours) the point is that the calorie expending effects of exercise are cumulative; *a caloric deficit of 3500 kcal is equivalent to a 1-pound loss of fat, whether the deficit occurs rapidly or systematically over a long time.*

In calculating the caloric cost of various physical activities, we must assume that the energy cost for people of a particular body size maintains a certain constancy. Recall that in Chapter 4 we pointed out that the values of energy expenditure determined for most physical activities were only averages based on few observations. Consequently a wide range of values may be possible because of individual differences in performance style and technique, and because of environmental factors such as terrain, temperature, and wind resistance, as well as the intensity of participation.

Two "average" golfers playing a typical course for 4 hours might expend considerably different amounts of energy. For that matter, the same golfer playing 2 or 3 consecutive days would never duplicate the same energy expenditure. This would also be true for most sports activities; however, under relatively constant exercise conditions the energy requirements will remain fairly stable and can be estimated with considerable accuracy.

The values of energy expenditure for physical activities presented in Appendix B should not be considered absolute. These are "average" values, applicable under "average" conditions when applied to the "average" person of a given body weight. However, these values do provide a *good approximation* of energy expenditure and are quite useful in establishing the appropriate caloric cost of an exercise program.

DIET PLUS EXERCISE: THE IDEAL COMBINATION

A negative caloric balance produced either by dietary restriction or by exercise can result in a desirable modification in body composition; that is, a *decrease* in body weight and percent body fat. Certainly, combinations of exercise and diet offer considerably more flexibility for achieving a negative caloric balance and accompanying fat loss than either exercise alone or diet alone. The question remains, however, is exercise combined with a reduced caloric intake more effective in fat loss and weight control than either dietary restriction alone or exercise alone? To provide insight into this complex question, many factors must be considered.

If weight reduction is attempted by simply reducing food intake, then one must consider how many calories to consume. While there are no hard and fast rules, considerable experimental data as well as clinical observations have shown that adverse changes in psychologic behavior can occur if caloric intake is reduced too much over an extended period of time. In addition, prolonged dieting greatly increases the chances of developing a variety of nutritional deficiencies. The obvious alternative to achieving a negative caloric balance through dieting is to blend diet with exercise to establish a caloric deficit. To create a daily caloric deficit of 1000 kcal, for example, a combination of diet and exercise would seem an easier method than either diet alone or exercise alone.

Most nutrition experts agree that a loss in body fat of up to *2 pounds each week* is within acceptable medical limits. This guideline is partially based on the fact that people who have been successful in achieving and maintaining a desirable body weight lost no more than 1½ pounds per week during the period of caloric deficit. A more conservative approach would establish a target loss of only 1 pound per week. Then even under the best circumstances the dieter would require 20 weeks to lose the 20 pounds of fat.

Suppose the target time selected to achieve a 20-pound fat loss is 20 weeks. The average weekly deficit must therefore be 3500 kcal; the daily caloric deficit is then 500 kcal (3500 ÷ 7). To achieve a daily deficit of 500 kcal by dieting, caloric intake must be reduced from 3000 kcal to 2500 kcal per day. Remember, this level of "semistarvation" needs to be maintained for 5 months to achieve the desired pound-per-week or total 20-pound fat loss. However, if the dieter performed a half hour of moderate exercise equivalent to 350 "extra" kcal 3 days a week, then the weekly caloric output would increase by 1050 kcal (3 days per week × 350 kcal per exercise session). With this additional exercise, the weekly caloric restriction necessary to lose the 1 pound of fat each week would now only have to reach 2450 kcal instead of 3500 kcal. The additional 1050 are "burned" during the weekly exercise. Instead of excluding 500 kcal from the daily diet, the caloric intake need only be restricted by 350 kcal, because the caloric contribution of the exercise averages 150 kcal a day (1050 kcal per week ÷ 7). If the same exercise were undertaken 5 days a week, the daily intake of food could be increased by an additional 100 calories and the pound-per-week fat loss would still be attained. If the *duration* of the 5 day-per-week workouts was extended from 30 minutes to 1 hour, then *no* reduction in food intake would be necessary to lose weight, because the required 3500 kcal caloric imbalance or deficit would have been created entirely through exercise.

If the *intensity* of the 1-hour exercise performed 5 days a week was then increased by only 10% (cycling at 22 miles per hour instead of 20 miles per hour; running a mile in 9 minutes instead of 10 minutes; swimming 50 yards in 54 seconds instead of 60 seconds), the number of calories burned each week through exercise would increase an additional 350 kcal (3500 kcal/week × 10%). This new weekly deficit of 3850 kcal or 550 kcal per day would actually permit the dieter to *increase* the daily food intake by 50 calories and still lose a pound of fat each week!

Clearly, physical activity can be used effectively by itself or in combination with mild dietary restriction to bring about an effective loss of body fat. Perhaps equally important, the feelings of intense hunger and other psychologic stresses may be minimal compared with a similar program of weight loss that relies exclusively on caloric restriction. Furthermore, exercise in a weight reduction program provides protection against the significant loss in lean tissue usually observed when weight loss is achieved by diet alone. The preservation of the lean tissue mass is partly due to aerobic exercise training that enhances the mobilization and breakdown of fat from the body's adipose depots. In addition, vigorous exercise tends to increase the rate of protein build up in skeletal muscle, while at the same time retarding its rate of breakdown. This protein-sparing effect causes a greater portion of the caloric deficit to be made up by the breakdown of *fat*.

Optimal Duration of Exercise Plus Diet Program

During the first few days of food restriction, when caloric intake is below the daily energy requirement, the observed decrease in body weight occurs primarily from a depletion of the body's carbohydrate stores and a corresponding loss in body water. As weight loss continues, a larger proportion of body fat is metabolized for energy to supply the caloric deficit created by food restriction.

Figure 7-3 shows the percentage composition of the average daily weight loss for water, protein, and fat that occurred during 24 days of a low-calorie diet consisting of 1000 kcal of carbohydrates per day. In addition to caloric restriction all subjects were exercised daily for 2½ hours in a prescribed activity program. During the first 3 days of the program, water loss represented 70% of the weight loss. The reduction of body water became progressively less as weight loss continued, and during days 11 to 13 water loss represented only 19% of the weight lost. In addition, the proportion of fat loss increased from 25 to 69% during this period. From day 21 to day 24, 85% of the weight loss was due to a reduction in body fat with no corresponding increase in water loss. The percentage of weight loss of protein increased from 5% initially to 12% during days 11 to 13 and to 15% by the end of the period of caloric restriction.

A relationship also exists between the proportion of water, protein, and fat lost and the amount of water consumed during the first few days of caloric restriction. Carefully conducted experiments have demonstrated that restricting water intake during the first 3 days of a diet significantly *increases* the proportion of water loss through dehydration and *decreases* the proportion of fat loss. The total *quantity* of fat lost was essentially the same regardless of the quantity of fluid ingested. It is therefore important to provide adequate hydration during the period of caloric restriction as water restriction in no way facilitates fat loss.

Figure 7-4 graphically displays the results of six experiments in terms of the caloric equivalent of each kilogram of weight loss. The important point to observe in this figure is that the caloric equivalent of each kilogram of weight loss increases substantially as the duration of caloric restriction increases. *This is the major reason why it is so important to maintain a caloric deficit for extended periods of time; shorter periods of caloric restriction result in a larger percentage of water and carbohydrate loss per unit of weight reduction with only a minimal decrease in body fat.* While the caloric equivalent of 1 kg of weight approaches only 3000 kcal during the first 4 or 5 days on a reduced caloric intake, the caloric equivalent more than doubles after 2 months of maintaining a caloric deficit.

The major findings of studies that evaluate the efficacy of various approaches to establishing a caloric imbalance are as follows:

1. Exercise combined with dietary restriction appears to be a more valid approach for achieving a negative caloric balance as compared with exercise or diet alone.

2. During the first few days of weight reduction, the rapid weight loss is due primarily to a loss in body water and carbohydrates; at least 2 months of weight reduction is associated with a substantially greater loss of fat per unit of weight loss.

3. Water intake should not be restricted when beginning a weight reduction program because this can precipitate dehydration but no additional fat loss.

4. Undesirable psychologic and medically related problems may occur with prolonged caloric restriction maintained below minimal energy requirements.

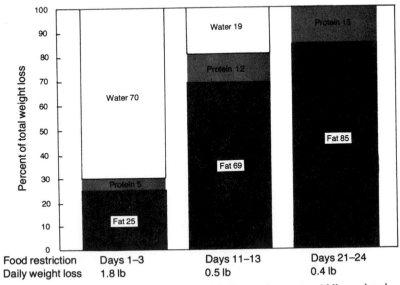

Figure 7-3. *Percentage composition of weight loss at the start, middle, and end of 24 days of food restriction (1000 kcal per day) plus enforced exercise of 2.5 hours per day. (From F. Grande, "Nutrition and Energy Balance in Body Composition Studies." In: Techniques for Measuring Body Composition. National Academy of Sciences–National Research Council, Washington, D.C., 1961.)*

5. Weight loss by diet alone also causes a significant loss of muscle mass. Exercise appears to protect against lean tissue losses; thus, more of the weight loss is fat loss.

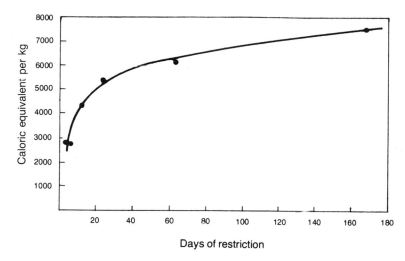

Experiment	Number of subjects	Duration (days)	Average weight loss (kg)	Total calorie deficit	Caloric equivalent
1	1	4	2.85	8,107	2,845
2	6	5	5.50	15,590	2,835
3	6	12	5.90	25,368	4,300
4	13	24	7.60	40,480	5,326
5	12	63	14.10	87,000	6,170
6	32	168	16.82	126,420	7,516

Figure 7-4. *Caloric equivalent of weight loss in relation to the duration of calorie restriction. Each data point represents an experiment as summarized in the accompanying legend. (Adapted from F. Grande, "Nutrition and Energy Balance in Body Composition Studies." In: Techniques for Measuring Body Composition. National Academy of Sciences–National Research Council, Washington, D.C., 1961.)*

8

Modification of Eating
and Exercise Behaviors

THE HUMAN ORGANISM is remarkably adaptable. People can modify existing food and exercise behavior patterns as long as they establish a clear-cut need for change and they have a good possibility of success. One of the techniques used to alter behavior is referred to by psychologists as *behavior therapy* or *behavior modification.* This approach helps the person to identify, control, and modify undesirable behaviors so they become desirable.

An excellent example of the application of behavior modification is the treatment of *anorexia nervosa,* a condition in which the person actually stops eating. As a result, body weight is reduced considerably, in some instances by as much as 50%. This disorder occurs mostly in young women and is associated with severe psychologic problems.

In one study women patients hospitalized for treatment of anorexia nervosa were found to walk considerable distances around the hospital (averaging 6.8 miles per day) compared to an average distance of 4.9 miles walked each day by women of normal body weight living at home. This hyperactivity was used as the behavioral modifier to induce patients to eat and subsequently gain weight. The patients were permitted to walk only if they made a daily gain in body weight. Any time the patient's body weight was at least a half pound above weight of the previous day, she was allowed 6 hours of unrestricted activity outside the hospital. Within 1 week, the patients' body weights increased significantly. On the average, body weight increased 4 pounds per week during the 6 weeks of hospitalization. Case studies of this type illustrate that a behavioral disorder (refusal to eat) can be altered by providing positive reinforcement (opportunity to engage in physical activity) once a permanent feature of the disorder is uncovered (hyperactivity).

Another application of eating behavior modification involved the treatment of a 17-year-old woman who weighed 50 pounds. The search for a potential positive reinforcer was unsuccessful until the young woman began to complain about the sedative effects of a particular drug that was administered as part of her treatment. The doctors used this aspect of her behavior (complaint) as the reinforcer. Following each day in which there was a further loss or no change in body weight, they administered a large dose of the sedative drug. On the other hand, a quarter-pound weight gain resulted in a smaller drug dose; for a half-pound weight gain, an even smaller dose was given, and if one pound was gained no drug was administered. The decrease in drug dosage served as the positive reinforcer, under which the young woman gained an average of 6 pounds each week. Ultimately, normal dietary patterns were established and a systematic weight gain occurred.

In the following sections we will present some basic principles of behavior modification, with special application to weight reduction by means of dietary modification and increased energy expenditure through physical activity. We use four basic steps in applying the principles of behavior modification to eating and exercise. These are: (1) description of the behavior to be modified, (2) replacement of established patterns of behavior with more desirable behaviors, (3) development of techniques to control behaviors, and (4) positive reinforcement or reward for controlling, altering, or modifying the undesirable behaviors.

Modification of Eating Behavior

While numerous treatment approaches have been used to rehabilitate obese people, none has been particularly successful in achieving long-term results. In fact, one doctor well known for his work in the treatment of obesity stated that "most obese patients won't even come for treatment. Those who do come often drop out, and the ones that don't drop out don't lose much weight. Finally, those who do lose weight usually regain it." The results of many studies provide ample support for this statement, especially with regard to long-term weight loss. The success record for weight loss in obese people is less than encouraging, and underscores the difficulties encountered with most traditional weight control programs in achieving either short-term or long-term results.

In 1967 an apparent breakthrough was made in the treatment of obesity when a behavioral psychologist reported the results of a 1-year treatment program for obesity using behavior modification techniques. Treatment sessions were conducted for 30 minutes, three times a week over a 4- to 5-week period. Subsequent sessions were conducted at 2-week intervals for 12 weeks; thereafter sessions were held only once a month or as needed. The total number of sessions attended by each person varied from 16 to 41 during the year. Of the eight obese women 3 lost more than 40 pounds and 5 lost more than 26 pounds. The magnitude of these changes was the highest ever reported for the treatment of obesity in a group of subjects not confined to a hospital or clinic environment. Figure 8-1 shows the results for the 8 women in the study. These results were impressive in view of the fact that no more than 1 of 4 obese subjects who seek treatment loses more than 20 pounds, and no more than 1 of 20 loses more than 40 pounds.

The following sections summarize the basic principles of eating behavior modification as applied to programs of weight control.

DESCRIPTION OF THE BEHAVIOR TO BE MODIFIED

The first step is to describe the various eating behaviors and habits of the dieter and *not* immediately to change the diet. The subject is asked to keep meticulous records to provide answers to the following questions:

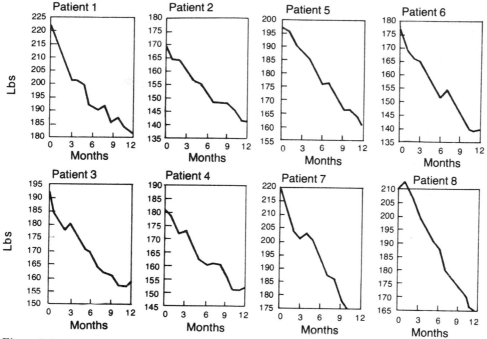

Figure 8-1. *Weight profile of eight women undergoing behavior therapy for overeating. (From R.B. Stuart,* "Behavioral Control of Overeating," Behavior Research and Therapy, 5:364, Fig. 1, 1967.)

1. Where are meals eaten?

2. When are meals eaten?

3. What is the mood, feeling, or psychological state during the meal?

4. How much time was spent at the meal?

5. What activities were engaged in during the meal (watching television, driving a car, sewing, etc.)?

6. Who was present during the meal?

7. What and how much food was eaten?

This time-consuming and often annoying record-keeping provides the dieter with objective information concerning personal eating behaviors. A careful examination of such records will reveal certain recurring patterns of behavior associated with eating. For example, the dieter may discover that feelings of depression are usually followed by eating candy; that he or she eats snacks while watching television, gets hungry at a particular time of day, goes on an ice-cream binge after an argument, or never eats breakfast or lunch at the kitchen table. Once an analysis is made of eating behaviors, the next step is to substitute alternate behaviors for the ones where a clear pattern has been established. Because circumstances intimately related to established eating patterns apparently signal the eating response, the objective is to eliminate or substitute these undesirable signals.

SUBSTITUTING ALTERNATIVE BEHAVIORS

Many alternate acceptable behaviors can be used to replace a particular set of environmental cues associated with eating. Below is a list of some examples of existing behaviors associated with eating, as well as possible substitute behaviors.

Established behavior patterns	Replacement behavior
1. Eating candy while driving	1. Singing along with the radio while driving
2. Eating snacks while watching television	2. Sewing, painting, or writing letters while watching television
3. Feeling hungry at 4:00 P.M.	3. Going for a walk at 4:00 P.M.
4. Eating ice cream after an argument	4. Doing 10 repetitions of an exercise after an argument
5. Never eating breakfast or lunch at the kitchen table	5. Eating breakfast and lunch only at the kitchen table

While we can give numerous other examples, the major aim of this approach is clear: *to create new associations to replace the old established patterns of behavior.*

DEVELOPMENT OF TECHNIQUES TO CONTROL THE ACT OF EATING

There are many useful techniques to gain control over eating habits once these undesirable environmental cues have been identified and replaced or eliminated. Examples include the following:

1. Make the act of eating foods a ritual; limit eating to one place in the house and no matter what foods you eat, follow a set routine. Use a place mat, set the table with silverware, and use the same dishes at each meal. Do this for main meals as well as for snacks. One dieter who continually snacked between meals curbed this habit by dressing up in a tuxedo and eating by candlelight for each meal and snack. Snacking between meals soon stopped. To discourage bread eating, take only one slice of bread at a time and toast it before eating. For each slice get up from the table, unwrap the loaf of bread from its package, take out a slice, rewrap the loaf and replace it in the cupboard, toast the slice and return to the table to eat it. Following an inconvenient routine to obtain some special food item often suppresses the desire for such food.

2. Use smaller dishes; the impetus to finish the meal may not be the food per se, but the desire to view an empty plate or glass.

3. Eat slowly, fight the urge to eat quickly by taking more time at meals. You can do this by cutting food into smaller pieces and chewing each piece 10 to 15 times before swallowing. Another technique is to place the knife, spoon, or fork back on the table after each two or three bites and allow for a 1- or 2-minute rest pause between mouthfuls.

PROVIDE POSITIVE REINFORCEMENT OR REWARDS

The ultimate long-term rewards of achieving the desired outcomes of a positive weight control program are threefold: (1) improvement in personal appearance, (2) subtle but observable changes in psychologic behaviors, and perhaps

(3) better health because of physiologic changes. Dieters can set up short-term goals to provide interim rewards. After you maintain a given amount of weight loss for several months (say, 5 pounds), buy a new article of clothing; after the next substantial weight loss (10 pounds), go on a trip. Continue to provide rewards until you reach the eventual goal. Another useful technique is to maintain a weight chart and plot changes in body weight. Keep separate charts for recording daily caloric intake from food and caloric expenditure due to exercise, as well as recording changes in various body dimensions such as the abdomen, buttocks, and thighs.

The positive and negative reinforcing power of money can also be used as an incentive. This may work better in a group situation, however. For example, a given amount of money is given to the group leader at the start of the program. A portion of the deposit is returned to the group members depending on the amount specified for a given weight loss (for example, $10 per pound). If a member quits the program or fails to maintain the weight loss for at least one week, the deposit is forfeited and divided equally among the remaining participants at the end of a specified time period. Many variations of such procedures are possible. Remember, though, that merely providing information about the techniques of eating behavior modification will not in itself ensure their continued use. *Encouragement* and *reinforcement* must be built-in features of the weight control program. They must continue until subjects establish mastery over eating behaviors and achieve a proper balance between energy input and energy output so that body size stays permanently reduced.

Modification of Exercise Behavior

In the past, it was generally accepted that the obese condition was the result of excessive food intake. Clearly, then, the effective approach to weight control would be some form of caloric restriction through dieting. However, research studies concerned with eating patterns and exercise behaviors of the obese show consistently that a low caloric output due to a lack of physical activity, rather than an inordinately high caloric (food) intake, is the prime factor associated with overfatness. *In fact, one is hard pressed for evidence that groups of overweight individuals actually eat more on the average than people of normal weight.* In the early 1940s, psychologists pointed out that only a small percentage of obese people participated in physical activities within the range usually observed for non-obese people of the same age and sex. This characteristic sedentary behavior pattern of the obese has been demonstrated in 6 of 9 studies conducted between 1953 and 1981. The surprising finding was that in all of the experiments, the food intake of the obese was *no greater* than for people of normal body size. In addition, the excess weight gain throughout life closely parallels reduced physical activity rather than reduced caloric intake. For example, obese infants do not characteristically consume more calories than either the recommended dietary standards or counterparts of normal weight. It is also noted that infant offspring of obese parents display less spontaneous movements than infants of normal weight parents. This suggests the possibility that such subdued movement patterns are abnormal and may reflect inherited characteristics.

It is of interest to point out that similar results of the relation between energy output and food consumption have been observed in genetically obese strains of mice and rats. Those strains of animals which fatten easily display significantly lower levels of motor activity than their relatively lean counterparts. Thus, in both obese humans and animals, physical inactivity appears to be a characteristic feature of their daily living habits.

Table 8-1 shows the results for one of the human experiments that compared the extent of participation in daily physical activities as well as average daily caloric intake of 28 obese and 28 normal high school girls. While time-in-motion analysis revealed that there was *little difference* between the two groups in the amount of time spent sitting, standing, grooming, baby-sitting, driving a car, or doing housework, a considerable difference was demonstrated in the extent of participation in active sports and other strenuous activities. "Extra" physical activity was engaged in for 4 hours a day on the average by the obese, while the nonobese girls were active for 11 hours during the day. In terms of caloric intake, the obese girls consumed 27% *fewer* calories each day than the nonobese girls; only 3 of 28 obese girls consumed more than 2500 kcal each day.

In a similar study conducted several years later with young boys, almost identical findings were observed; obese boys consumed fewer calories each day than a group of nonobese boys. Daily food intake averaged 3011 kcal for the obese and 3476 kcal for the nonobese boys during the school year, and 3430 kcal and 4628 kcal for the obese and lean boys, respectively, during an 8-week summer camp. Researchers observed little difference between the groups in the amount of time they participated in light and moderate exercise; however, the degree of participation by the obese boys in more strenuous activities was generally less than for the nonobese.

This observation that fat people often eat the same or even less than thinner ones is also true for adults as they become less active and slowly begin to add weight. In one experiment, the physical activity levels were compared for a group of obese and nonobese men and women who were matched for age, occupation,

Table 8-1. *Physical activity and calorie intake of obese and nonobese adolescent girls.*

WEEKLY PHYSICAL ACTIVITY (HOURS)

GROUP	SLEEP, LYING STILL AWAKE	SITTING	STANDING	GROOMING	BABY-SITTING	PLAYING PIANO, DRIVING CAR	HOUSEWORK	ACTIVE SPORTS AND OTHER VIGOROUS ACTIVITY
Obese	61	81	1	7	1	1.4	3.6	4
Nonobese	63	75	3	10	1	1.2	3.3	11

DAILY CALORIE INTAKE (KCAL/DAY)

GROUP	2500	2500–2000	2000	AVERAGE
Obese	3	6	19	1,965
Nonobese	15	10	3	2,706

Source: M.L. Johnson et al., "Relative importance of inactivity and overeating in the energy balance of obese high school girls," *American Journal of Clinical Nutrition,* 4:37–44, 1956.

and socioeconomic background. Physical activity expressed in miles walked each day was assessed by means of *pedometers*. These small precision instruments are usually hooked from a belt worn around the waist. The pedometer is calibrated to the person's stride length and is operated by an internal pendulum that registers each stride. Total mileage walked was recorded daily for 1 week by the women and for 2 weeks by the men.

The results for the women were unequivocal; the average distance walked by the obese women was about 41% shorter than that walked by the nonobese women. Total miles walked each day averaged 2.0 miles for the obese and 4.9 miles for the nonobese. A comparison of the data for the men showed a similar pattern with regard to distance walked; the obese men walked an average of 39% less than their nonobese counterparts.

The data from the above studies illustrate clearly that inactivity is a major behavioral characteristic that distinguishes overfat from nonobese people. *Individuals who maintain physically active lifestyles or who become involved in appropriate exercise programs generally maintain a desirable level of body composition.* Consequently the obese must not only relearn or modify existing eating behaviors, but also reverse the existing syndrome of insufficient caloric output due to a sedentary life style. Learning how to replace daily periods of relative inactivity (low caloric output) with more strenuous activity requiring a greater energy expenditure may seem a difficult task. Experiencing *enjoyment* and *success* in a given activity is the most important aspect of this relearning process. Only a few people will continue to participate in exercise that is so taxing from a physiologic standpoint that little or no enjoyment is possible. A good example is running. It is not much fun to run for a minute or two when the end result is shortness of breath, wobbly legs, and a "stitch" in the side. All the personal motivation you can muster cannot overcome the genuine discomfort you feel when you pursue unrealistic goals. Even jogging for 5 minutes at a relatively slow pace is not easy, especially for people who have previously been sedentary. If there is little chance for enjoyment and success, then most people will become discouraged and discontinue participation. In psychologic behavior terms, they have received negative reinforcement from the activity participation. However, walking and jogging as well as other programs of vigorous activities *can be enjoyable* if the probability of success is maximized. This necessitates a carefully planned, systematic approach with long-term rather than short-term goals. If the long-term goal is to jog continuously for 30 minutes each day, then the beginning jogger should plan to achieve this goal over a period of weeks or months, rather than trying to run this distance on the first or second day.

DESCRIPTION OF THE BEHAVIOR TO BE MODIFIED

The first step is to determine the daily pattern of physical activity, including such minimal daily requirements as sleeping, eating, going to the bathroom, and bathing. An activity profile can be constructed by keeping a daily record of the actual time allotted for the various activities for seven consecutive days. The activity profile for a physically active college teacher during a typical day of summer vacation is presented in Table 8-2. This record includes a description of the activity, its duration, and its classification into one of three broad categories of energy expenditure: light exercise (under 150 kcal per hour), moderate exercise (150 to 250 kcal per hour), and heavy exercise (over 250 kcal per hour). The actual caloric

Table 8-2. *Detailed record of physical activity for one day.*

ACTIVITY	BEGIN ACTIVITY	END ACTIVITY	TOTAL TIME, MINUTES	CLASSIFI-CATION
1. Wake up	6:45 A.M.			
2. Use bathroom	6:45	6:53 A.M.	8	Light
3. Go back to bed	6:53	7:30	37	Light
4. Eat breakfast	7:30	7:50	20	Light
5. Use bathroom	7:50	8:00	10	Light
6. Dress	8:00	8:06	6	Light
7. Drive to school	8:06	8:17	11	Light
8. Walk to office	8:17	8:25	8	Light
9. Work in office	8:25	10:00	95	Light
10. Pick up mail—walk up and down stairs	10:00	10:10	10	Light
11. Work in office and lab	10:10	12:10 P.M.	120	Light
12. Go to locker room— get dressed	12:10 P.M.	12:16	6	Light
13. Walk to track	12:16	12:20	4	Light
14. Wait for friend	12:20	12:30	10	Light
15. Run to park and back	12:30	2:00	90	Strenuous
16. Walk to locker room	2:00	2:04	4	Light
17. Shower and dress	2:04	2:20	16	Light
18. Walk to office	2:20	2:24	4	Light
19. Have student confer- ence (eat lunch)	2:24	3:00	36	Light
20. Work in office	3:00	5:05	125	Light
21. Walk to library	5:05	5:12	7	Light
22. Work in library	5:12	6:05	53	Light
23. Walk to dean's office	6:05	6:10	5	Light
24. Meet with dean	6:10	6:35	25	Light
25. Walk to office	6:35	6:43	8	Light
26. Walk to car	6:43	6:51	8	Light
27. Drive home	6:51	7:03	12	Light
28. Change clothes	7:03	7:07	4	Light
29. Wash up	7:07	7:11	4	Light
30. Play with baby	7:11	8:00	49	Light
31. Watch TV	8:00	8:30	30	Light
32. Eat dinner	8:30	9:00	30	Light
33. Mail letter	9:00	9:05	5	Light
34. Listen to stereo	9:05	9:30	25	Light
35. Watch TV	9:30	10:30	60	Light
36. Wash up	10:30	10:38	8	Light
37. Read in bed	10:38	11:15	37	Light
38. Turn off lights	11:15	6:45 A.M.	450	Light
		Total	Light	1350
			Moderate	0
			Strenuous	90

values of energy expenditure for various physical activities are included in Appendix B.

The results present a fairly detailed picture of the variations in caloric output during a work day. For the teacher, the following results are clear: an average of 1350 minutes each day were spent in relatively sedentary activities, and 90 minutes per day were for activities requiring a relatively high energy output. If it were not for the hour and a half devoted to strenuous activities, the energy output level for this teacher would be classified as sedentary.

Any hope of changing the pattern and quantity of daily physical activity is predicted on an accurate appraisal of the energy cost of the activities that make up a person's life style. Once this has been determined, the next step in exercise behavior modification is to substitute more strenuous activities for those that rate low on energy expenditure.

SUBSTITUTING ALTERNATE BEHAVIORS

Moderate to strenuous physical activity can easily replace the more sedentary activities only when the dieter is willing to become more physically active. This substitution process should begin after an analysis is made of the amount of time devoted to the various daily activities.

There are many ways to increase energy expenditure within the time allotted to daily routines. The important considerations are to determine *when* and *how* to make changes. For example:

1. When driving to work, park a half mile away and walk the remaining distance. Brisk walking to and from the car each day, 5 days a week, will burn up the caloric equivalent of about seven pounds of fat in 1 year.

2. When taking public transportion, get off 8 or 10 stops early and walk the remaining distance.

3. When traveling relatively short distances, walk instead of taking a cab or bus.

4. Don't go to a restaurant for lunch; participate in some form of physical activity, such as walking, which you can continue for 30 to 45 minutes.

5. Wake up an hour early and take a brisk walk, cycle, or swim before breakfast.

6. Replace the cocktail hour with 20 minutes of exercise.

7. Replace coffee breaks with exercise breaks.

8. Walk up and down several flights of stairs after each hour of work.

9. Sweep the sidewalks in front of your house or apartment. One of our dear colleagues, a world-renowned 80-year-old scientist, sweeps the perimeter of a four-square-block park in San Francisco, 2½ hours a day, 5 to 6 days a week! He does this not only as a public service, but to augment his generally sedentary life style with physical demanding tasks to maintain his arm and leg strength.

10. When going on a family outing, allow time for exercise: (a) Get out of the car before reaching your destination; let your family drive the rest of the way while you walk. (b) Instead of eating at half-time or intermission at sports events,

walk around the stadium or arena. Climb up and down stairs instead of using elevators or escalators.

11. Replace the hired help and undertake some of these tasks yourself:
    a. Gardening
    b. Mowing the lawn
    c. Painting
    d. Washing and waxing the car
    e. Walking the dog

12. During television commercials, run in place, jump rope, jog up and down stairs, or perform vigorous calisthenics.

13. Replace power tools and appliances with manually operated devices:
    a. Lawn care equipment
    b. Automatic household appliances such as vacuum cleaners, eggbeaters, ice cream maker, juicers.
    c. Saws
    d. Drills
    e. Snow shovelers
    f. Garage doors

14. Play golf without a golf cart or caddy.

15. Walk or jog up and down the beach in addition to sun bathing.

The most difficult task in rearranging a daily routine is to replace conveniences with tasks requiring more effort. Identifying possible areas for activity modification is easy because twentieth-century men and women have become accustomed to an automated, labor-saving society. Humans are slaves to machines; we have learned to live the "easy life." Learned behaviors, however, *can* be changed or modified; the major requirement is a willingness to commit yourself to a new life style that incorporates more vigorous activities within the fabric of the daily routine. Unless a person makes this commitment he or she will be unable to modify a sedentary life style. Unfortunately, most of us are too "locked into" daily routines even to try to modify existing behaviors. There may be a few things we are willing to do, such as use a hand lawnmower now and then or go for a brisk walk at lunchtime. However, it takes a real commitment to sweep the streets, jog around the block, bicycle to and from work, or walk up and down stairs without feeling embarrassed or self-conscious. People must overcome social pressures and constraints to attain permanent changes in life style.

DEVELOPMENT OF TECHNIQUES TO MAXIMIZE EXERCISE SUCCESS

Several techniques can be used to maximize the "fun" potential of exercise. These techniques may not apply to team or individual sports in which skill or competition are the key elements (tennis, badminton, basketball, golf, racquetball, squash) but to activities such as jogging, bicycling, swimming, and calisthenic exercises.

1. Progress slowly: People who have not exercised for a long time should progress slowly and not try to accomplish too much in the first few weeks. Instead of running 1 mile initially, run or even walk 1 block; instead of trying to cycle 10 miles, cycle 3 miles; instead of trying to do 100 sit-ups, do 15 to 25.

2. Include variety: Rather than perform the same exercise over and over again within a given time period, alternate exercises as well as the number of repetitions. For example, instead of jogging continuously around the track, intersperse other forms of exercise: Jog for 2 minutes—skip for 1 minute—hop on the right foot 20 times—hop on the left foot 20 times—jump up and down 20 minutes—skip 1 minute—jog 3 minutes—and so on, until you reach the desired end-point.

3. Become goal oriented: There are three ways to exercise using goal-oriented behavior: (1) Exercise for a certain amount of time; (2) continue to exercise until you reach a predetermined number of repetitions or distance; (3) combine both of the preceding approaches. Select one of these three methods depending on your personal preference. If a track is available, then total distance run becomes a convenient guide. One limitation with this approach, however, is the tedium of running the same route, over and over again, with little or no change in scenery. An alternative is to mark off a given distance (your house to the store, the store to the playground, the playground to the house), and then run this route.

   If exercise for a specific time is the goal, then run a predetermined route such as around a track or through the neighborhood. The latter alternative has the advantage of changing sceneries. For the novice jogger who may only run continuously for a minute or two between rest intervals, the goal should be to cover a given distance, such as running from a big tree to the fence post, the fence post to the green car, and the green car to the stop sign. Mastery of preset goals provides immediate positive reinforcement and minimizes chances of failure. At the same time the fun aspect of the activity is maximized because of the feeling of personal achievement.

4. Be systematic: Set aside certain times during the day to exercise. Don't permit outside factors such as watching television, shopping, and doing housework to interfere with *your* daily activity.

5. Wear clothes conducive to exercise: You need not be concerned with what clothes to wear while swimming or skiing, as the choices are limited and obvious. Many activities have no established patterns of dress, and people should follow their personal preferences. On hot and humid days, wear light clothing to permit rapid heat loss.

PROVIDE POSITIVE REINFORCEMENT OR REWARD

   Positive reinforcement should be intimately tied to exercise, especially for the beginner.

1. Keep charts to record progress. Fill in the chart as soon as you achieve the preset goal. Such charts provide immediate feedback and serve the important purpose of helping to maintain motivation and interest.

2. Exercise with a "buddy" or in small groups. Exercising may be more enjoyable when performed in small groups of two or three people. Having to make commitments with others can be a subtle form of motivation, and can help to ensure exercise on a regular schedule.

3. Provide rewards. Self-made competition can be an effective means for achieving preset goals. This is especially true for people who are just beginning an exer-

cise program and need some incentive. We have found that a simple game is effective in helping many people maintain a high degree of self-motivation. The game can be played by as many persons as desired. The object is to perform a given amount of exercise, and a painted button is awarded when the exercise goal is achieved. A predetermined reward is given for accumulating 10 buttons. To start, obtain 16 white shirt buttons. Then paint 10 of them a favorite color. Each of the remaining white buttons is equal to a given number of minutes of exercise. We make a 5-minute exercise period equal to 1 white button. When a person accumulates 6 white buttons (equal to 30 minutes of exercise), they are traded in for a painted button. When the person secures 10 painted buttons, he or she has won the game and receives a reward. The reward is chosen in advance, and can be anything the participant wants. We suggest that the painted buttons be stored in a prominent place in the house, where family members can keep track of progress and provide encouragement and support. For people just beginning an exercise program, the goal is to achieve 5 painted buttons each week. The exercise equivalent for each button can be increased as exercise capacity improves. For purposes of illustration, suppose 30 minutes of exercise is made to equal 1 painted button. For the person who weighs 200 pounds and accumulates 5 painted buttons each week by walking briskly, the "extra" caloric expenditure due to walking would be equal to approximately 1200 kcal per week, 4800 kcal per month, *or the equivalent of 16.5 pounds of fat per year.* It should be obvious that if the reducer achieved a corresponding decrease in calorie intake, the rate and quantity of fat loss would double!

While this particular game may at first seem inappropriate for both younger and older adults, its underlying principle provides for ample positive feedback and reinforcement. As long as the player places value on the reward, the process of striving to achieve it takes on new meaning and offers at least a fighting chance for *success.*

III

Physiologic Conditioning for Total Fitness

The Concept of Total Fitness

To some, physical fitness reflects the trim legs and waist of the model demonstrating stretching exercises in the popular glamour magazines. To others, fitness means superior strength with its accompanying large muscular development. In the past, the popularity of many health clubs, spas, and other exercise facilities has flourished in this image. At the other extreme the fit individual is exemplified by the lean, rather frail-looking competitive marathoner running at a 5-minute per mile pace for 26 miles.

The housewife, business executive, or college student may take a more moderate view and consider themselves physically fit by successfully completing a set of tennis, a round of golf, a game of racquetball, or climbing several flights of stairs without fatigue. This perspective places fitness on a continuum, with the necessary level of fitness being determined by the physical requirements of one's daily life. While this may be a practical view, medical evidence suggests that evolution has not kept pace with automation—our bodies need *regular, vigorous aerobic exercise*, especially if our jobs are sedentary and our life styles inactive.

While it is difficult to formulate a precise definition of fitness, it is appropriate to view *total fitness* as a state of physical well-being that incorporates a balance between several well-developed fitness components. More specifically, total fitness requires adequate muscular strength and endurance, reasonable joint flexibility, an efficient cardiovascular system with a good level of aerobic fitness, and favorable body composition with acceptable control of body weight. Within this framework, exercise programs must be formulated on an individual basis using research-proven training principles and techniques with regular adjustments made

187

to keep pace with the participant's changing level of fitness. *The approach to physiologic conditioning for men is basically the same as the approach to physiologic conditioning for women.*

General Principles of Physiologic Conditioning

The term *physiologic conditioning* refers to a planned program of exercise directed toward improving the functional capacity of a particular bodily system. This improvement does not occur haphazardly; you must incorporate a basic training principle into an exercise program for physiologic adaptations to occur. This principle is overload.

OVERLOAD PRINCIPLE

Although programs of exercise differ considerably depending on a person's specific goals and expectations, any effective exercise program must be based on the proper application of physiologic stress or *overload.* By exercising a system of the body at a level above that at which it normally operates, that system will adapt and function more efficiently. The method and extent of the overload will directly affect the conditioning of the particular system involved. Overload can be accomplished in several ways:

1. Increase the *frequency* of exercise.

2. Increase the *intensity* of exercise within a given time period.

3. Increase the *duration* of exercise at a specified intensity.

Consider the following example of a woman who wishes to use jogging to train her cardiovascular system and thus improve her aerobic exercise capacity. If this woman jogged one block twice a week at a slow pace for 1 year, there is no doubt there would be some increase in exercise capacity. However, the improvement would be minimal. To more effectively use exercise for improving cardiovascular capacity above some minimal level, a person must select one of the preceding three methods of implementing the overload. The jogger could elect to speed up her running pace, which in the case of jogging would directly increase the intensity of exercise. Other alternatives for overload would be periodically to increase the distance run or to increase the frequency of exercise to 5 days a week. The relative importance of frequency, duration, and intensity in physiologic conditioning will be developed more fully in the sections that follow. *The important point is that to ensure continued improvement in physiologic capacity during training, the relative degree of overload must keep pace with the adaptive changes that occur both in physiology and performance.* This concept of individualized and progressive overload applies to the athlete, the sedentary person, and even the cardiac patient.

A good example of the positive results of progressive overload is the cardiac patient who completely recovered from a heart attack and through training was able to run a 26-mile marathon in 4 hours. This extraordinary capability in exercise capacity did not occur within a few months. At first, walking for just a few minutes was strenuous. Soon, functional capacity improved and the patient could walk longer distances. In a short time the patient reached a plateau where further improvements in cardiovascular capacity and performance did not take place until additional overload was applied. Walking was replaced by slow jogging, which in turn was replaced by jogging at faster speeds. Simultaneously, distance gradually and systematically increased from a few yards to several blocks, to miles, and finally to a point that was personally rewarding. Of course, this can be carried to spectacular extremes: The world record for continuous swimming is 168 hours; the record for walking nonstop is 47 hours and 42 minutes (215 miles, 1670 yards); for running nonstop, the record is 22 hours and 27 minutes (121 miles, 440 yards); for hiking, the record is 32 miles a day for 81 consecutive weeks over a distance of 18,500 miles.

SPECIFICITY PRINCIPLE

The important principle of *training specificity* will be expanded in the following two chapters. In a general sense, however, training specificity refers to adaptations in the *metabolic* and *physiologic* systems depending on the type of overload imposed. Exercise that develops one aspect of fitness generally contributes little to other fitness components. It is known that a specific exercise stress such as strength-power training induces specific strength-power adaptations. However, such strengthening exercises per se offer little stimulus for increasing the flow of blood through the body and provide only a minimal effect in terms of calories expended.

Recent research has indicated there is also a high degree of specificity in terms of improving a particular physiologic capacity. Evidence from these studies suggests strongly that a person should perform the training exercises in a manner as close as possible to the way he or she wishes to use this improved capacity. Developing the cardiovascular system for swimming, bicycling, or rowing, for example, can be achieved more readily when the exerciser works with the specific muscles involved in the particular activity. Consequently, fitness for bicycling is best achieved through cycling exercise, those desiring fitness for swimming should swim, while the runner is best conditioned through specific programs of run training. The same is true for improving the muscular system; performing an exercise with the arms in one pattern of movement, as in lifting a weight with two hands from the waist to a position above the head, does not necessarily mean that improvement in this specific type of lifting strength "transfers" to another arm movement such as the shot-put, even though both movements may use the same muscles. *Specific exercise elicits specific adaptations creating specific training effects.*

INDIVIDUAL DIFFERENCES PRINCIPLE

Many factors contribute to individual variation in training response. Of considerable importance is the person's relative fitness level at the start of training. It is unrealistic to expect different people to be in the same "state" of training at the same time. Consequently, it is counterproductive to insist that all individuals train the same way or at the same work rate. It is also unrealistic to expect all individuals to respond to a given training dosage in precisely the same manner. *Training benefits are optimized when programs are planned to meet the individual needs and capacities of the participants.*

PRINCIPLE OF REVERSIBILITY

Another important principle of physiologic conditioning is *reversibility*. The functional capacity of a bodily system is determined by the current level of overload. Once a person reaches a certain level of conditioning, a regular program of activity must be maintained to prevent deconditioning or a loss in functional capacity. When the normal level of exercise can no longer be applied, as occurs when an arm or leg is placed in a cast or when someone adopts a sedentary life style, the current level of physiologic capacity will regress to a lower level. For this reason the muscles of a limb immobilized in a cast will atrophy to a size much smaller than the weight-bearing or opposite limb.

Some researchers estimate that once a conditioning program is discontinued, the improvements gained during the conditioning process are lost in 5 to 10 weeks. This is one reason why athletes in various sports begin a reconditioning program a month or two prior to the start of the competitive season. Many ex-athletes are in poorer physiologic condition several years after they retire from active participation than the 50-year-old business executive who has played handball 1 hour a day, 3 days a week, since college days.

An optimal state of functional capacity can be developed and maintained through activities such as tennis, handball, swimming, bicycling, volleyball, vigorous dancing, or backpacking, as well as through organized programs of jogging and calisthenics. In fact, the simple and practical activity of skipping rope or exercising to music can be easily adapted to formulate a program of aerobic conditioning. Many programs will work; the important point is to select a group of activities that blend with your personality and life style.

A Word of Caution Before You Begin

Before beginning a program a *medical checkup* is recommended. A sudden burst of vigorous exercise could be dangerous to some people. For example, intense physical activity coupled with certain environmental conditions may aggravate an existing asthmatic condition. People with a tendency toward high blood pressure should refrain from heavy lifting or straining exercises that may cause temporary yet rapid increases in blood pressure above a safe level. Those over the age of 35 and certain "coronary-prone" younger people who possess a cluster of risk factors such as overweight, hypertension, diabetes, sedentary life style, cigarette smoking, and a family history of early heart disease are urged to obtain an electrocardiogram, preferably one administered during increasing levels of exercise.

There is no evidence that participation in intense physical exercise will damage a normal heart. In fact, the circulatory system adapts to exercise by an increase in its performance capacity. The exercise or *stress electrocardiogram*, however, may pick up subtle changes in the heart muscle that indicate the early development of coronary heart disease. Seemingly healthy people may seriously harm themselves if after years of sedentary living, they decide suddenly to become active by running a mile, climbing a mountain, or shoveling the snow from the front walk. This does not mean that the coronary-prone or those with existing coronary heart disease should avoid exercise. On the contrary, with objective medical advice, different forms of exercise can properly be prescribed to improve capacity for exercise. Such programs may also have a positive effect in retarding the progression of the cardiovascular degenerative process. For this reason exercise "cardiac clubs" are flourishing throughout the country. Such groups engage in regular *aerobic exercise* at the proper intensity for the purpose of improving fitness and possibly reducing the risks of a heart attack.

9

Conditioning for Muscular Strength

IN TRAINING for muscular strength the overload principle is applied by the use of weights (dumbbells or barbells), immovable bars, straps, pulleys, or springs. There is nothing unique in the use of a barbell or spring, or any heavy object to improve muscular strength. In each case the muscle responds to the *intensity* of the overload rather than to the actual method of overload. A barbell of known weight is convenient because resistance can be adjusted quantitatively in small increments. This is not usually the case with a spring, cement blocks, or pieces of iron.

In general, the muscular overload is created by either increasing the load or *resistance* to be lifted, increasing the number of times or *repetitions* the exercise is performed, increasing the *speed* of muscular contraction, or by various combinations of these.

Three exercise systems are commonly used for developing muscular strength: (1) *weight training*, (2) *isometric training*, and (3) *isokinetic training*.

Types of Strength Training

WEIGHT TRAINING

This is the most popular system of strength training and involves the use of barbells and dumbbells or a variety of special exercise machines in which the muscles exert tension to overcome a fixed or variable resistance during muscular contraction. There are three types of muscular contractions: *eccentric, concentric,* and *isometric.*

1. Eccentric contraction: This occurs when a muscle *lengthens* at a controlled rate as it contracts under tension. Figure 9-1A illustrates an eccentric muscular contraction. The weight is lowered but at a speed that acts against the force of gravity. The muscles of the upper arm increase in length as they contract eccentrically in an attempt to prevent the weight from crashing to the floor.

2. Concentric contraction: This is the most common type of muscular contraction and occurs in rhythmical activities where the muscle *shortens* as it develops

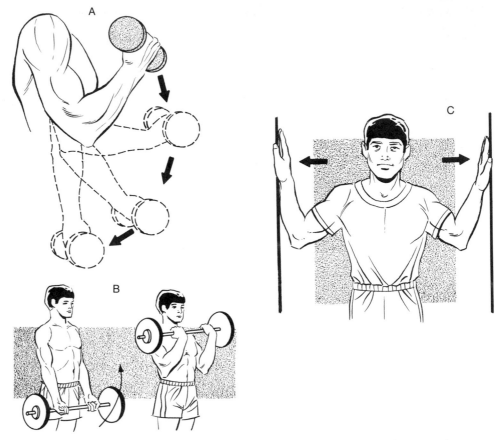

Figure 9-1. *A. Eccentric contraction; B. Concentric contraction; C. Isometric contraction.*

tension. The muscles contract concentrically in most sports activities. Figure 9-1B illustrates a concentric muscular contraction during weightlifting.

3. Isometric contraction: This occurs when a muscle attempts to shorten but is unable to overcome the resistance. Considerable muscular force may be generated during an isometric contraction with *no noticeable shortening* of the muscle. Figure 9-1C illustrates an isometric muscular contraction.

Both eccentric and concentric contractions are commonly referred to as *isotonic* because in both cases movement occurs. With such contractions, muscular force is developed either to overcome or to control the resistance during movement. The term isotonic is derived from the Greek word *isotonos* (*iso*, the same or equal; *tonos*, tension or strain). Actually, the use of this term is imprecise when applied to most muscular actions involving movement because muscular tension does not remain constant but varies as the joint angle changes.

ISOMETRIC TRAINING

This system of strength training was popular in the decade from 1955 to 1965. Research in Germany during this time showed that an increase in isometric strength of about 5% a week could be achieved by performing a single, maximum contraction of only 1 second's duration each day! Repeating this contraction between 5 and 10 times daily produced even greater increases in isometric strength. Although isometric training can provide a quick and convenient method for overloading and strengthening the muscular system, certain limitations make this means of strength training less than desirable, especially for most sport activities.

One major drawback of the isometric method is the difficulty of obtaining knowledge of results concerning the effectiveness of the program. Because there is almost no muscular movement, it is difficult to determine if the person's strength is actually improving, or if she or he is exerting an overload force. The measurement of isometric force requires specialized laboratory equipment not available at most exercise facilities. Another basic limitation is that isometric strength development is *specific* to the angle at which the isometric force is applied and developed. In other words, pushing against an immovable object as illustrated in Figure 9-1C will develop isometric strength at the particular joint angle at which the force is applied. The greatest increases in isometric strength will then occur when the strength is measured in nearly the exact position at which isometric training took place. There is little if any transfer of isometric strength developed at one joint angle to other body positions, even when the same muscles are involved! Thus the muscle trained isometrically is stronger when measured isometrically, especially when measured at the specific joint angle at which the isometric overload was applied.

Isometric exercise can be effective for developing the "total" strength of a particular muscle or group of muscles if the isometric force is applied at four or five angles in the joint range of motion. This can be time-consuming, especially if conventional isotonic methods are available. Isometric training may be desirable and beneficial for special orthopedic applications requiring accurate strength assessment and specific rehabilitation. With isometric training, the exact area of muscle weakness can be isolated and strengthening exercises administered at the proper joint angle.

ISOKINETIC TRAINING

Isokinetic exercise training is quite different from both the conventional isotonic and isometric systems. Recall that isotonic training occurs against an external load that generally remains constant throughout the movement, while isometric or static training is performed against an immovable load. In contrast, isokinetic exercise works against a resistance that permits movement at a preset, fixed speed, and enables the muscle to mobilize its maximum tension-generating capacity throughout the full range of movement *while contracting*. This is done with the aid of a mechanical device containing a speed-controlling mechanism that accelerates to a preset speed when force is applied. Once this constant speed is attained, the isokinetic loading mechanism accommodates to provide a counterforce equal to the force generated by the muscle.

We can make a distinction between a muscle loaded isotonically and one loaded isokinetically. In isotonic or weightlifting exercises the inertia or initial resistance of the load must be first overcome; then the execution of the movement progresses. The weight of the resistance can be no heavier than the maximum strength of the weakest muscle acting in the particular movement. Otherwise the movement would not be completed. Consequently the amount of force generated by the muscles during an isotonic contraction does not attain maximum levels throughout *all* phases of the movement. In an isokinetically loaded muscle the desired speed of movement occurs almost immediately, and the muscle is able to generate a peak power output at a specific but controlled speed of contraction.

The application of the isokinetic principle for overloading muscles to achieve their maximum power outputs has direct application in the fields of sports medicine and athletic training. Many rehabilitation programs utilize isokinetic training to recondition injured limbs in their full range of motion.

Muscular Adaptations with Strength Training

The gross structural and microscopic changes that occur within muscle tissue as a result of overload training are fairly well documented. Considerable attention has also focused on the role of psychologic and learning factors in determining and modifying the expression of muscular strength.

PSYCHOLOGIC FACTORS

The importance of psychologic factors in the acquisition of muscular strength was clearly illustrated in a unique series of experiments conducted in 1961. The strength of the arm muscles was determined for 17 male and 8 female subjects prior to various psychologic treatments. These strength scores served as the baseline for all subsequent comparisons. In one series of experiments the researchers measured arm strength while intermittent gunshots were fired behind the subjects just before their exertions. At another time they instructed the subjects to shout or scream loudly at the moment force was exerted. Following the "shoot and shout" experiments, the experimenters measured subjects' strength under the influence of two disinhibitory drugs, alcohol and amphetamines or "pep pills." They also measured strength while subjects were in a posthypnotic state and were told their strength would be greater than ever before and they should have no fear of injury. In almost all of the "psychologic" conditions, arm strength was significantly greater than under normal conditions. The greatest strength increases were observed under hypnosis, the most "mental" of all the treatments. To explain these observations the researchers suggested that physical factors such as the size and type of muscle fibers and the anatomical lever arrangement of bone and muscle ultimately determine a person's capacity for muscular strength. They took the position that psychologic or mental factors within the central nervous system exert neural influences that prevent most people from achieving this strength capacity. *Inhibitions* within the central nervous system might be the result of social conditioning, unpleasant past experiences with physical activity, or an overprotective home environment. When performing under intense emotional conditions, such as athletic competition, an emergency situation, or posthypnotic suggestion, the inhibitory neural mechanisms may be reduced so much that the person is often capable of a "super performance" that more closely matches the physiologically determined capacity.

Observations such as these help to explain the apparent beneficial effects of "psyching" or the almost self-induced hypnosis of athletes before competition. Excellent examples of such *disinhibition* can be observed in weightlifters, high-jumpers and other track and field competitors, and self-defense experts who perform nontraditional skills such as smashing cement bricks with their hands and feet. The great feats of strength observed during emotionally laden emergency situations also fit nicely into this explanation. In addition, the rapid improvements in muscular strength made during the first few weeks of a strength training program may largely be due to a learning phenomenon as well as to the lessening of fear and psychologic inhibition as the person becomes more accustomed to performing in the strength activity.

MUSCULAR FACTORS

Although psychologic inhibitions as well as learning factors greatly modify ability to express muscular strength, the ultimate limit of strength development is determined by anatomic and physiologic factors within the muscle. These factors are not immutable and can be modified with strength training. The gross structural and microscopic changes in muscles that occur as a result of strength training are usually accompanied by substantial increases in muscular strength.

The large size of the skeletal muscles of weightlifters results from hypertrophy of individual muscle cells. Research has indicated that hypertrophy is due to an increase in the size of the already existing small muscle fibers in relation to the cross-sectional size of the larger fibers. This growth results from an increase in the cellular materials within the muscle cell; there is an increase in the contractile proteins, actin and myosin, as well as an increase in enzymes and nutrients. There is no definitive evidence to indicate that muscular overload significantly stimulates the development of new muscle fibers. In addition to enlarging the existing muscle fibers, muscular overload thickens and strengthens the connective tissue surrounding the muscle, the tendons that attach the muscle to the bone, and the ligaments that attach bones to bones.

Strength Training for Women

Until recently the only physical conditioning activities viewed as socially "acceptable" for women and encouraged by the media and through organized classes were the bending and stretching flexibility exercises. Pseudo-conditioning programs of this type have been camouflaged under titles such as "slimnastics" and "figure control" in order to appear more attractive to the socially conditioned expectations of most women. Times have changed, however. One of the more vivid and positive illustrations of the redefinition of women's roles in society has been their present attitude toward and participation in a wide range of competitive sports and physical activity experiences. Women now compete routinely for positions on athletic teams instead of just the cheerleaders' club. Most jogging clubs and physical conditioning classes are no longer sexually segregated; if they are, they shouldn't be.

Some women are still concerned, however, about the expected "masculinizing" effects of some activities. This is particularly true in the area of strength development by use of weight training procedures. Although muscular strength appears to be a major factor in achieving optimum performance in many sport activities, many women have shied away from strength training exercises for fear of developing the enlarged or bulging muscles that are so commonly observed for men. This is unfortunate, because the failure of many women to learn the basic skills and improve in activities such as tennis, golf, dance, and gymnastics can be directly attributed to a lack of sufficient muscular strength, especially upper-body strength. A proper program of strength training can usually improve such muscular weakness.

Recent research indicates that women who participate in weight training programs are capable of making strength improvements similar to men's *without* the accompanying excessive muscular hypertrophy. In one series of studies, changes in the size and strength of 47 untrained college-aged women and 26 untrained college-aged men were evaluated during a 10-week weight training program.

Before training, the men's strength was about 28 and 26% greater than that of the women for muscle groups of the upper and lower body, respectively. These strength differences were due entirely to the larger body size of the men, since when strength was expressed in relation to body weight (strength per pound of body weight), *no sex differences in strength appeared.* After completing 10 weeks of weight training, both men and women showed significant and almost equal improvement in muscular strength, with improvements of approximately 30% in some areas of the body. It should be noted that the differences in muscular strength between the sexes observed at the beginning of the program still existed. However, after training the strength of the women was greater than that of the men as measured at the start of the program! While the muscles of the men became significantly enlarged with training, there was no increase in muscle size for the women. The authors suggested that hormonal differences between the sexes, especially in the male hormone *testosterone*, account in part for the differences in muscular enlargement during strength training. Although more extensive data on this topic are needed, it appears that women can significantly increase their present level of muscular strength with conventional weight training procedures with little fear of developing bulging or overdeveloped muscles.

Metabolic Stress of Strength Training

Numerous claims have been advertised concerning the physical benefits to be derived from various strength training programs. These include the promise of improved "organic vigor," reduced body fat, and improved cardiovascular functioning. Although a properly planned program of isometric, isokinetic, or weight training can provide an effective means for developing and maintaining muscular strength, there is little information as to how these three systems of strengthening exercises affect the metabolic rate and ventilatory and cardiovascular systems.

In a series of experiments in one of our laboratories, we studied the effects of isometric and weight training exercises on overall cardiovascular functioning. The weightlifting exercises were performed with a weight that enabled the students to complete eight repetitions of a particular movement. A 6-second isometric contraction was performed against a bar placed in a position halfway through the range of motion of the corresponding weightlifting exercise. In this experiment we studied the two-arm curl, two-arm press, bench press, and squat.

The results we obtained for heart rate and oxygen consumption indicated that both isometric and weightlifting exercises would be classified as *light to moderate* in terms of energy expenditure, even though considerable stress is placed on the involved muscle groups. The rate of oxygen consumed during weight training was equivalent to walking at a pace of 4 miles per hour, gardening, or swimming at a slow speed. Although a person may perform 15 or 20 different exercises during a 1-hour weight training session, the amount of time devoted to the exercise per se is short, usually no longer than 6 or 7 minutes. This short activity period, which produces only mild circulatory and metabolic stress, indicates that traditional isometric and weightlifting programs would *not* be effective for improving circulatory capacity for activities like running or swimming. Furthermore, they would not be effective as major activities in weight-reducing programs because the caloric expenditure during an exercise session is so low.

CIRCUIT WEIGHT TRAINING

By modifying the approach to standard strength training methods so that heavy muscle overload is deemphasized, it is possible to increase the caloric cost of exercise and bring about improvements in more than one aspect of fitness. Current research has focused on the energy cost and cardiorespiratory effect of *circuit weight training.* In this form of training, different weight lifting exercises are performed in a preestablished exercise-rest sequence. In most programs, the circuit consists of 8 to 12 exercise stations with a prescribed number of repetitions, usually 15 to 20, performed for each exercise. The person performs an exercise that usually is between 40 and 50% of his or her maximum force generating capacity.

In one experiment, the energy expended during circuit weight training was determined for 20 men and 20 women. They performed three exercise circuits (10 stations per circuit utilizing weight machines); there was a 15-second rest interval between exercises. The total time to perform the three circuits was 22.5 minutes. The net amount of energy expended, which excluded the resting metabolism, was 129 kcal for the men and 95 kcal for the women for the total exercise period. At this level of energy expenditure, the heart rate averaged 142 (72% maximum heart rate) and 158 beats (82% max heart rate) for the men and women, respectively. This corresponded to an exercise intensity of about 41% of maximum oxygen uptake capacity for the men and 45% of maximum for the women. Because the rate of energy expenditure for this weight training circuit was related to an individual's body weight, the results in Table 9-1 for net energy expenditure are presented in terms of body weight. On the average, the level of energy expended for circuit weight training was approximately the equivalent of a slow jog (11 minutes:30 seconds per mile or 5.2 mph pace), hiking in the hills at a moderate pace, or playing in a basketball game, a tennis match, or leisurely swimming the crawl stroke. At this energy output, for example, a 130-pound woman working for 22 minutes per workout would expend an additional 1000 kcal a month if she performed the total circuit three times a week. At this rate, providing food intake and other physical activities remained unchanged, it would require about 14 weeks to reduce body weight the equivalent of 1 pound of fat. Her 170-pound male counterpart would burn 1500 extra kcal per month or the equivalent of 1 pound of fat every 9 to 10 weeks.

In terms of improving the cardiovascular system, there are conflicting reports concerning the improvements to be expected. While one experiment concluded that circuit weight training that made use of weight machines had a negligible

Table 9-1. *Net energy expenditure of circuit weight training in men and women.*

	KCAL EXPENDED PER MINUTE[a]											
BODY WEIGHT, POUNDS	100	110	120	130	140	150	160	170	180	190	200	210
Men			4.1	4.4	4.8	5.1	5.4	5.7	6.0	6.4	6.7	7.0
Women	3.4	3.6	3.7	3.9	4.1	4.3	4.4	4.6	4.8			

[a]Calculated from the data of Wilmore, J.H. and others. Energy cost of circuit weight training. *Medicine and Science in Sports 10:75*, 1978. To determine the total number of calories expended during workouts (over and above rest), multiply the value in the column that corresponds to your body weight by the duration of the circuit. For example, a 163-pound male who exercises on the circuit for 43 minutes would expend 232 kcal (5.4 kcal/min × 43 min).

effect on improving cardiovascular function and did little to improve flexibility, other studies report more positive results for both aerobic fitness and body composition. Clearly, more research is needed in this area, particularly for comparisons of different ways of measuring improvements and the various types of exercise circuits and equipment such as free weights, pulley and cam devices, hydraulic cylinders, isotonic-type machines, and especially the new generation of computer controlled, force and power resistive equipment.

Physiologic Experiments Utilizing Hydraulic Resistive Equipment

Two recent experiments in one of our laboratories have focused on the cardiovascular and metabolic response to a new form of exercise training, termed *omnikinetic* by the manufacturer,* that relies on hydraulic cylinders to provide resistance to movement.

Experiment 1. *Pulse rate response during a 13-week circuit-type training program.* Pulse rate response was measured during and immediately following 11 different exercises that were performed in circuit fashion utilizing a *20-second exercise* and *30-second rest* period between exercises. Two circuits (22 exercises) were performed; the first at what would be classified as moderate resistance while the second was relatively hard exercise. Pulse rate was monitored daily in 15 college men and 13 women who participated in the 13-week, thrice weekly training program. The results for heart rate displayed in Table 9-2 have been expressed in relation to the maximum pulse determined before and after training on an ergometer test of maximal aerobic capacity. In addition to higher pulse counts for men compared to women on all exercises at both resistive settings, the average pulse

* Omnikinetic is total dynamic accommodating resistive training which emphasizes double concentric (positive) reciprocal muscle work. Hydra-Fitness Industries, Belton, Texas.

Table 9-2. *Percentage of maximum pulse rate achieved throughout 13 weeks of hydraulic resistive circuit exercise training in men and women.*

ORDER OF EXERCISE	RESISTANCE 3 (MODERATE)		RESISTANCE 5 (HARD)	
	MEN	WOMEN	MEN	WOMEN
1. Bench press	76	71	71	68
2. Hip adduction/abduction	76	71	73	71
3. Biceps/triceps curl	74	70	72	70
4. Squat	85	84	81	78
5. Neck-side/side	75	71	70	69
6. Unilateral quad/ hamstring	80	74	76	73
7. Incline shoulder press/lat pull	78	72	74	68
8. Neck-front/back	73	67	69	65
9. Hip flexion/extension	75	73	72	72
10. Sit ups	79	76	78	76
11. Upright row- triceps extension	79	76	77	73

for both groups throughout the training period, including the rest pauses, exceeded 70% of maximum pulse. For exercise on some machines, notably the squat, the pulse averaged 85% of maximum for men and 84% of maximum for women.

Experiment 2. *Heart rate and metabolic response to three modes of hydraulic resistive exercise.* Twenty college males were evaluated for the heart rate (HR) and metabolic response to three modes of concentric (positive) reciprocal resistive exercise performed on the single unit, hydraulic exercise machine shown in Figure 9-2. Exercise was performed on two separate days; there were three sets of leg exercise (LE), chest exercise (CE), and shoulder exercise (SE). The duration of exercise was 20 seconds with a 20-second rest interval and 5-minute rest pause between each exercise mode. The average oxygen consumption based on the average of three sets for each exercise mode was 1.7 (LE), 1.6 (CE), and 1.5 (SE) liters/minute. In relation to the maximal aerobic capacity, the oxygen consumption was 57.4% (LE), 51.9% (CE), and 49.2% (SE) of the maximum response. In terms of caloric expenditure, the values were 7.5, 6.8, and 6.2 kcal/min for the leg, chest, and shoulder exercises, respectively. The average heart rate response in relation to the maximum heart rate for LE was 85.4%, 85.2% for CE, and 83.1% for SE. These findings demonstrate that leg, chest, and shoulder concentric reciprocal exercise performed on a single unit hydraulic resistive device significantly augments energy expenditure and heart rate response above the minimum threshold level required to promote improvement in cardiorespiratory function. Similar observations have also been noted with other forms of standard weight training equipment that follow a similar circuit training protocol.

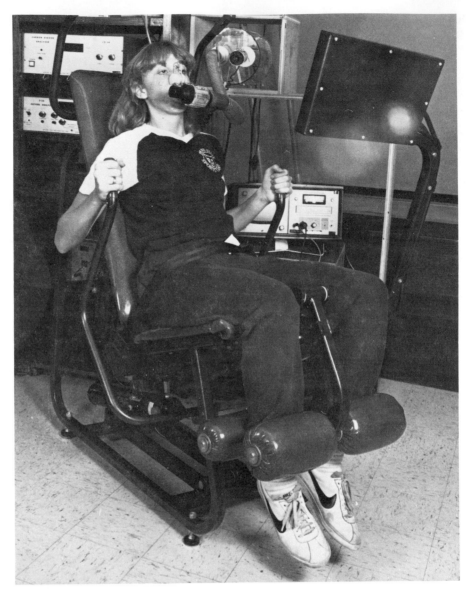

Figure 9-2. *Subject exercising on a 3-station, hydraulic resistive exercise machine. (Photo courtesy of Exercise Science Department, University of Massachusetts, Amherst. Total power exercise machine provided by Hydra-Gym Athletics, Belton, Texas.)*

Specificity of Strength

The correct application of force in relatively complex, learned movements such as the tennis serve or the shot-put depends on a series of coordinated neuromuscular patterns and not *just* the strength of the muscle groups recruited during the movement. The complex interaction between the nervous and muscular systems provides some explanation for the observation that the leg muscles, when strengthened in an activity like squats or deep knee bends, do not usually show improved force capability when used in another leg movement such as jumping. In fact, a group of muscles strengthened with weights does not generate an equal improvement in force when measured isometrically. Consequently strengthening muscles for use in a specific activity such as golf, rowing, swimming, or football requires more than just identifying and overloading muscles involved in the movement. It requires that training be specific with regard to the exact movements involved. Training the muscles of the arms to become stronger by weightlifting does not necessarily mean that the performance of all subsequent arm movements will be improved. Generally there will be little transfer of this newly acquired strength to other types of movements, even though the same muscles are involved. *To improve a specific performance by the strengthened musculature, you must train the muscles with movements as close as possible to those used in the desired movement or actual skill.*

An intelligent application of the principle of specificity of strength training is used by football linemen who develop specific leg "strengths" by pushing weighted blocking sleds in a position and movement pattern similar to the act of blocking during a football game. Swimmers apply specific overload to their back and shoulder muscles by using "swimming machines" that enable them to train their muscles in a manner reasonably similar to the muscular action involved in a particular stroke. Leg strength for jumping in basketball would probably best be developed by applying overload in the movement pattern of the actual jump.

Organizing a Strength Training Program

In this section we will present basic guidelines concerning strength training. Men and women without previous experience in strength training should follow a program designed to produce all-around improvements in muscular strength. We also include exercises that people can do at home without special equipment.

THE WARM-UP

The value of warm-up or preliminary exercise in preventing muscle and joint injuries as well as in improving performance has been frequently and perhaps justifiably challenged over the years. Although the scientific basis for recommending a warm-up is not conclusive, we feel it would be unwise to completely ignore warm-ups until there is more substantial evidence justifying their elimination. Any sequence of calisthenic and flexibility exercises can be used as a warm-up, as well as running in place or other vigorous exercises. The warm-up exercises illustrated in Figure 9-3 serve this purpose and can be completed in a few minutes. These exercises will gradually increase circulation, will improve body flexibility, and may help prevent painful muscle and joint injury.

The stretching or flexibility exercises should be done slowly and smoothly until you feel a mild tension on your muscles. The goal is not to complete many repetitions of the particular exercise, but rather to hold the stretching movement. A reasonable goal to achieve is to hold the stretch for about 10 seconds in the beginning; as flexibility improves, individuals should increase the duration of the

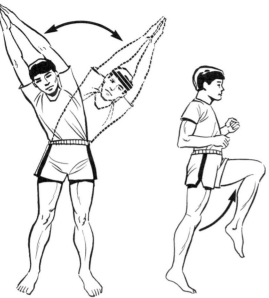

Side bender
Stretch arms straight up, hands together.
Sway from side to side.

Jogging in place
Lift knees to waist level

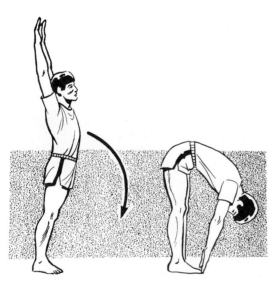

Toe touch—Lock knees, keep hands together, and touch toes.

Single leg raises

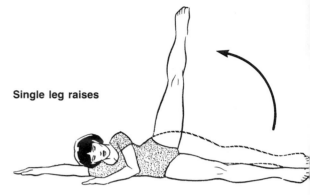

Lying first on one side, then on the other, raise leg sideways.

Simultaneous leg raises

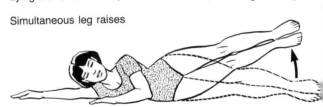

Lying first on one side, then on the other, raise both legs sideways.
Keep legs straight.

Back extensions

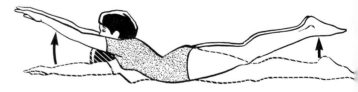

Lie flat. Arch back and lift arms and legs off the ground. Keep arms stretched, legs straight.

Figure 9-3. *Selected calisthenic and flexibility exercises that can be performed as part of a "warm-up" prior to muscle training.*

Simultaneous knee raises

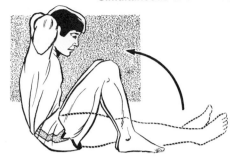

Sitting with hands clasped behind neck, bring both knees toward the chest, then return to the starting position.

Bent knee sit-up

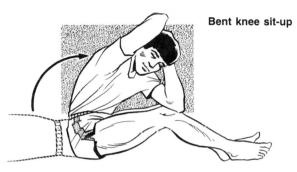

With hands clasped behind head, curl up and touch elbow to opposite knee. Keep knees bent.

Figure 9-3. Continued

static stretch to 30 seconds. Remember, stretching that employs fast bouncing and jerky movement that use the body's momentum can strain or tear muscles and may actually set up a reflex action that will resist the muscle's stretching.

THE LOWER BACK

One of the areas of the body most susceptible to injury is the lower back. Many people lose considerable time at work, suffer chronic discomfort, and spend large amounts of money on orthopedists and chiropractors in an attempt to alleviate the pain caused by low back strain. The causes of this malady are not always apparent and the cure is elusive. However, many orthopedists feel that the prime factors in the low back syndrome are *muscular weakness*, especially in the abdominal region, *and poor joint flexibility* in the back and legs. Both strengthening and flexibility exercises are commonly prescribed for the prevention of and rehabilitation from chronic low back strain.

The use of strength training exercises poses a dilemma. If done properly, such training can provide an excellent means for strengthening the muscles of the abdomen and lower back. As is often the case, however, many people, attempting to lift too much weight, perform the exercises improperly. As a result additional muscle groups are recruited, the spinal column is placed in improper alignment, especially with the arching of the back, and low back strain results. A seemingly simple exercise such as a sit-up, if done improperly with the legs stiff, the back arched and the head thrown back, can place considerable strain on the lower spine. Pressing and curling exercises, if performed with excessive hyperextension or arch to the back may cause a muscle strain or spinal pressure that can trigger low back pain. For these reasons, those who begin a program of strengthening exercises are urged to do all exercises correctly in the manner described. Do not sacrifice proper execution in order to lift a heavier load or "squeeze out" an additional repetition. The extra weight lifted through improper technique will not facilitate strengthening the desired muscle groups and may cause injury to the lower back.

SELECTING THE PROPER WEIGHT

In the beginning stages of a program, people should *not* attempt to see how much weight they can lift. This serves little purpose in improving strength and greatly increases the likelihood of muscle or joint injury. *It is unnecessary to exercise at maximum levels to develop muscular strength.* A resistance or load that represents between 60 and 80% of a muscle group's maximum strength is sufficient overload to produce gains in strength. Generally such a resistance permits the completion of between 6 and 8 repetitions of a particular exercise. Our experience has shown that beginners should attempt to complete 12 repetitions of an exercise. The amount of weight lifted during 12 repetitions will not place an excessive strain on the muscles during the beginning phase of the muscular conditioning program. If the weight selected for the 12 repetitions feels "too easy," a heavier weight should be used. If the exerciser cannot do 12 repetitions, the weight is too heavy. This is a trial and error process and it may take several exercise sessions before a proper starting weight is selected.

After 5 or 6 exercise sessions the muscles will have adapted to the exercise, and the exerciser will have learned the correct movements involved in lifting. The number of repetitions should now be reduced to between 6 and 8 and the resistance increased accordingly. When the exerciser can complete 8 repetitions, add more weight. This additional weight will undoubtedly reduce the number of repetitions he or she can do. This is exactly the desired outcome. Eight repetitions should be achieved within several exercise sessions, and again, you will need to add more weight. This is one overload method that is generally used in weight training to increase the strength of a particular group of muscles. For a general strength conditioning program, select exercises that overload a variety of muscle groups. If strength training is geared to sports performance, choose specific exercises that closely resemble the movements in the particular skill.

The exercises should be performed in the same order on each workout day. This is because many exercises involve more than one muscle group, and some fatigue may result from a previous exercise. By maintaining the same order of exercise, the cumulative fatigue effect should remain relatively constant. In scheduling workouts, consistency is the key to achieving a successful training effect. This does not mean that workouts should be scheduled every day. *From the relatively limited information available, it appears that at least 2 or 3 exercise sessions each week are necessary to continue strength improvements.* Some people exercise 5 or 6 days a week. However, with this protocol different muscle groups are usually exercised on alternate days, so in reality, a specific muscle group is still only trained 2 or 3 days a week.

The *first step* in planning a workout is to establish the primary aims and objectives of the strength training program. Strengthening exercises are performed for many different reasons: improved sports performance, development and maintenance of muscular tone and firmness, aesthetic enhancement, or fun and pleasure. Whatever the reason, include exercises that will help meet personal objectives. You should use a variety of exercises for an all-around strength conditioning program, with exercises for the neck, arms, forearms, shoulders, abdomen, back, chest, buttocks, and legs.

The *second step* is to determine the length of time available for exercise. Work schedules and other restraints often pose limitations on the number of exercises that someone can complete during a workout. A minimum of about 15 minutes is usually required to complete a series of basic exercises. This includes the rest intervals as well as the time spent in actual exercise.

The *third step* is to determine the available facilities and equipment. It is not necesssary to purchase expensive equipment; many household items can be used to provide muscular overload, and often people can construct equipment with minimal expense. Figure 9-4 shows common household and store items that can be used to construct strength training equipment. Weights can be made by filling plastic cleanser containers with water or filling socks and other clothes with sand. A broom or mop handle can serve as a bar to which these heavy objects can be attached. Ski boots, telephone books, bricks wrapped in a towel, and other objects can also provide the resistance to muscular contraction. Of course, barbells and dumbbells are the easiest to use and are relatively inexpensive. Chairs, table tops, and other household furniture items can take the place of standard gymnasium equipment. A piece of clothesline can be used as a jump rope.

The *fourth step* is the selection of the exercises. A variety of exercises for strengthening the large muscle groups of the body are presented in Figure 9-5. These exercises represent a variety of basic isotonic exercises that should meet the needs of most people interested in improving muscular strength. The exercises have been placed into one of three groups: (A) exercises for the neck, arms, and shoulders, (B) exercises for the chest, abdomen, and back, and (C) exercises for the buttocks and legs. In cases where exercises are illustrated without equipment, adaptations can be made by including weights. The shaded areas within each figure denote the muscle groups primarily affected by the exercise.

Once the exercises have been selected, the *fifth step* is to arrange an *exercise circuit*, similar to that described for circuit weight training. When arranging the exercises in a proper sequence, it is important not to perform consecutively two exercises that involve the same muscle groups. This way the possible transfer of fatigue effects will be minimized. For example, two exercises for the arms should be separated by other exercises that do not require the use of the arms in the same pattern of movement. Figure 9-6 illustrates the basic model of the circuit. In this example, there are 10 different exercise stations, with one exercise performed at each station.

Each exercise may consist of any number of repetitions desired. Initially, when working with weights, 12 repetitions of each exercise are done until the proper load or resistance is established. After several weeks, add additional weights until a target number of 6 to 8 repetitions is achieved. The goal of this circuit could be simply to complete the desired exercises in the time available for the workout. When the target number of repetitions is achieved, add more weight. Another objective might be to perform the required number of repetitions of each

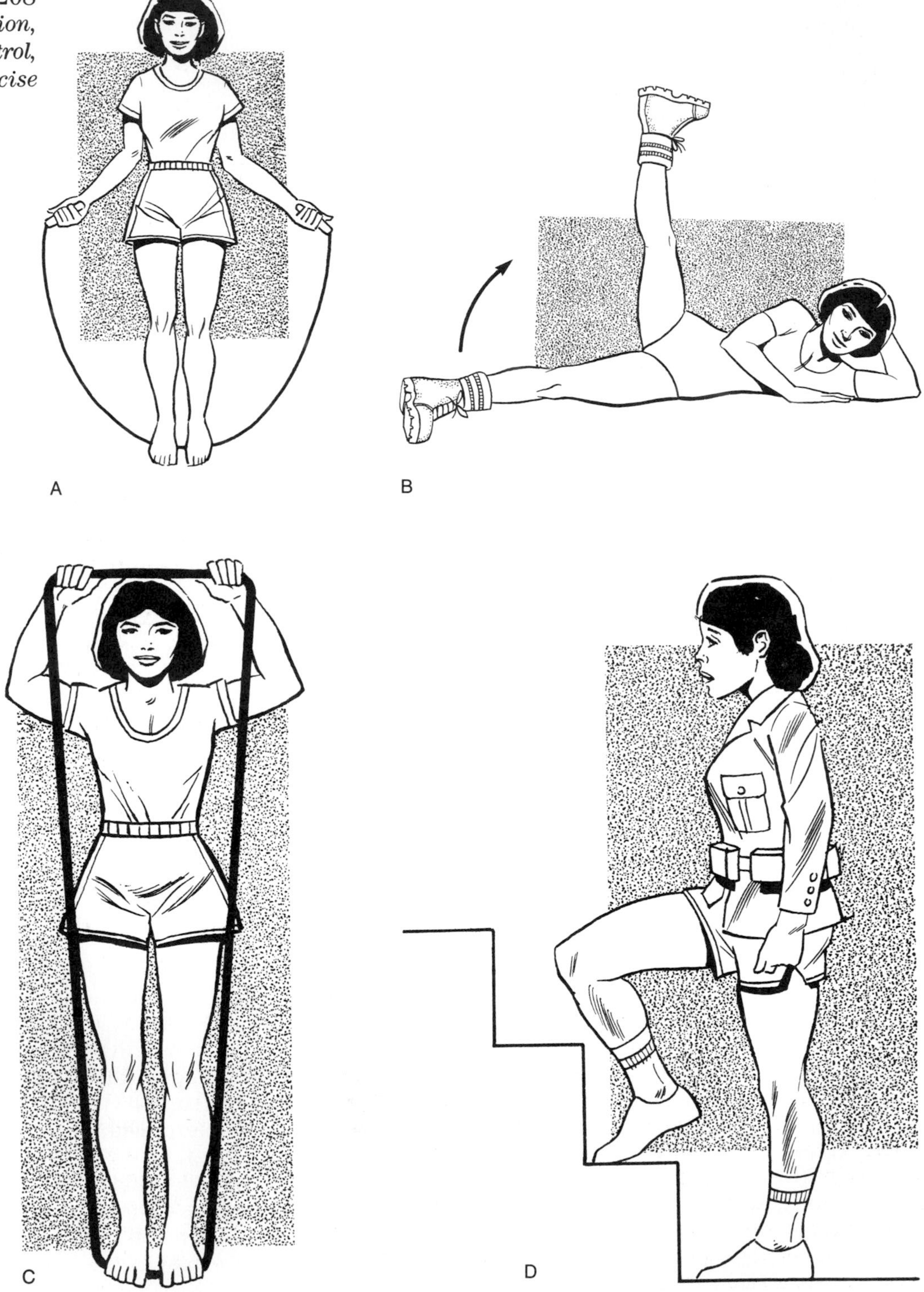

Figure 9-4. *Household items incorporated into a strength development program.*

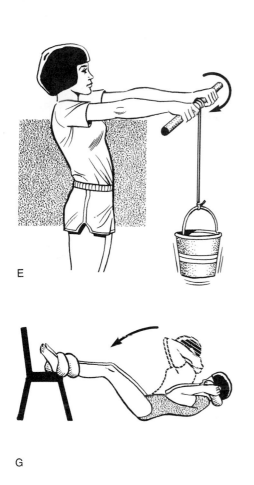

E

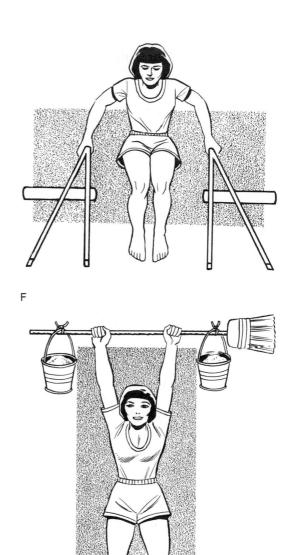

F

G

H

exercise in the sequence within a *target time* previously established according to individual needs. For example, suppose the 10 exercise stations, each with one exercise to be performed 12 times, are to be completed twice. Initially, it may require 20 minutes to complete two circuits. This would then become the target time, and each exercise day the objective would be to complete two circuits within this time limit. As physiologic conditioning progresses, the target time will be achieved more easily. Once this occurs, several methods can be used to maintain a *progressive overload*. For example, a faster target time might be established. Other modifications could include the use of heavier weights while maintaining the 20-minute target time, or attempting to complete one additional circuit during the

A

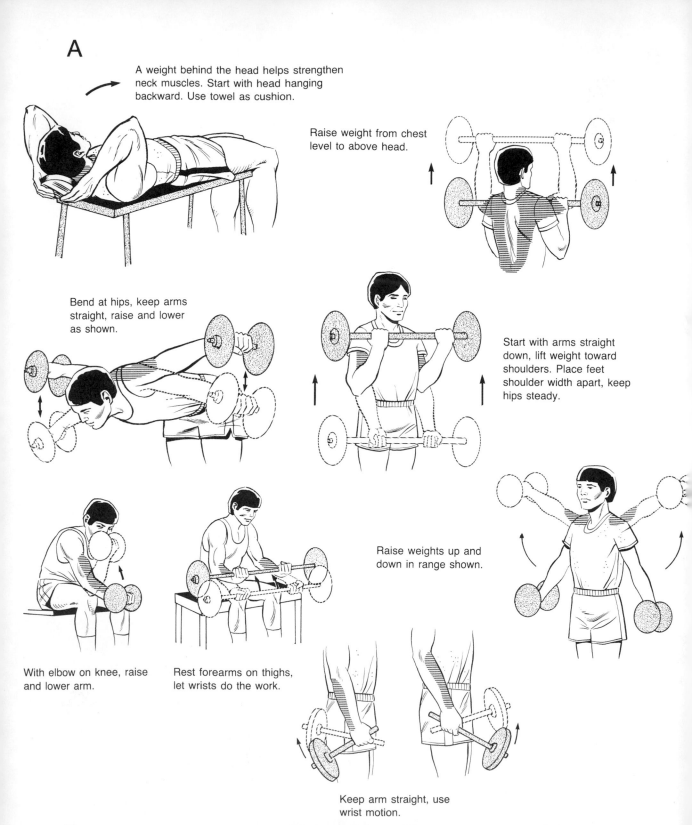

A weight behind the head helps strengthen neck muscles. Start with head hanging backward. Use towel as cushion.

Raise weight from chest level to above head.

Bend at hips, keep arms straight, raise and lower as shown.

Start with arms straight down, lift weight toward shoulders. Place feet shoulder width apart, keep hips steady.

With elbow on knee, raise and lower arm.

Rest forearms on thighs, let wrists do the work.

Raise weights up and down in range shown.

Keep arm straight, use wrist motion.

Figure 9-5. *A. Exercises to strengthen the neck, arms, and shoulders. B. Exercises to strengthen the chest, abdomen, and back. C. Exercises to strengthen the buttocks and legs.*

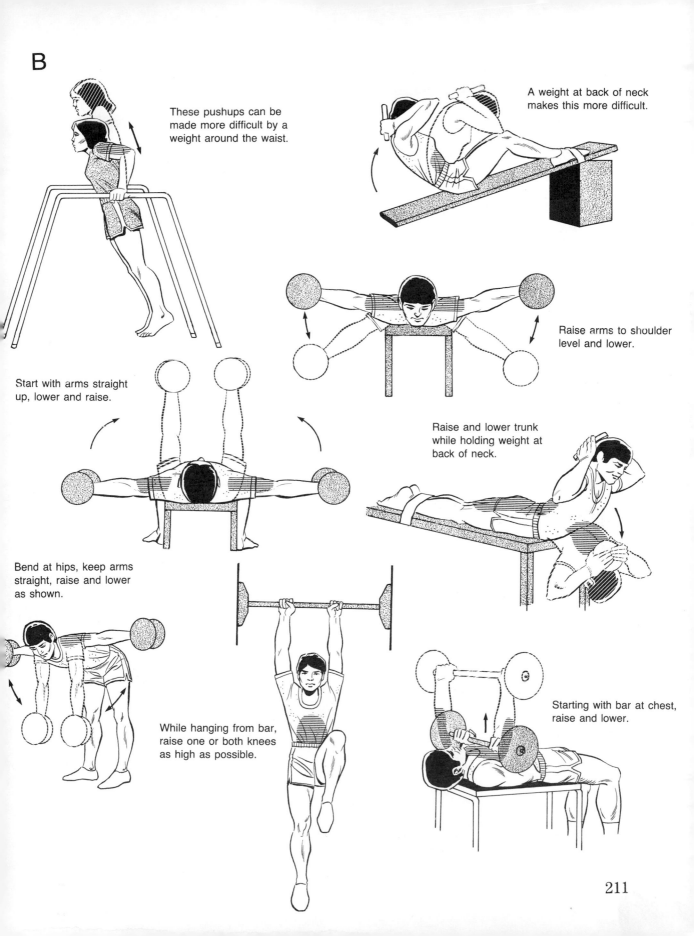

B

These pushups can be made more difficult by a weight around the waist.

A weight at back of neck makes this more difficult.

Raise arms to shoulder level and lower.

Start with arms straight up, lower and raise.

Raise and lower trunk while holding weight at back of neck.

Bend at hips, keep arms straight, raise and lower as shown.

While hanging from bar, raise one or both knees as high as possible.

Starting with bar at chest, raise and lower.

C

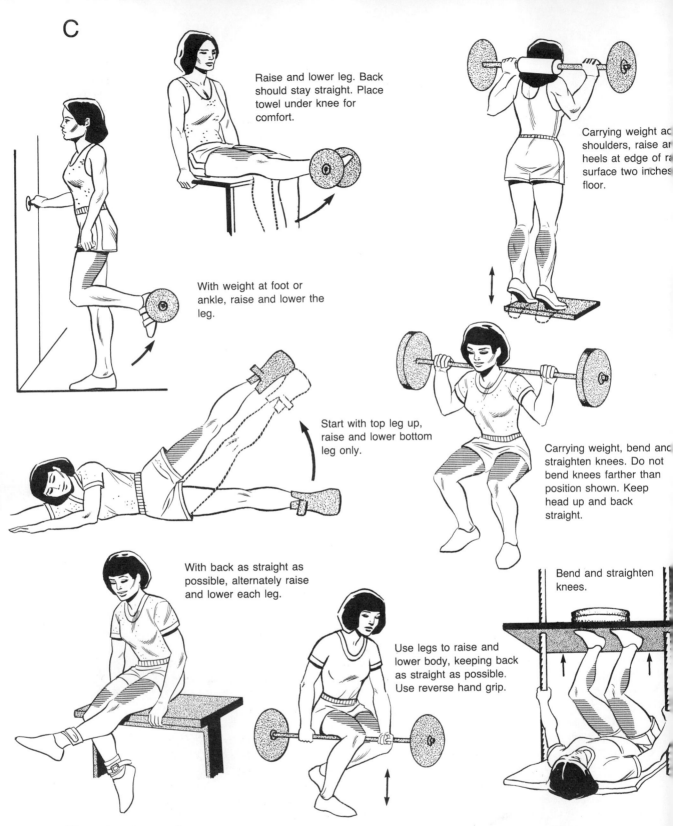

Raise and lower leg. Back should stay straight. Place towel under knee for comfort.

Carrying weight across shoulders, raise and lower heels at edge of raised surface two inches off floor.

With weight at foot or ankle, raise and lower the leg.

Start with top leg up, raise and lower bottom leg only.

Carrying weight, bend and straighten knees. Do not bend knees farther than position shown. Keep head up and back straight.

With back as straight as possible, alternately raise and lower each leg.

Use legs to raise and lower body, keeping back as straight as possible. Use reverse hand grip.

Bend and straighten knees.

Figure 9-5. *Continued*

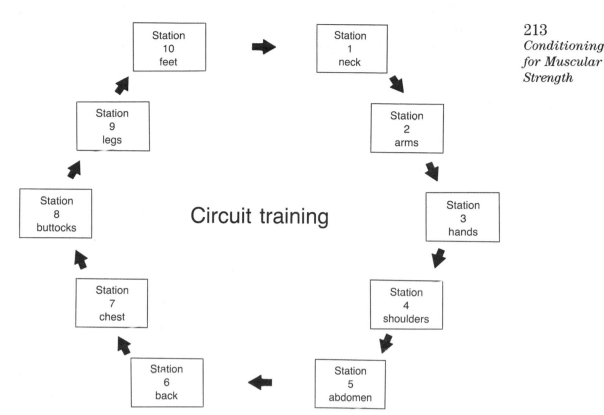

Figure 9-6. *Arrangement of an exercise circuit. Ten exercises of a general nature are performed, with each exercise designed for a different group of muscles. After completing an exercise at one station, the exerciser performs the next exercise in the circuit.*

20-minute exercise period. Thus circuits for the development of muscular strength can achieve overload by the manipulation of three variables: increase the load or resistance, increase the repetitions of exercise in the circuit, or decrease the target time. Each variable can be manipulated separately or in combination to ensure progressive overload.

It is also possible to apply the principle of overload to exercises that require little or no equipment. This is done by increasing the difficulty and thus the strenuousness of the exercise. For example, the conventional push-up can be made more difficult by changing the body position from horizontal (starting position on the level) to a slant by placing the feet on a 12 to 16 inch bench. The same can be done for sit-ups. Place the feet on the seat of a chair; hands are clasped behind the neck. Attempt to curl up until the elbows touch the knees, and then return to the starting position. This type of "incline" sit-up can be made even more strenuous if a weight is held behind the head. A dumbbell, weight plate, or any other object that can be conveniently held will provide additional resistance to movement, and hence, will serve as an appropriate overload as fitness improves.

The sixth and *last step* in planning the exercise workout involves the most efficient use of the available facilities. This is usually not a problem in gymnasiums or health clubs where specialized equipment and facilities are available. For those who exercise in their homes the situation is quite different and necessitates other solutions. Figure 9-7 shows the organization of "exercise stations" in a high-rise building. In small or confined areas, progressing from one station to the next may not be possible. In this case, many exercises would have to be performed in one or two small areas. Sometimes, however, the constraints of exercising in a limited space makes a person more aware of the potential for using other available facilities, such as hallways, staircases, washrooms, garages, or nearby parks and walkways.

We are aware of a muscular training and cardiovascular conditioning circuit arranged by a 62-year-old man who lived in an apartment in New York City. From his home, he exercised 4 days a week, completing three circuits, each circuit con-

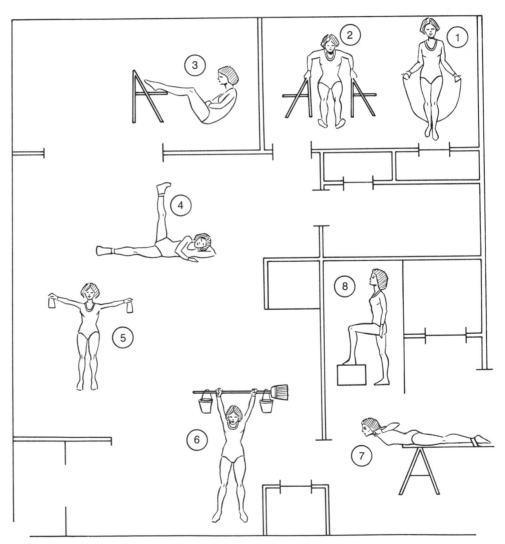

Figure 9-7. *Floor plan of a high-rise apartment and the efficient use of space for arranging an exercise circuit.*

sisting of eight stations and 10 repetitions per station. Station 1 was sit-ups, done on the bedroom floor with knees bent and feet supported under the bed. He held a 10-pound weight behind his head. Station 2 consisted of pull-ups on a bar in the bathroom doorway. The exerciser wore a jacket filled with 20 pounds of sand. Station 3 was rope skipping in the hallway. To increase the intensity of this cardiovascular exercise, the exerciser wore ski boots while jumping. Station 4 involved raising and lowering the body with the arms supported between two kitchen chairs, wearing the 20-pound jacket. Station 5 was performed on the living room floor. The exercise consisted of raising and lowering each leg while lying supported on the side, with a knee-high sock filled with 15 pounds of sand attached around the ankle. Station 6 was a chest press performed while lying supine on the floor, using a broom barbell with weights of plastic containers filled with 26 pounds of cement. Station 7 consisted of back extensions performed while lying face down over the edge of a coffee table with the feet secured under a rope tied around the table top, with a 10-pound weight held behind the head. Station 8 involved quickly descending and then ascending five flights of stairs. On the first and second circuit, stair climbing was done as fast as possible. Going up the stairs on the last circuit, the man hopped up each stair keeping his feet together, with only a minimal rest between floors!

10

Conditioning for Anaerobic and Aerobic Power

A N IMPORTANT ASPECT of many forms of physical activity is the necessity to generate energy rapidly. Because such energy release is almost instantaneous, sufficient oxygen cannot be delivered to the muscles quickly enough to match the energy requirements. Even if oxygen was available immediately, it could not be metabolized fast enough to be of much use. Thus success in sprinting through the line in football, "spiking" in volleyball, or beating out an infield hit in softball depends in part on the capacity to generate energy anaerobically.

The importance of this capacity for rapid energy metabolism is clearly seen in a sport like football, where each play requires short periods of all-out, intense effort. Likewise, a maximum effort is required in sprint running and swimming, weightlifting, and during the "kick" phase of a middle distance run or swim. The apparent steady state sports such as basketball, tennis, field hockey, lacrosse, and soccer also involve sprinting, dashing, darting, and stop-and-go, in which the capacity to generate short bursts of anaerobic power plays an important role. Too often, coaches of sports such as basketball or soccer place considerable importance on the development of cardiovascular or aerobic capacity in their conditioning programs at the sacrifice of vigorous anaerobic conditioning. It is true that these sports require a relatively steady release of energy for a considerable period of time. However, in those crucial situations that demand an all-out effort, the relative capacity of the athlete's anaerobic energy system may be poor and the player or team will be unable to perform at full potential. On the other hand, training the anaerobic capacity of endurance athletes such as marathon runners or channel swimmers would be wasteful, because the contribution of these energy systems to successful performance is minimal. Success in endurance activities necessitates a highly trained oxygen transport or aerobic energy system and a well-conditioned heart and vascular system capable of circulating large quantities of blood for long durations.

Figure 10-1 summarizes the predominant energy systems required in the more common physical activities. Keep in mind that the three energy systems, the ATP-CP system, the lactic acid system, and the oxygen or aerobic system are often

217

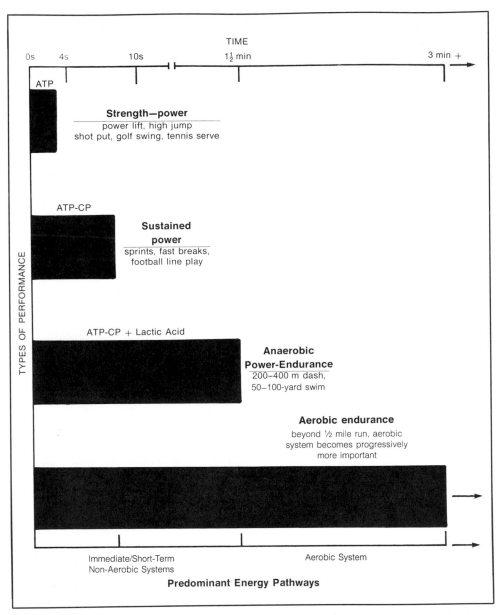

Figure 10-1. *Classification of activities based on duration of performance and the predominant energy pathways. (McArdle, W.D., Katch, F.I., and Katch, V.L.: Exercise Physiology, Lea & Febiger, 1981.)*

operative during physical activity. However, their relative contributions to the energy requirement during an exercise may differ markedly. This contribution in the energy continuum is directly related to the length of *time* and *intensity* a specific activity is performed. With an intense, maximum burst of energy such as occurs in the tennis serve, golf swing, volleyball spike and even the 60- or 100-yard dash, the energy is provided anaerobically and supplied almost exclusively by the stored high energy phosphates, ATP and CP. In a performance lasting between 10 and 90 seconds, as in a 100-yard swim or 220-yard run, the energy is still supplied predominantly by anaerobic reactions. In this case, however, the energy from lactic acid production plays a much more important role, and the training program for such activities must be of sufficient intensity and duration to stimulate lactic acid production as well as to overload the ATP-CP energy system. As the intensity of an activity diminishes somewhat and the duration extends to between 1½ and 4 minutes, dependence upon energy from the phosphate stores decreases, while energy release from aerobic or oxygen-consuming reactions becomes more important. In wrestling, boxing, ice hockey, an 880-yard or 1-mile run, or a full-court press in basketball, the portion of energy required from anaerobic sources depends predominantly on a person's capacity and tolerance for lactic acid. In these activities aerobic energy metabolism occupies a role of equal importance. After 4 minutes of continuous exercise, an activity becomes more dependent on aerobic energy; in a marathon run or long-distance swim, the body is powered almost exclusively by the energy from aerobic reactions. It is clear, therefore, that in training for a particular sport or fitness goal, the activity must be evaluated in terms of its energy components. After this careful analysis, a proportionate allocation of time should be devoted to the overload or training of the particular energy systems.

Anaerobic Conditioning

The capacity to perform all-out exercise of up to 90-second duration depends mainly on anaerobic energy metabolism. As was the case with training to improve muscular strength, you must apply the overload principle in conditioning the anaerobic energy systems to improve this energy-generating capacity significantly.

THE ANAEROBIC ENERGY SYSTEMS

In Chapter 3 we presented the energy reactions at rest and during exercise in some detail. Recall that anaerobic energy is generated from the breakdown of the high-energy phosphates ATP and CP, as well as in the reactions of glycolysis, where glucose is ultimately transformed into lactic acid.

The Phosphate Pool

During the first 6 seconds of all-out exercise, energy is made available from the breakdown of the energy currency ATP and the energy reservoir CP. Energy is released almost immediately in these reactions and does not require oxygen. Sports such as football and weightlifting rely almost exclusively on energy derived from the phosphate pool. In these kinds of activities, developing the capacity of the ATP-CP energy system to the fullest should be of paramount importance.

Maximum overload of the phosphate pool can be achieved by engaging specific muscles in maximum bursts of effort for 5 to 10 seconds. A sprint swimmer might swim intervals of 20 to 25 yards, while the sprint runner could achieve a similar overload in the leg muscles by running sprints of 60 to 100 yards. A football lineman, on the other hand, might sprint for only 5 to 30 yards on any one play. To increase the intensity of the overload during this relatively short but intense exercise period, the player might run with a weighted belt or vest or sprint up hills or stairs. Because the high energy phosphates supply the energy for such intense, intermittent exercise, only small amounts of lactic acid will be produced and recovery will be quite rapid. Thus a subsequent exercise bout can begin after only a brief rest period. In training to enhance the ATP-CP energy capacity of specific muscles the individual should undertake numerous bouts of intense, short-duration exercise. *The training activities selected* must *engage the muscles for which the person desires improved anaerobic power.*

Lactic Acid

As the duration of all-out effort extends beyond 10 seconds, dependence on anaerobic energy from the phosphates decreases, while the quantity of anaerobic energy generated in the reactions of glucose to lactic acid increases. To improve capability for more prolonged anaerobic energy release via the lactic acid energy system, the physiologic conditioning program must provide for increasing the degree of overload on this means of energy metabolism. This form of training is physiologically and psychologically taxing and requires considerable motivation. Repeat bouts of up to 1 minute of maximum running, swimming, or cycling, stopped 30 to 40 seconds before exhaustion, will cause lactic acid to increase to near maximum levels, and will overload this energy system. To assure that maximum levels of lactic acid are produced during each training session, the exercise bout should be repeated several times after 1 to 2 minutes of recovery. Each repeated work level will cause a "lactate stacking" that will result in higher levels of lactic acid than just one bout of all-out effort to the point of voluntary exhaustion. Of course, it is critical to use the specific muscle groups that need this enhanced anaerobic capacity. A backstroke swimmer should train by swimming backstroke, a cyclist must bicycle, and the basketball or football player must rapidly perform various movements and direction changes that are similar to those required by the demands of the sport.

When the body produces large amounts of lactic acid, the time necessary to recover from the exercise can be considerable. For this reason, this form of anaerobic power training should occur at the end of the conditioning session. Otherwise, fatigue from the high intensity, anaerobic training would carry over and perhaps hinder the efficiency of aerobic training.

Aerobic Conditioning

The current interest in physiologic conditioning has resulted to a large degree from the desire of many people to improve their ability to sustain physical activity without fatigue. In most instances this desire is directed toward sports participation, although a variety of recreational, leisure, household, and occupational activities require a continuous and fairly high level of energy expenditure. Participation in swimming, jogging, tennis, hiking, bicycling, and many other forms of activity all require a cardiovascular system conditioned to supply adequate oxygen to the exercising muscles.

In the following discussion of aerobic conditioning we present a relatively simple method for evaluating a person's present physiologic status. Also, we present a program of activities that can be used to overload the aerobic energy systems.

THE AEROBIC ENERGY SYSTEM

Continuous exercise performed for longer than 2 minutes requires energy from both anaerobic and aerobic metabolic reactions. In the early stages of exercise the energy demands are met by the anaerobic breakdown of the high energy phosphates and by the initial phase of carbohydrate metabolism in which glucose is transformed into pyruvic acid. However, the energy liberated from these anaerobic reactions is quite limited, supplying only enough energy to power an all-out run or swim for about 60 to 90 seconds. If exercise continues beyond this time, additional energy for the resynthesis of the phosphates must be supplied by reactions requiring *oxygen*. Under these aerobic conditions the pyruvic acid from carbohydrate metabolism, as well as the food fragments from fat and protein, are changed into various substances with the resulting formation of carbon dioxide, water, and large amounts of energy. This energy released from the complete breakdown of food is used to resynthesize the high energy phosphate ATP. If the supply of oxygen is adequate to meet the energy requirements, then exercise can be continued in a steady state and the feelings of discomfort from fatigue are minimal. On the other hand, if oxygen delivery or utilization is inadequate, anaerobic energy metabolism will exceed the energy generated from aerobic reactions, lactic acid will quickly accumulate, and fatigue will set in. Therefore the intensity at which exercise can be sustained for relatively long periods of time depends on the body's capability for aerobic metabolism. This capacity depends in turn on the functional capacity of the support systems for oxygen transport, that is, the heart, lungs, and vascular system. The terms "endurance fitness," "cardiovascular fitness," and "aerobic fitness" refer to the body's ability to generate ATP aerobically.

A METHOD TO EVALUATE CARDIOVASCULAR CAPACITY

As we discussed in Chapter 3, a low heart rate during exercise and a small increment in heart rate with more vigorous exercise generally reflect a high level of cardiovascular fitness; this can be attributed to a large stroke volume of the heart. Because more blood can be pumped with each heart beat, a smaller increase in heart rate is required to deliver a specific quantity of blood with its complement of oxygen to the exercising muscles. The *step test* provides a convenient means by which heart rate can evaluate the efficiency of the cardiovascular response to aerobic exercise. Suppose, for example, three people perform 3 minutes of step up exercise on a bench to the cadence of a metronome. Figure 10-2 illustrates the heart rate response of each subject during the 3 minutes of stepping.

During the first minute of stepping the heart rate increases rapidly and then starts to level off. Subject A, a varsity basketball player, reaches a heart rate of 120 beats per minute at the end of 3 minutes, while the heart rate of subject B, a physical education major, is 142 beats per minute. For subject C, a sedentary college student, the heart rate response to the metabolic demands of this exercise is 170 beats per minute. It is clear that the cardiovascular stress of bench stepping for student C is considerably greater than for the other two students, especially student A, whose increase in heart rate is minimal. It would be reasonable to conclude that cardiovascular capacity is greatest for the athlete, less for the physical education major, and relatively poor for the sedentary student.

One problem in applying the principles discussed above to a nonlaboratory situation is the determination of exercise heart rate. The accurate way to obtain

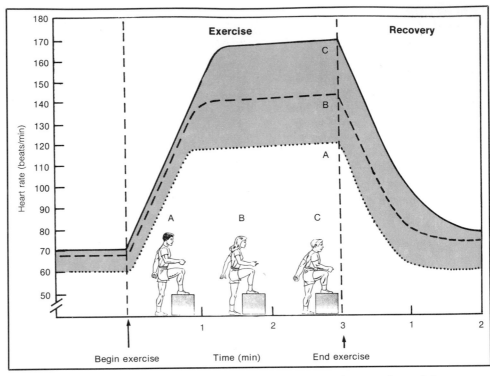

Figure 10-2. *Heart rate response of three people during a stepping exercise and in recovery. (McArdle, W.D., Katch, F.I., and Katch, V.L.: Exercise Physiology, Lea & Febiger, 1981.)*

heart rate during exercise is to monitor the electrical activity of the heart preceding each beat with specialized equipment. An alternative is to record the heart rate during recovery, when the subject stops stepping. Figure 10-2 also shows the pattern of heart rate recovery of the three subjects for the 2 minutes immediately following the bench-stepping exercise. Notice that on completion of exercise, heart rate decreases rapidly during the first 30 seconds of recovery. Following this, the heart rate continues to decline but at a much slower rate. After 2 minutes heart rates have essentially returned to resting values. The most noticeable differences in heart rate between subjects A, B, and C are observed in the period immediately following exercise. Thus if recovery heart rate is measured soon after exercise, it is still fairly easy to discriminate between subjects in terms of their heart rate response to the stress of the exercise test.

THE QUEENS COLLEGE STEP TEST

Using a simple step test, we have measured cardiovascular capacity in thousands of male and female college students at Queens College in New York. In order to measure large numbers of students at the same time, stepping was done using the bottom step of the gymnasium bleachers, which was 16¼ inches high. For women, the stepping cadence was set by a metronome at 88 beats per minute, or 22 complete step-ups; for men, it was set at 96 beats or 24 steps per minute. One complete stepping cycle on the bench represented 4 beats on the metronome, "up-up-down-down." Following a demonstration, students were given 15 seconds of practice stepping to adjust to the cadence of the metronome. The test was then begun and continued for 3 minutes. On completion of stepping the students remained standing while the pulse was counted at the carotid artery for a 15-second interval beginning 5 seconds after the end of stepping. This 15-second pulse rate value was then multiplied by 4 to give the heart rate score in beats per minute. The percentile rankings for the various heart rate scores for men and women are presented in Table 10-1. Accompanying these scores are the corresponding values for maximal oxygen consumption that were *predicted* from the heart rate values. We will present the basis for this prediction of aerobic capacity shortly.

It is important to note that in comparing someone's cardiovascular response to the stepping exercise to that of the students measured at Queens College, you must follow the exact procedures for administering the test. The stepping cadence *must* be 22 steps per minute for women and 24 steps per minute for men. The bench height *must* be 16¼ inches and recovery heart rate *must* be measured during the 5- to 20-second interval at the end of exercise. You can easily construct the bench from plywood, or make a modification with an old end table or foot locker.

Table 10-1. *Percentile rankings for recovery heart rate and predicted maximal oxygen consumption for male and female college students.*

PERCENTILE RANKING	RECOVERY HR, FEMALE	PREDICTED MAX $\dot{V}O_2$ (ml/kg · min)	RECOVERY HR, MALE	PREDICTED MAX $\dot{V}O_2$ (ml/kg · min)
100	128	42.2	120	60.9
95	140	40.0	124	59.3
90	148	38.5	128	57.6
85	152	37.7	136	54.2
80	156	37.0	140	52.5
75	158	36.6	144	50.9
70	160	36.3	148	49.2
65	162	35.9	149	48.8
60	163	35.7	152	47.5
55	164	35.5	154	46.7
50	166	35.1	156	45.8
45	168	34.8	160	44.1
40	170	34.4	162	43.3
35	171	34.2	164	42.5
30	172	34.0	166	41.6
25	176	33.3	168	40.8
20	180	32.6	172	39.1
15	182	32.2	176	37.4
10	184	31.8	178	36.6
5	196	29.6	184	34.1

MEASUREMENT OF PULSE RATE

The accurate measurement of heart rate is essential in evaluating cardiovascular response to the step test and comparing scores to established norms. Locating the pulse at rest requires some practice. The pulse can be easily located after exercise, however, by pressing softly at the carotid artery along the trachea in the neck. Do not press too hard, for this can slow your actual heart rate. Following exercise, the surge of blood from the heart distends this artery and the pulse is easily located. The recovery pulse rate can also be used to estimate the heart rate *during* exercise. In this case you should use the *immediate* 10-second recovery period. Then multiply the number of beats counted during the 10-second interval by 6 to express the heart rate per minute. The heart rate measured during the 10 seconds immediately after exercise only decreases by about 3%, or the equivalent of 4 to 6 beats per minute if the exercise heart rate is between 160 and 180 beats per minute.

PREDICTION OF MAXIMAL OXYGEN UPTAKE

On the basis of the previous discussion, it is reasonable to expect that a person with a low heart rate during the step test would be further from his or her maximal oxygen consumption than someone whose heart rate on the same test was relatively high. To evaluate the validity of this expectation, laboratory studies were conducted on a sample of men and women who were part of the larger study in which the norms of the Queens College Step Test were developed. Maximal oxygen consumption was measured for each subject using treadmill test procedures. Each subject's maximal oxygen consumption was then plotted in relation to the corresponding recovery heart rate score obtained on the step test. Figure 10-3 illustrates these results for the sample of women.

It was clear that a definite relationship existed. Subjects with higher maximal oxygen uptakes tended to have lower heart rate recovery scores on the step test. Although there was considerable variability about a line drawn through these points, it did appear that a knowledge of maximal oxygen consumption could be obtained from recovery heart rate on the step test. We therefore derived the mathematical equation to describe the "best fit" line that passed through the scores for recovery heart rate and maximal oxygen consumption. The equations predicting maximal oxygen consumption from heart rate recovery for the men and women were as follows:

$$\text{Men: max } \dot{V}O_2 = 111.33 - (0.42 \times \text{step-test pulse rate, beats} \cdot \text{min})$$
$$\text{Women: max } \dot{V}O_2 = 65.81 - (0.1847 \times \text{step-test pulse rate, beats} \cdot \text{min})$$

The predicted maximal oxygen uptake value is expressed in relation to body weight as milliliters of oxygen consumed per kilogram of body weight. This is written as ml/kg · min.

The above equations provide a reasonably accurate method for predicting maximal oxygen consumption from step test recovery heart rate for *college-aged* men and women. For example, suppose recovery heart rate following the Queens

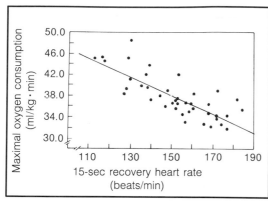

Figure 10-3. *Scattergram and line of "best fit" relating
step-test heart rate score and maximal oxygen consumption in college women. (From McArdle, W.D. et al.:
Reliability and interrelationships between maximal
oxygen uptake, physical work capacity, and step test
scores in college women.* Medicine and Science in
Sports, 4:*182, 1972.*)

College Step Test for a woman was 156 beats per minute. Substituting this heart
rate score in the equation would predict a maximal oxygen consumption of 37.0
ml/kg · min. A heart rate value of 172 beats per minute for a college-aged male
results in a predicted maximal oxygen uptake of 39.1 ml/kg · min. To simplify these
conversions Table 10-1 presents the predicted maximal oxygen uptake values determined from recovery heart rate scores.

Ideally, the most accurate measurement of maximal oxygen uptake would
take place in the laboratory, where fairly sophisticated equipment is used. This
type of test would require near maximal physical effort from the subject. While the
step test prediction method certainly does not possess the accuracy required for
research purposes, it does provide a valid method for classification purposes. The
step test method presented in this section gives as good an estimate of maximal
oxygen consumption as that obtained with other submaximal tests that require the
bicycle ergometer or treadmill, or performance in a running test on a track. You
can evaluate the predicted maximal oxygen uptake score by comparing this value
with the aerobic capacity classifications in Table 10-2. Although such classifications are subjective, they have been constructed from average values for aerobic
capacity of hundreds of trained and sedentary men and women measured in this
country and abroad.

THE TECHUMSEH STEP TEST: A VALID ALTERNATIVE

A step test has been developed for use with adult men and women of all ages.
While a heart rate score on this test cannot be transposed into a value for maximal
oxygen uptake, the recovery heart rates are valid for showing relative fitness for
aerobic exercise. The fitness classifications have been constructed from average
values based on a large sample from Techumseh, Michigan, a representative mid-
western community. Aside from the fact that the norms are applicable to a broad

Table 10-2. *Aerobic capacity classification based on sex and age.*

AGE	MAXIMAL OXYGEN CONSUMPTION (ml/kg · min)				
	LOW	FAIR	AVERAGE	GOOD	HIGH
Women					
20–29	28	29–34	35–40	41–46	47
30–39	27	38–33	34–38	39–45	46
40–49	25	26–31	30–37	38–43	44
50–65	21	22–28	27–34	35–40	41
Men					
20–29	37	38–41	42–50	51–55	56
30–39	33	34–37	38–42	43–50	51
40–49	29	30–35	36–40	41–46	47
50–59	25	26–30	31–38	39–42	43
60–69	21	22–25	26–33	34–37	38

age range, the test is attractive from a practical standpoint because the work level is relatively moderate and the stepping surface is the approximate height of most stairs.

The test can be performed alone, but it is much easier with a partner. Find a stair or stool *8 inches high.* The correct stepping height can easily be achieved by adjusting the stepping or floor surface with a board or similar hard, flat object. As with all standardized step tests, the correct stepping cadence is important, so practice briefly to make sure that you step up and down *twice* within a 5-second span, or *24 complete step-ups each minute for 3 minutes.* You can have your partner chant "Up, up; down, down; up, up; down, down" within a 5-second span to establish the proper cadence. Each new sequence starts at second 5, 10, 15, 20, and so on. For more precision, set a metronome at *96 beats per minute* giving one footstep per beat.

Once you master the cadence, either time yourself or have someone else signal you when to begin and stop. At the completion of 3 minutes of stepping, remain standing and locate your pulse. Exactly 30 seconds after stopping, measure your pulse for 30 more seconds. The number of pulse beats, from 30 seconds after stepping to the 1-minute post-exercise period, is your heart rate score. Refer to Table 10-3 to obtain your cardiovascular fitness classification for your age and sex.

Although a bench of different height than that used in either the Queens College or Techumseh step tests will not permit the comparison of heart rate scores with the norms, you can still determine a person's cardiovascular response to a standard exercise stress. This heart rate response can then serve as the frame of reference for evaluating cardiovascular adaptation to a particular program of physiologic conditioning. As the circulatory system becomes more efficient in delivering blood and oxygen, the exercise heart rate as well as the heart rate in recovery will decrease. *The important consideration is that the procedures for administering a step test prior to the start and during the program must be identical each time the test is taken.*

Table 10-3. *Step test classifications based on 30-second recovery heart rate for men and women.*

CLASSIFICATION	AGE			
	20–29	30–39	40–49	50 & OLDER
Men	**Number of Beats**			
Outstanding	34–36*	35–38	37–39	37–40
Very good	37–40	39–41	40–42	41–43
Good	41–42	42–43	43–44	44–45
Fair	43–47	44–47	45–49	46–49
Low	48–51	48–51	50–53	50–53
Poor	52–59	52–59	54–60	54–62
Women				
Outstanding	39–42*	39–42	41–43	41–44
Very good	43–44	43–45	44–45	45–47
Good	45–46	46–47	46–47	48–49
Fair	47–52	48–53	48–54	50–55
Low	53–56	54–56	55–57	56–58
Poor	57–66	57–66	58–67	59–66

*Thirty-second heart rate is counted beginning 30 seconds after exercise stops.
Based on information in H.J. Montoye, Physical Activity and Health: An Epidemiologic Study of an Entire Community (Englewood Cliffs, N.J.: Prentice-Hall, 1975).

FACTORS AFFECTING AEROBIC CONDITIONING

As shown in Figure 10-4, there are two major goals of aerobic conditioning: (1) to enhance the capacity of the central circulation for delivering blood, and (2) to develop the "metabolic machinery" to consume oxygen within the specific muscles.

To achieve success in aerobic conditioning you must consider several factors: (1) the person's initial level of cardiovascular capacity, (2) the frequency of training, (3) duration of training, (4) intensity of training, (5) the application of proper overload to the specific muscles to function under improved aerobic conditions, and (6) muscle fiber type.

Initial Level of Cardiovascular Capacity

As a general rule, the amount of improvement through physiologic conditioning depends largely on the person's initial state of cardiovascular capacity. Stated in simple terms, if you rate low at the start, there is room for significant improvement. On the other hand, if your aerobic capacity is already close to that of a world class endurance athlete, there is relatively little room to advance and the absolute amount of improvement may be small. However, a 5% improvement in physiologic function for an elite athlete is just as important as a 40% increase for a sedentary person. As a broad guideline, individuals classified as average in terms of maximal oxygen consumption generally show an improvement of about *10 to 15%* from an aerobic conditioning program. Although few studies have been conducted with

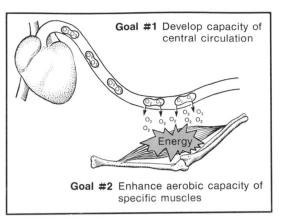

Figure 10-4. *The two major goals of aerobic conditioning. (McArdle, W.D., Katch, F.I., and Katch, V.L.: Exercise Physiology, Lea & Febiger, 1981.)*

women, it appears that the amount of improvement in aerobic capacity that can be
expected from training is similar to that of men.

The preceding discussion represents a generalization based on average values
for cardiovascular improvement reported in the literature. Individual differences
determined by genetic factors also play an important role in influencing the
amount of improvement in aerobic capacity as a result of training. This makes it
quite difficult to predict exactly how much improvement can be expected based on
a subject's pretraining test results. Due to inherited traits, some people possess a
relatively high aerobic capacity without having had any previous experience in
physiologic training or conditioning programs. Some physiologists contend that
a highly developed and efficient aerobic capacity is as much determined by
the "choice" of parents as by participation in programs of rigorous aerobic conditioning.

Frequency of Training

In general, it is necessary to exercise *at least* 2 days a week to bring about
adaptive changes in the aerobic systems. This was also true in training for muscular strength. Of course, it is possible to locate one or two research studies that
report a significant improvement in cardiovascular capacity as a result of training
only 1 day a week. The subjects in those studies, however, had been quite sedentary prior to training and for them any form of overload, even though infrequent,
would stimulate cardiovascular improvement. In contrast, the majority of experiments dealing with the optimal frequency of training indicates that a training response occurs if exercise is performed 2 or preferably 3 times each week for at
least 6 weeks. Interestingly several studies have shown that the improvements
resulting from running or cycling 4 or 5 times a week were either no greater or only
slightly greater than when the same exercise was performed only 3 times a week. It
seems that an extra investment of time may not be that profitable in terms of
producing changes in physiologic function. *On the other hand, if exercise is used
as a means for weight control, you should give strong consideration to exercising
5 or 6 days a week because this frequency of exercise can represent a considerable
caloric expenditure when compared with training only 2 days a week.*

Duration of Training

One of the most common inquiries concerning exercise participation deals with the optimal duration of the daily workout. For example, are 10 minutes twice as beneficial as 5 minutes of jogging? Would a relatively fast run of 2 or 3 minutes that is repeated several times be recommended over a run performed at a slightly slower pace yet continued for 20 to 30 minutes? Precise answers to these questions are difficult because the mechanisms underlying the improvement in aerobic capacity are still not clearly understood. What is known, however, is that both *continuous* as well as *intermittent* overload are effective in improving aerobic capacity. Even a single 3- to 5-minute bout of vigorous exercise performed three times a week will improve aerobic capacity. Similarly, performing less exhausting but steady-state exercise for 20 minutes or longer will also increase the pumping ability of the heart as well as the metabolic capacity of specific muscles. Most competitive endurance runners and swimmers spend from 2 to 5 hours or more per training session in activities geared to enhance the capacity of their physiologic systems.

Intensity of Training

Intensity of training is the most critical factor related to successful aerobic conditioning. The intensity of exercise reflects both the caloric requirements of the activity and the specific energy sources required. Intensity can be expressed in several ways: (1) as calories consumed, (2) as a percentage of maximal oxygen consumption, and (3) as a particular heart rate or some percentage of maximum heart rate, or (4) in terms of multiples of the resting metabolic rate required to perform the work. *By far, the most practical means of assessing and understanding the strenuousness of exercise is by means of the exercise heart rate.* Many researchers have used exercise heart rate to structure a training program and evaluate the effectiveness of various training intensities. In general, for college-age people the exercise must be of sufficient intensity to produce an increase in heart rate to at least 130 to 140 beats per minute. This is equivalent to about 50 to 55% of the maximum aerobic capacity or about *70% of the maximum exercise heart rate.* This intensity of exercise appears to be the minimal stimulus required to provide cardiovascular improvement. Although this level of cardiovascular stress represents the threshold intensity for training improvement, more intense exercise is even more effective.

In one study, subjects who trained at a heart rate of 180 beats per minute made greater gains in endurance capacity than groups that trained at heart rates of 150 and 120 beats per minute. This does not mean that exercise *must* be strenuous in order to obtain positive results. On the contrary, an exercise heart rate of 140 beats per minute (70% of maximum heart rate for young adults) represents only moderately intense exercise that can safely be continued for a long period of time with little or no discomfort. This training level is frequently referred to as "conversational exercise"; it is sufficiently intense to stimulate a training effect yet not so strenuous that it limits a person from talking during the workout. *It is unnecessary to exercise above this heart rate in order to improve physiologic capacity.* Recall that as cardiovascular capacity improves heart rate gradually becomes reduced. Consequently the intensity of exercise will have to increase periodically to achieve a threshold heart rate, or whatever target heart rate has been selected.

Within the framework of available research as well as the recommendations of the American College of Sports Medicine, it appears that an aerobic training program should be conducted 3 days a week utilizing 20 to 30 minutes of continuous exercise of sufficient intensity to expend about 300 kcal. This is usually assured by exercising at a pulse rate of about 70% of maximum pulse.

Specificity of Training

Another common inquiry concerning exercise participation deals with the question of whether swimming, cycling, or running is most effective in developing aerobic capacity. The usual answer is that each would probably be equally effective as a training stimulus, since all three provide an adequate overload to the central circulation. In fact, champion athletes in each of these activities are noted for their high maximal oxygen uptakes. Recall, however, that *two* physiologic capacities must be developed through an aerobic conditioning program. The first is the central circulation (heart and vascular system), which can be trained in a variety of "big muscle" activities such as running, swimming, rowing, and bicycling, *as long as a threshold heart rate is achieved during the training.* The second and equally important factor is the development of the aerobic metabolic capacity of the specific muscles. Activities like jogging, walking, and running *broadly* meet the two requirements of aerobic training for those activities that require a predominant use of the legs; that is, the central circulation can be overloaded and the lower leg musculature is used. One could raise the question, however, of whether training in running would improve one's aerobic capacity for swimming, or vice versa. Although the answers are far from definitive, the results from recent experiments have shown that improvement resulting from aerobic training is not as general as once thought.

In a study conducted in one of our laboratories, 20 men trained on a bicycle ergometer 20 minutes a day, 3 times a week, for 8 weeks. The training intensity was set at 85% of maximum heart rate. Each subject's maximal oxygen consumption was determined in the laboratory on both the treadmill and bicycle ergometer before and after the training program. Maximal oxygen uptake improved 7.8% as a result of the conditioning program of bicycle exercise when the subjects were measured on the bicycle test. However, when the subjects were measured during treadmill running, the improvement in aerobic capacity averaged only 2.6%. These results indicated that improvement in physiologic capacity was specific to the mode of exercise; there was little improvement in aerobic capacity when measured running, but a significant improvement when the test apparatus was the same as that used during training.

In another experiment of a similar nature, swimming was used as the means for aerobic conditioning. Fifteen men trained 1 hour a day, 3 days a week for 10 weeks. Training heart rates averaged between 85 and 95% of each subject's maximum heart rate. All subjects were measured during treadmill running, an exercise involving predominantly the leg muscles, and swimming, which uses the muscles of the arms and upper body. The results indicated complete specificity in the *improvement* in aerobic capacity with swim training. While improvements in maximal oxygen consumption averaged 11% when the subjects were measured while swimming, no improvement was demonstrated while running on the treadmill. This was surprising, since we had expected at least a minimal improvement on the running test due to the intense nature of the overload placed on the central circulation during the swim training. Apparently, there was no "transfer" in aerobic capacity from swim training to running.

At our present state of knowledge it is reasonable to advise that in training the aerobic systems for a specific activity such as rowing, swimming, or cycling, the method of training *must* overload the appropriate muscles required by the activity as well as provide an exercise stress for the heart and vascular system. In each of the above examples, the appropriate overload would consist of training in the actual activity.

Muscle Fiber Type

As we pointed out in Chapter 3, two distinct fiber types have been identified in human skeletal muscle. One type, the fast-twitch fiber, has a high capacity for the anaerobic production of ATP through the breakdown of carbohydrates to pyruvic acid and ultimately to lactic acid. The slow twitch fiber, on the other hand, is distinguished by its ability to generate ATP aerobically.

In terms of physiologic conditioning, several interesting questions arise concerning fast- and slow-twitch muscle fibers. First, does the distribution of each fiber differ significantly among people, especially among people who are successful in various sports? Second, can the metabolic capacity of each fiber be improved through a specific program of physiologic conditioning? Third, can fast-twitch fibers be changed into slow-twitch fibers through aerobic training, and conversely, would an anaerobic conditioning program develop predominantly fast-twitch fibers?

The answer to the first question is a definite yes. The average percentage of slow-twitch fibers in sedentary men is about 45 to 50%, but the variation is large. Even within an individual, the distribution pattern of fiber types can vary considerably from muscle to muscle. It would thus seem logical that those people with a large proportion of slow-twitch fibers in the leg muscles would be successful in endurance running, while those runners with a distribution favoring a predominance of fast-twitch fibers would tend to excel in sprint activities. Muscle biopsies from trained athletes support this contention (Figure 10-5). Successful endurance runners and cross-country skiers possess between 80 and 90% slow-twitch fibers in their leg muscles, while sprint-type athletes possess a predominance of fast-twitch fibers. As might be expected, athletes who perform in middle-distance events have an approximately equal percentage of the two types of muscle fibers. In an experiment designed to answer the question of whether fiber type can be changed with training, 6 men were trained for 1 hour a day, 4 days a week for 5 months. The exercise intensity required 75 to 90% of each subject's maximal oxygen consumption. Muscle biopsies from the leg were obtained and fiber type determinations were made before and after training. Although the work capacity of all subjects increased, training did *not* change the relative distribution of the fast- and slow-twitch muscle fibers in the leg muscles.

In summary, the percentage distribution of muscle fibers differs significantly among people and among the various muscles in the same person. Although the metabolic capacity of both fiber types can be increased through training, it appears that the distribution of these fibers is determined by the genetic code and largely fixed before birth or early in life. The distribution of fiber types probably cannot be greatly changed through physiologic conditioning, at least not in male adults. It also appears that a certain percentage of each fiber type is associated with success in certain types of sports activities, depending on their specific energy requirements. Although this suggests an obvious genetic predisposition to success in sports and to some degree in conditioning, training can improve the metabolic capacity of both slow- and fast-twitch fibers significantly.

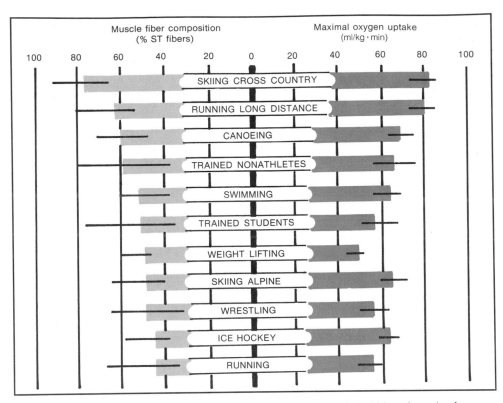

Figure 10-5. *Muscle fiber composition (percent slow-twitch fibers) (left side) and maximal oxygen uptake (right side) in athletes representing different sports. The dark horizontal bar denotes the range. (From Bergh, U. et al.: Maximal oxygen uptake and muscle fiber types in trained and untrained humans.* Medicine and Science in Sports, 10:*151, 1978. Copyright 1978, the American College of Sports Medicine. Reprinted by permission.)*

Developing an Aerobic Conditioning Program

In this section we present a method for gauging the intensity of training. We will also discuss the advantages and possible limitations of aerobic conditioning through intermittent and continuous training procedures.

Regardless of your present physical condition, there are some basic guidelines to follow as you begin your aerobic exercise program. These guidelines are based on both research and common sense, and are designed to help you achieve fitness effectively and enjoyably. The person who "pulls" a muscle or develops painful cramps early in an exercise program usually has violated one of the rules of intelligent conditioning.

1. *Start Slowly:* It is important to emphasize this point. Any sudden burst of vigorous activity following a few years of sedentary living can be dangerous. While it is normal to experience minor muscle aches and twinges of joint pain with the initiation of an exercise program, it is not normal to experience severe muscular discomfort or excessive cardiovascular strain. Anyone who has experienced

such discomfort knows that there is no greater discouragement to a program of regular exercise.

2. *Warm-Up:* Before you start any exercise program, it is important to stretch your muscles gently and limber up for at least several minutes. There are numerous warm-up and calisthenic exercises you can do (your own favorites included), to limber up joints and stretch muscles. You should also run in place, jog on a treadmill, skip rope, or cycle on a stationery bicycle. The important point is to perform a variety of big muscle exercises in a rhythmic, moderate, and continuous manner so your pulse attains between 50 and 60% of its maximum. This will help ease your cardiovascular system into the more vigorous exercise that is to follow.

3. *Dress Sensibly:* Wear loose-fitting, light cotton exercise attire (T-shirt, shorts, sweat socks and running shoes). Above all, be comfortable and allow sweat to evaporate freely from your body.

4. *Allow a Cool-Down Period:* After having exercised for 30 minutes or so, allow 5 to 10 minutes to gradually slow down before stopping. This allows metabolism to slowly progress back to normal levels. More importantly, however, a gradual cool down prevents blood from pooling in the large veins of the previously exercised muscles. Such *venous pooling* will bring about a drop in blood pressure to cause less blood to circulate to the brain and heart. Insufficient blood flow can cause dizziness, nausea, and even fainting, while a reduction in blood to the heart muscle may precipitate a series of irregular heart beats and trigger a dangerous cardiac episode.

DETERMINATION OF TRAINING INTENSITY

The intensity of training is probably the most important factor for increasing aerobic capacity. The term "intensity" is quite relative, however. What could pose a considerable exercise stress for one person might well be below the threshold intensity of 70% of maximum heart rate for the marathon runner. Thus it is necessary to evaluate a particular exercise task in terms of the stress it places on each person's aerobic systems. Several methods have been proposed for this purpose.

In one method the actual oxygen consumption during exercise is determined. For example, if jogging at 5.5 miles per hour requires an oxygen consumption of 33 ml/kg · min and the jogger's maximal oxygen consumption is 60 ml/kg · min, this particular exercise would represent an aerobic stress of 55% of the maximal aerobic capacity. For another person with a lower aerobic capacity of 40 ml/kg · min, the oxygen cost of jogging at 5.5 miles per hour would still be approximately 33 ml/kg · min, yet this person would be exercising at 83% of maximum. To provide a similar overload for the first jogger, the pace of jogging would have to be increased to about 8.6 miles per hour (48 ml O_2/kg · min). The strenuousness of any exercise is relative and depends on the present level of physiologic condition.

Although the assessment of exercise intensity by the direct measurement of oxygen consumption is quite accurate, it is impractical to measure oxygen consumption without a fairly extensive laboratory. An alternative is to use *exercise heart rate* to classify an exercise in terms of its relative intensity or strenuousness. This makes it possible to personalize an exercise program and regulate the intensity of exercise to keep pace with changes in physiologic capacity.

Train at a Percentage of Maximum Heart Rate

To train at a predetermined percentage of maximum heart rate requires a knowledge of what the heart rate would be during near-exhausting exercise. Someone's *actual* maximum heart rate can be determined immediately following 3 or 4 minutes of all-out running or swimming. Generally this procedure is inadvisable because such intense exercise is difficult and requires considerable motivation and could be dangerous for people predisposed to coronary heart disease. For this reason we recommend that people consider themselves "average," and use the age-predicted average maximum heart rates shown in Figure 10-6. As a general rule, maximum heart rate is approximately 220 beats per minute minus the person's age. In addition to the average age-adjusted maximum heart rates, Figure 10-6 illustrates the "training sensitive zone" that represents the threshold level of 70% and the upper level of 90% of maximum heart rate for each age group. *Conditioning of the aerobic systems will occur as long as the exercise heart rate is within this zone.*

Suppose a 30-year-old man wishes to train at moderate intensity, yet still be at or above the threshold level. A training heart rate would be selected that is equal to 70% of the age-predicted maximum heart rate, or a target exercise heart rate of 133 beats per minute (0.70 × 190). For a 54-year-old woman, on the other hand, the target heart rate would be 116 beats per minute (0.70 × 166). By trial and error each person can arrive at a walking, jogging, or cycling speed that would produce the desired target heart rate.

In carrying out this trial-and-error procedure, the person should exercise moderately for 3 to 5 minutes, counting pulse rate for 10 seconds immediately afterwards. If the exercise is not intense enough to produce the target heart rate, he repeats the same exercise but at a faster pace: jogging instead of walking, pedaling faster or switching to a lower gear while cycling, or swimming faster, covering a

Table 10-4. *Age-predicted maximum heart rate and "training sensitive zone" for submaximal exercise.*

AGE, YEARS	AGE-PREDICTED MAXIMUM HEART RATE	TRAINING SENSITIVE ZONE	
		LOWER LIMIT 70% HEART RATE	UPPER LIMIT 90% HEART RATE
15	210	147	189
20	200	140	180
25	195	136	175
30	190	133	171
35	185	129	166
40	180	126	162
45	173	121	156
50	166	116	149
55	160	112	144
60	155	108	139
65	150	105	135

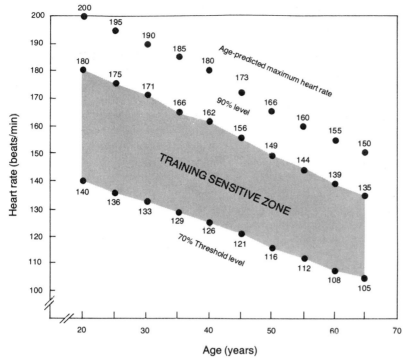

Figure 10-6. *Maximal heart rate and target zone for use in aerobic exercise
training programs.*

greater distance within a specified time. If the 30-year-old man wants to increase
his training intensity to 85% of maximum, his exercise heart rate would have to be
increased to 161 beats per minute in order to work at the same relative training
intensity of 85% of maximum (0.85 × 190) as the "typical" 30-year-old man.

In one of our laboratories we compared the cardiovascular response to running and swimming in trained and untrained subjects. In both activities the cardiovascular and metabolic adjustments to exercise were quite similar. The maximum
heart rate of swimming, however, averaged about 13 beats per minute lower than
that of running. This occurred in both trained and untrained subjects, and could
probably be attributed to the influence of the horizontal body position during
swimming and the cooler temperature of the water. Therefore if you select swimming as the training exercise consider the decrease in maximum heart rate that
occurs in this form of work in establishing the appropriate exercise intensity. We
recommend that an average of 13 beats per minute be subtracted from the age-
predicted maximum heart rate values in Figure 10-6. Consequently, a 25-year-old
person wishing to swim at 80% of maximum heart rate would select a swimming
speed that produced a heart rate of about 146 beats per minute (0.80) × (195 − 13).
This represents more accurately the appropriate training heart rate for swimming.

CONTINUOUS EXERCISE TRAINING

Continuous training involves steady state exercise performed at either moderate or high intensity for a sustained period. With this form of training it is only

necessary to exercise at least 15 minutes at or above the threshold heart rate. This can be done by swimming, cycling, stationary and forward running, rope skipping or stepping up and down on a bench. By its very nature, continuous exercise training is submaximum and can be engaged in for considerable time in relative comfort. This form of training is therefore suitable for people just beginning an exercise program. It is certainly a pleasanter method of training the oxygen transport system than the more intense interval training discussed in the next section. Continuous exercise training can be maintained at the threshold intensity of 70% maximum heart rate or increased to 85 or even 90% of maximum heart rate.

Continuous exercise training is desirable for endurance athletes because it allows them to train at nearly the same intensity as in actual competition. A champion middle-distance runner may run 5 miles continuously in 26 minutes during workouts at a heart rate of 180 beats per minute; this pace would not be exhausting but would still nearly duplicate race conditions. By finishing each exercise session with several all-out sprints stopped 30 to 40 seconds before exhaustion, the athlete can also train the anaerobic system that does play a small role in such middle-distance events, especially at the race's finish. The marathon runner will train at a slightly slower pace than the middle-distance champion because much longer distances must be run in practice as well as in competition. To provide some relief from this relatively high-intensity, continuous running, exercise can also be performed continuously at a lesser intensity but for longer durations. In this way distance runners can run between 100 to 200 miles during a week of training.

INTERVAL EXERCISE TRAINING

Many activities carried out in daily life in general, and in sports in particular, are intermittent and characterized by periods of intense activity interspersed with periods requiring only a moderate to low level of energy expenditure. Interval training is based on the concept that the correct spacing of work and rest periods enables someone to accomplish a tremendous amount of exercise over a considerable period of time with minimal fatigue. The rest-to-work intervals can vary from a few seconds to several minutes or more. The training prescription can vary in terms of the intensity and duration of the exercise interval, the length of the recovery period, and the number of repetitions. The apparent value of interval training is that intermittent exercise permits high intensity training for long periods of actual exercise at a given intensity. For example, running continuously at a "4-minute mile" pace would exhaust most people within 1 or 2 minutes. However, running at this speed for only 15 seconds followed by a 30-second rest period would enable many people to run 4 minutes at this near record pace. Of course this is not equivalent to a 4-minute mile; but during 4 minutes of running, 1 mile would have been run even though the combined work and rest intervals would have taken 11 minutes and 30 seconds.

The rationale for interval training also has a sound basis in physiologic fact. In the above example of the continuous run at a 4-minute mile pace a major portion of energy would be supplied through the anaerobic production of lactic acid. Within a minute or two the lactic acid levels would rise precipitously and cause exhaustion. On the other hand, intermittent exercise performed for 20 seconds or less would allow a severe load to be imposed on the muscles and oxygen transport systems before lactic acid accumulates appreciably. In this way the oxygen debt incurred during the work interval would be predominantly "alactic" in nature and recovery would take place quickly. The work interval could then begin again after only a brief rest period.

In interval training as in other forms of physiologic conditioning, *the intensity of exercise should be geared to the particular energy systems the person desires to train.* Sprint runners and swimmers should train by running or swimming for short distances at maximum intensity and near race pace. In training for longer distances the exercise interval should be at least 1 minute. A longer work interval will engage the aerobic systems, while shorter exercise intervals place a greater overload on the anaerobic energy systems. Generally you can use pulse rate to gauge the intensity of exercise as well as the length of the recovery period. Fast running for about 1 minute will elevate heart rate close to maximum levels. When heart rate decreases to 120 beats per minute after exercise, physiologic recovery is sufficient to begin another exercise. Only a short rest period should be used when the exercise intervals are less than 90 seconds because during this brief exercise period, oxygen consumption does not have enough time to adjust to the demands of the exercise. For this reason the succeeding exercise interval should begin before recovery is completed. This will ensure that the circulatory and metabolic stress will reach maximum levels even though the exercise intervals are short. With longer periods of intermittent exercise there is sufficient time for metabolic and circulatory adjustments; thus the duration of the rest interval is not as crucial.

At present there is insufficient evidence for a claim as to the superiority of either continuous or interval exercise training for enhancing aerobic capacity. Either training procedure will succeed; they can probably be used interchangeably.

11

Aging, Exercise, and Cardiovascular Health

THERE IS NO QUESTION that the physiologic and exercise performance capabilities of older people are generally below those of younger counterparts. What is uncertain, however, is the degree to which these differences are attributable to true biologic aging or simply the result of environmental factors and disuse brought on by social constraints that alter the lifestyles and activity opportunities for people as they grow older. No longer can older men and women be stereotyped as sedentary with little or no initiative to pursue active lifestyles. The past decade has seen a tremendous upswing in participation by so-called "senior citizens" in a broad range of physical activity experiences and exercise programs. Research clearly demonstrates that if an active lifestyle is continued into later years, a relatively high level of function is retained and vigorous activities can be engaged in safely and successfully.

Aside from the positive effects of exercise in maintaining physiologic function, it now appears that physical activity is protective against the ravages of this nation's greatest killer, *coronary heart disease*. It is well documented that individuals in physically active occupations have a two- to three-fold lower risk of heart attack than those in sedentary jobs. Furthermore, the chances of surviving a heart attack are much greater for those with a physically demanding job or life-style that includes frequent, vigorous physical activity.

Despite the inherent problems in heart disease research, there is considerable evidence to support the contention that evolution is not keeping pace with automation. Regular physical activity can modify some of the important risk factors related to heart disease. Elevated blood pressure can be lowered by participation in a regular program of aerobic conditioning; body weight, body fat, and elevated blood lipids can be favorably modified with prudent exercise and diet; the blood clotting mechanism can become normalized with exercise training, which might reduce the chances of a blood clot forming on the roughened surface of the coronary arteries. Research with animals has demonstrated an improved blood supply to the heart muscle as a result of regular exercise. If such an adaptation in the heart's circulation actually takes place in humans, then regular exercise may retard the heart disease process or maintain an adequate supply of blood to the heart muscle to compensate for those channels already narrowed by fatty deposits on the vascular walls. More than likely, these vascular adaptations would reduce the chance of heart attack and decrease the severity of damage to the heart muscle should a vessel become clogged.

From a practical standpoint, a lifestyle that includes vigorous physical exercise may be effective in preventing or at least slowing down the cumulative effects of the highly atherogenic American diet and a sedentary and stressful environment. Regardless of genetics, age, and life circumstances, individuals can significantly enhance their chances for a healthy life by adapting sound health habits that include regular exercise. In the sections that follow, we explore several aspects of the aging process with special emphasis on exercise and its relation to cardiovascular disease.

Aging and Bodily Function

As shown in Figure 11-1, the various measures of bodily function generally improve rapidly during childhood to reach a maximum between age 20 and 30 years; thereafter, there is a gradual decline in functional capacity with advancing years. While the trend with age is quite similar for the physically active person, physiologic function is attained at about 25% higher levels for each age category, so that a 50-year-old active man or woman may attain the functional capabilities of a 20-year-old counterpart. Although all measures eventually decline with age, not all decline at the same rate and considerable variation is noted from person to person and from system to system within the same person. Nerve conduction velocity, for example, declines only 10 to 15% from 30 to 80 years of age, whereas resting

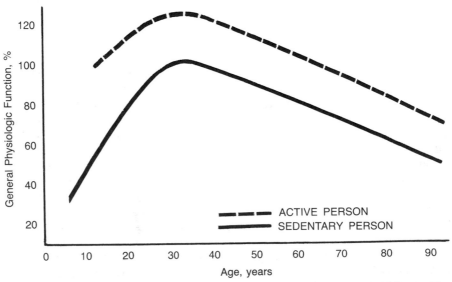

Figure 11-1. *Generalized curve to illustrate changes in physiologic function with age. All comparisons are made against the 100% value achieved by the 20- to 30-year-old sedentary person.*

cardiac index (ratio of cardiac output to surface area) declines 20 to 30%; maximum breathing capacity at age 80 is about 40% that of a 30-year-old. Brain cells die at a constant rate until age 60, while the liver and kidneys lose about 40 to 50% of their function between ages 30 and 70. By age 70, the average female has lost about 30% of her bone mass, while men at this age have lost only about 15%.

Because longitudinal exercise studies on the same subjects are lacking, it is not known whether long-term exercise participation can change the actual rate of decline in physiologic function or "override" deterioration in function that normally occurs with increasing age.

MUSCULAR STRENGTH

Maximum strength of men and women is generally achieved between the ages of 20 and 30 years when muscular cross-sectional area is usually the largest. Thereafter, there is a progressive decline in strength for most muscle groups so that between age 20 to 70 years there is a 30% reduction in overall strength. This is due primarily to a 3 to 5% reduction in muscle mass each decade due to a loss of total muscle protein brought about by inactivity, aging, or both. Indirect evidence indicates that habitual physical training facilitates protein retention and strength maintenance. Research *clearly shows* that older adults can greatly increase muscular strength and endurance with regular overload, strength-type training.

FLEXIBILITY

With advancing age, connective tissue (cartilage, ligaments, and tendons) becomes stiffer and more rigid and reduces joint flexibility. What is not certain, however, is the degree to which biologic aging per se causes these changes or the impact with which sedentary living or degenerative disease affects the tissues that comprise a specific joint. What is clearly known is that appropriate exercises that move joints through their full range of motion can increase flexibility in men and women at all ages.

NERVOUS SYSTEM

The cumulative effects of aging on central nervous system function are exhibited by a 37% decline in the number of spinal cord axons, a 10% decline in nerve conduction velocity, and a significant loss in the elastic properties of connective tissue. These changes may partially explain the age-related decrements in neuromuscular performance. When reaction time is partitioned into a central processing time and muscle contraction time, it is the central processing time that is most affected by the aging process. Thus, aging largely affects the ability to detect a stimulus and process the information to produce a response. Since reflexes, such as the knee jerk reflex, do not involve processing in the brain, they are less affected by the aging process than voluntary responses. While there appears to be a definite aging effect on the nervous system in terms of reaction time, *physically active groups (be they young or old) move significantly faster than a corresponding age group that is less physically active.* These observations suggest that an active life-style may *significantly* and *positively* affect movement function at any age. It is tempting to speculate that the biologic aging of certain neuromuscular functions can be somewhat retarded by regular participation in physical activity.

CARDIOVASCULAR FUNCTION

Maximal oxygen consumption and endurance performance show a steady decline in men and women after age 20 and by age 65, aerobic endurance has decreased by about 35%. The heart's ability to pump blood decreases about 8% per decade during adulthood. This is due largely to various age-related decrements in physiologic functions related to oxygen transport. One well-documented change is a progressive decline in the maximal heart rate. A rough approximation of the change in maximal heart rate with age is expressed by the following relationship:

$$\text{max HR (beats/min)} = 220 - \text{age (years)}$$

Also contributing to a reduced blood flow capacity with age is a reduction in the heart's stroke volume, which may reflect changes in myocardial contractility. Other age-related changes in the cardiovascular system include a reduction of blood flow capacity to peripheral tissues, a narrowing of the arteries that supply blood to the heart, and a decrease in the elasticity of major blood vessels.

Whether the preceding changes in cardiovascular function are a direct result of the aging process per se or of a lack of habitual physical activity has not been determined. *In fact, sedentary living may bring about losses in functional capacity that are as great as the effects of aging itself!* Results from training studies show no loss in aerobic capacity over a 10-year period for middle-aged men who were regular participants in running and swimming programs. In fact, at age 55, these active men had maintained the same values for blood pressure, body weight, and maximal oxygen consumption they had when measured at age 45.

BODY WEIGHT AND BODY FAT

The accumulation of excess fat usually begins early in childhood or develops slowly in adulthood. Middle-aged men and women invariably weigh more than college-aged counterparts of the same height—and this weight difference is due to differences in *body fat*. In the Western world, the average 20-year-old male will gain between one-half to one pound of fat each year until the sixth decade of life. In one study, the fat content of 27 adult men increased an average of 14 pounds over a 12-year period, from age 32 to 44. This was equal to the group's total gain in body weight over the duration of the study. The extent to which such gains in body fat during adulthood represent a normal biologic pattern is unknown. However, observations of older individuals who maintain physically active lifestyles suggests that this pattern can be reduced significantly.

After age 60, there is a reduction in total body weight despite increasing body fat. This is partly explained by the fact that in the upper age group many of the grossly overweight people have died, so there are just not many heavy subjects to be measured. Also, lean body weight does tend to decrease with age. This is largely due to the aging skeleton becoming demineralized and porous; concurrently, the quantity of muscle mass is reduced. Whether or not regular physical activity can retard these changes in body density with age is also unknown.

A major limitation of age-trend studies is that the same subjects are not followed over time, but rather different subjects in different age categories are evaluated at the same time. From these cross-sectional data, one attempts to generalize as to expected age-related changes for an individual. Sometimes these generalizations are misleading. For example, today's 70- and 80-year-olds are generally shorter than 20-year-old college students. This does not necessarily mean that we get shorter as we grow older (although this does happen to some extent). Rather, the young adults of this generation are better nourished than their 80-year-old counterparts were at the age of 20 and thus achieve optimal growth. In terms of body fat changes, the limited longitudinal data from the same subjects tend to support the trends noted in cross-sectional studies.

Does Exercise Extend Life?

Because older fit individuals have many of the functional characteristics of younger people, one could argue that improved physical fitness and a vigorous lifestyle may retard the aging process and thus offer some protection to health in later life. In an early study of exercise and longevity, it was shown that former Harvard oarsmen exceeded their predicted longevity by 5.1 years per man. While other research supported these findings, these studies were plagued with methodologic problems, including inadequate record keeping, small sample size, improper statistical procedures for estimating expected longevity, and an inability to account for other important factors such as socioeconomic background, body type, cigarette smoking, and family background.

One group of researchers attempted to overcome many of the limitations of earlier research in their study of the diseases and longevity of former college athletes. Because collegiate athletes usually have a longer involvement in habitual physical activity prior to entering college than non-athletes, and since they *may* remain more physically active after college, this seemed to be an excellent group to study to provide insight concerning exercise and longevity.

Figure 11-2 shows there was essentially no difference in the longevity of the ex-athletes compared to non-athletes. Some degree of equality in genetic background existed between the groups because the average age at death of grandpar-

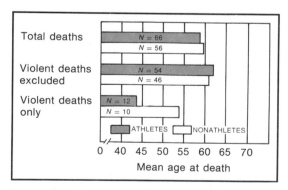

Figure 11-2. *Age at death of athletes and nonathletes. None of the differences between the groups are statistically significant. (From Montoye, H.J. et al.: The Longevity and Morbidity of College Athletes. Indianapolis, Ind., Phi Epsilon Kappa, 1957.)*

ents, parents, and siblings of ex-athletes and non-athletes was similar. These findings suggest that participation in athletics as a young adult does not necessarily ensure increased longevity in later years. It is still possible, however, that *regular* physical activity practiced *throughout life* offers protection in terms of health and longevity. Certainly, if aerobic exercise can reduce the risk of early heart disease, then regular physical activity should have a positive effect on longevity.

Coronary Heart Disease

Diseases of the cardiovascular system have reached epidemic proportions in the United States and other affluent, high-technology industrialized nations. Figure 11-3 illustrates that 53% of the total deaths in the United States are caused by diseases of the heart and blood vessels of which coronary heart disease (CHD) accounts for about 75% or nearly 800,000 deaths yearly. Between ages 55 and 65, about 13 of every 100 men and 6 of every 100 women die from CHD. While the death rates for women lag about 10 years behind those of men, the gap is closing fast, especially with the upswing in cigarette smoking by women. Although recent years have shown a slight decline in mortality from CHD, it is still the greatest single killer and the most common cause of premature death. It is estimated that 40 million Americans have cardiovascular disease. For every American who dies of cancer, 3 die of heart-related disease. The economic cost attributable to such health disasters—medical costs, loss of earnings and productivity—is estimated at more than 40 billion dollars a year, not to mention the emotional impact of a loss of a loved one in the prime of life!

THE HEART'S BLOOD SUPPLY

Although literally tons of blood may flow through the heart each day, none of its nourishment passes directly into the heart muscle. This is because there are no direct circulatory channels to the cardiac muscle within the heart's chambers. Instead the heart muscle has an elaborate circulatory network of its own. As shown in Figure 11-4, these vessels form an especially visible, crownlike arterial network, called the *coronary circulation*, on top of the heart. Openings for the two coronary arteries are situated in the aorta at a point where the fresh, oxygenated blood leaves the left ventricle to be distributed through the body. These arteries then curl around the heart's surface; the *right coronary artery* supplies predominantly the right atrium and ventricle, whereas the greatest volume of blood flows in the *left coronary artery* to supply the tissue of the left atrium and ventricle and a small part of the right ventricle. These vessels divide and eventually form a dense capillary network within the heart muscle.

The driving force of the heart pushes a portion of blood into the coronary arteries with each heartbeat. This blood is distributed throughout the heart's dense vascular network to the individual muscle fibers. The blood supply to the heart is so profuse that at least one capillary supplies each of the heart's muscle fibers. After the blood passes through the capillaries, it returns to the right atrium via the coronary veins. Exercise produces increased pressure in the aorta, which causes a greater flow of oxygenated blood to be forced into the coronary circulation.

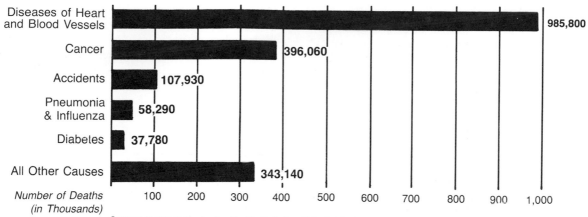

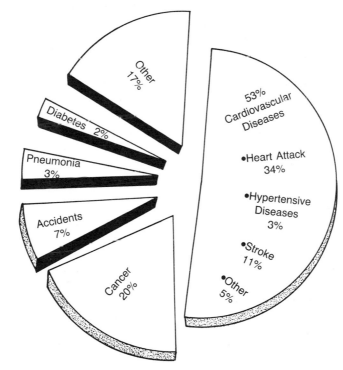

Figure 11-3. *Leading causes of death in the United States: 1978 Estimates.*

A LIFE-LONG PROCESS

As shown in Figure 11-5, CHD involves long-term degenerative changes in the inner lining of the arteries that supply the heart muscle. These vessels become congested with either lipid-filled plaques or fibrous scar tissue or both. Almost all people show some evidence of CHD, and it can be quite severe in seemingly healthy young adults.

245

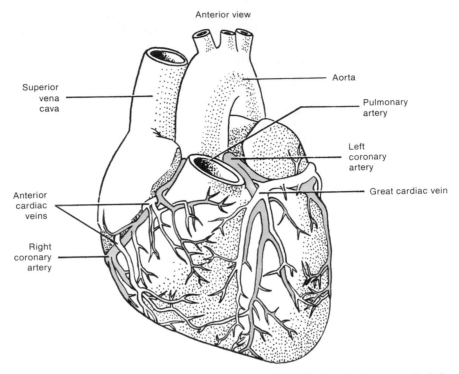

Anterior view

Aorta

Pulmonary artery

Left coronary artery

Great cardiac vein

Superior vena cava

Anterior cardiac veins

Right coronary artery

Figure 11-4. *The coronary circulation. Arteries are shaded dark and veins are unshaded. (McArdle, W.D., Katch, F.I., and Katch, V.L.: Exercise Physiology, Lea & Febiger, 1981.)*

The degenerative process of *atherosclerosis* begins in childhood and progresses silently for decades. There seems to be little harm, however, until there is marked arterial narrowing and the heart becomes poorly supplied with oxygen. The roughened, hardened lining of the coronary artery frequently causes the slowly flowing blood to clot. This blood clot may plug one of the smaller coronary vessels. In such cases, a portion of the heart muscle dies and the person is said to have suffered a heart attack or *myocardial infarction*. If the blockage is not too severe, but blood flow is still reduced below the heart's requirement, the person may experience temporary chest pains termed *angina pectoris*. These pains are usually felt during exertion, because this causes the greatest demand for myocardial blood flow. Such anginal attacks provide painful and dramatic evidence of the importance of adequate oxygen supply to this vital organ. Generally, death occurs from CHD when there is advanced obstruction in several major blood vessels supplying the heart muscle.

The mechanism by which fatty-type deposits or plaques develop is poorly understood. Many feel this lumpy thickening of the arterial wall begins as a fatty streak on the vessel's inner lining. It is often argued that this process is in some way facilitated by consuming a diet high in cholesterol and saturated fat. The deposition of fatty material eventually leads to calcification and fibrotic changes so that the arterial walls become narrower, rigid, and hard, making blood flow more difficult. It has also been suggested that changes in cellular characteristics of the vessel's smooth muscle wall initiate the athersclerotic process. These changes cause cellular mutation of smooth muscle cells and proceed in a manner similar to

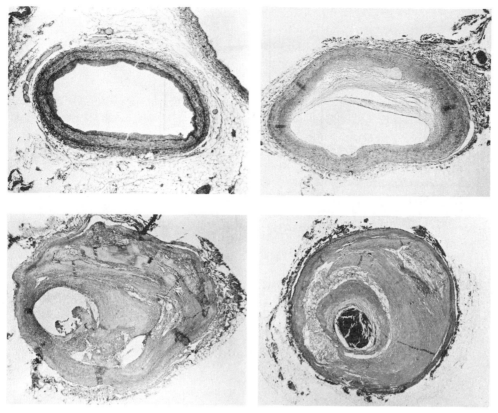

Figure 11-5. *Progressive narrowing of a normal coronary artery. During this degeneration process fatty deposits accumulate on the arterial wall. The wall becomes roughened and loses its elasticity, and the size of the opening becomes smaller. If the opening becomes too narrow, blood flows so slowly that it coagulates forming a clot. This plugs the artery depriving the heart muscle of vital blood to cause a heart attack.*

the development of a benign tumor. This abnormal cell division may be triggered by a sequence of repetitive injury to the arterial wall brought on by environmental factors such as diet, cigarette smoking, and high blood pressure.

RISK FACTORS FOR HEART DISEASE

Significant information has been gathered over the past 30 years on the natural history and dynamics of heart disease. By studying the incidence of heart attacks, chest pain, and sudden death in previously healthy people in large representative communities such as Framingham, Massachusetts, scientists have uncovered specific factors that contribute either directly or indirectly to the probability of getting this disease. From this, the relative importance of each factor has been established. *In general, the greater the risk factor the more likely it is that the coronary arteries are diseased or will become diseased in the near future.* This is not to say that a specific risk factor is the *cause* of the disease, as numerous factors may be acting and interacting in a cause and effect manner. However, based on the total evidence presently available it is prudent to assess these factors on a personal basis and make efforts to modify each within reasonable limits. In fact, part of the reason for the decline in CHD since the mid 1960s may be that people are taking charge of their lifestyles and modifying risk factors in favorable directions. The following is a list of the more frequently implicated CHD risk factors: (1) age and sex; (2) elevated blood lipids; (3) hypertension; (4) cigarette smoking; (5) physical inactivity; (6) obesity; (7) diabetes mellitus; (8) diet; (9) heredity; (10) personality and behavior patterns; (11) high uric acid levels; (12) pulmonary function abnormalities; (13) race; (14) electrocardiographic abnormalities during rest and exercise; and (15) tension and stress.

It is difficult to determine quantitatively the importance of a single CHD risk factor in comparison to any other because many of the factors are interrelated. For example, blood lipid abnormalities, diabetes, heredity, and obesity often go hand-in-hand. Compounding such observations is the often observed finding that physical training generally lowers body weight and body fat. Also, certain groups are generally exposed to less psychologic stress because of the nature of their occupation or cultural setting.

The factors of age, sex, and heredity are predetermined and cannot be controlled or remedied. Based on careful risk factor evaluation, however, three "treatable" factors—serum lipids, blood pressure, and cigarette smoking—stand out as potent, consistent CHD risk factors. Of somewhat less predictive value than these three *primary risk factors* are the risk factors of obesity, personality type, and physical inactivity. It must be noted that although these factors are closely associated with CHD, the associations do not necessarily infer causality. It still remains to be shown that risk factor modification offers effective protection from the disease. Until definite proof is demonstrated, however, logic causes us to assume that elimination or reduction of one or more risk factors will cause a corresponding decrease in the probability of contracting CHD.

AGE, SEX AND HEREDITY

The likelihood of developing CHD generally increases rapidly with age. For a white American male between the ages of 25 and 35 the chances of dying from heart disease is 10 in 100,000; this increases to 1000 in 100,000 between the ages of 55 and 64. At most ages women fare much better than men. For example, a middle-aged man stands about 6 times the chances of dying from a heart attack as a woman of similar age. However, American women still lead all other countries in heart disease rates and the specific sex advantage is reduced greatly in older age. This has led some to speculate that some of this CHD protection for women may be provided by hormonal differences between the sexes. The age risk factor is due in large part to the fact that other associated risk factors such as hypertension, elevated blood lipids, and glucose intolerance become more prevalent in older years. Although the cause is not known, heart attacks that strike at an early age appear to run in families.

BLOOD LIPIDS

The precise mechanism by which elevated blood fats (lipids) affect the development of CHD is almost totally unknown. Nevertheless, the overwhelming evidence links high levels of blood lipids with increased incidence of CHD. For example, the American Heart Association estimates that a man with a blood cholesterol level above 250 milligrams per 100 milliliters of blood (mg/dl) has about 3 times the risk of heart attack as a man with cholesterol below 200 mg/dl. In many cases, these elevated lipids are related to consuming diets high in saturated fats and cholesterol as well as to excess body fat and lifestyles that are physically inactive.

Cholesterol and triglycerides are the two most common lipids associated with CHD risk. These fats are not soluble in water so they do not circulate freely in the blood plasma. Rather, they are transported in combination with a carrier protein to form a *lipoprotein*. This lipoprotein can vary in size depending on how much protein and fat it contains. Serum cholesterol represents the total cholesterol contained in the different lipoproteins. Although it is proper to refer to an elevation in blood lipids as *hyperlipidemia*, it is more meaningful to evaluate and discuss the different types of *hyperlipoproteinemia*.

The distribution of cholesterol among the various *types* of lipoproteins is a more powerful predictor of heart disease than simply the total *quantity* of plasma lipids. This partially explains how one person with a high total serum cholesterol may not develop CHD, while another with a lower cholesterol level develops the disease. As shown in Figure 11-6, a high level of *high-density lipoproteins* (HDL, which comprise the smallest portion of lipoproteins but contain the largest quantity of protein and least amount of cholesterol) is associated with a lower heart

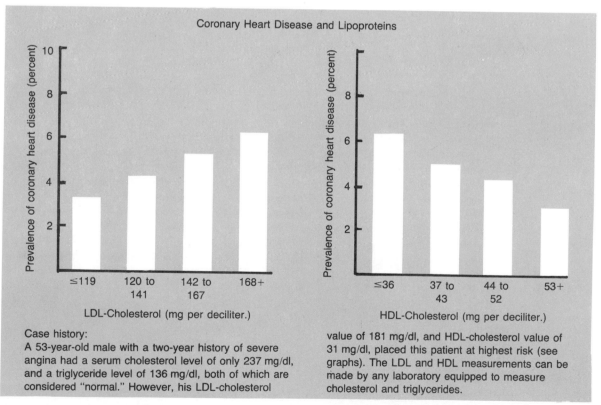

Figure 11-6. *Coronary heart disease and lipoproteins. (Courtesy CPC International. Best Foods Division.)*

disease risk, whereas elevated levels of the cholesterol-rich, *low-density lipoproteins* (LDL) represent an increased risk. In fact, data from the Framingham study suggest that high levels of HDL may actually confer longevity.

Although much controversy exists as to the precise role of lipoproteins in heart disease, it is generally believed that the LDL are the means for transporting fat throughout the body for delivery to the cells, including those of the smooth muscle walls of the arteries. Here it ultimately becomes involved in the artery-narrowing process of atherosclerosis. Whereas LDL carries cholesterol to the tissues, HDL may act as a scavenger gathering cholesterol from cells (including arterial walls) and returning it to the liver where it is metabolized and excreted in the bile. It is also possible that HDL may retard cholesterol buildup in the cells by interfering with the binding and subsequent uptake of LDL at the cell membrane of the peripheral tissue.

Research is currently progressing to clarify whether HDL is truly protective and what factors can raise them. For one thing, cigarette smoking has adverse effects on the HDL pattern while moderate alcohol consumption may improve the lipoprotein profile. *It is encouraging from an exercise perspective that HDL levels are elevated in endurance athletes and may be favorably altered in sedentary people who engage in vigorous aerobic training.* Concurrently, the LDL are lowered so the net result is a considerably improved ratio of HDL to LDL or HDL to total cholesterol. This exercise effect appears to be independent of whether or not the diet is low in fat or whether or not the exerciser is overweight. The effect of regular aerobic exercise on the blood lipid profile is certainly a strong argument for incorporating vigorous physical activity into a total program of health maintenance and preventive medicine.

HYPERTENSION

For individuals whose arteries have become "hardened" because fatty materials have deposited within their walls (or because the vessel's connective tissue layer has thickened), or whose arterial system offers excessive resistance to blood flow in the periphery due to nervous strain or kidney malfunction, systolic pressure at rest may be as high as 250 or even 300 mm Hg. The diastolic or run-off pressure may also be elevated about 90 mm Hg. Such high blood pressure, called *hypertension*, imposes a chronic, excessive strain on the normal functioning of the cardiovascular system. It has been estimated that one out of every five persons will have abnormally high blood pressure sometime during their lives. Presently, more than 24 million Americans have systolic pressures over 140 mm Hg or diastolic pressures over 90 mm Hg. These values form the *borderline* limits for the classification of high blood pressure. Uncorrected chronic hypertension can lead to heart failure, heart attack, stroke, or kidney failure.

Hypertension is often called the silent killer because it generally progresses unnoticed for decades before it deals its deadly blow. It is also a mysterious killer because the cause is unknown in more than 90% of the cases. Statistics indicate that the optimal blood pressure for longevity is 110 mm Hg systolic and 70 mm Hg diastolic. Anything higher results in an increased risk for disease. For example, a man with a systolic blood pressure above 150 mm Hg has more than 2 times the risk of heart disease as a man with 120 mm Hg.

Hypertension can often be reduced by altering factors over which we have direct control. If you are overweight, reduce; if you smoke, stop, for the nicotine may constrict peripheral blood vessels and elevate pressure. Reduce salt intake as sodium causes the body to retain fluid which boosts blood pressure. High blood pressure can also be effectively treated by relatively safe drugs (diuretics) that reduce fluid volume.

Further encouraging news is that *both systolic and diastolic blood pressure can be significantly lowered with a regular program of exercise*. In patients with documented coronary artery disease and in "borderline" hypertensive patients, the effects of exercise training on blood pressure were impressive. For middle-aged male patients resting systolic pressure decreased from 139 to 133 mm Hg following 4 to 6 weeks of training. In addition, during submaximal exercise, systolic pressure fell from 173 to 155 mm Hg, whereas diastolic pressure was also reduced from 92 to 79 mm Hg. Consequently, mean arterial blood pressure during exercise was reduced by approximately 14% following training. Based on available evidence, a prudent recommendation is to have your blood pressure checked periodically and include exercise in most therapeutic programs to manage hypertension.

CIGARETTE SMOKING

In terms of health status, the more a person smokes the less healthy he or she is likely to be in the future. Cigarette smoking may be one of the best predictors of CHD. In fact, the probability of death from heart disease for smokers is almost twice as great as for non-smokers. Essentially, the more you smoke, the deeper you inhale, the stronger the cigarette in terms of tars and noxious byproducts, the greater your risk. In addition, smokers are nearly 5 times as likely to have a stroke as non-smokers. The increase in death rate from heart disease among women in this country almost parallels their increased consumption of cigarettes. Surprisingly, this CHD risk for men and women is associated with 2 to 3 times more deaths than the excess mortality of cigarette smokers due to lung cancer!

It is generally observed that the smoking risk acts independently of other risk factors. At the same time, however, if other risk factors are present, the multiple risks interact in an *additive* way and cigarette smoking may even accentuate the influence of other risks. The interaction of the three primary CHD risk factors when elevated in the same person is shown in Figure 11-7. With one risk factor, a 45-year-old man's chances of CHD during the year is about 2 times that of a man with no risks. With three risk factors present, however, the man's chance of chest pain, heart attack, or sudden death is 5 times higher than if there were no risk factors present.

OBESITY

Approximately 40% of all Americans are considered too heavy in that their body weight is at least 10% above their ideal weight. This is not necessarily an adult problem as, for many, the onset of obesity begins in the first and second decades of life. The average male and female in the United States is 8 and 6 pounds heavier, respectively, than their 1960 counterparts. This is in spite of the fact that the nation's per capita caloric intake has steadily *decreased* over this 20-year period. Such facts further support the position that the "creeping obesity" in our society may be more due to physical <u>inactivity</u> than overeating.

It is difficult to determine quantitatively the importance of excess body fat per se as a risk to good health. While the death rate for men who weigh 30% more

**The Danger of Heart Attack
Increases with the Number of Risk
Factors Present**

(example: 45-year-old male)

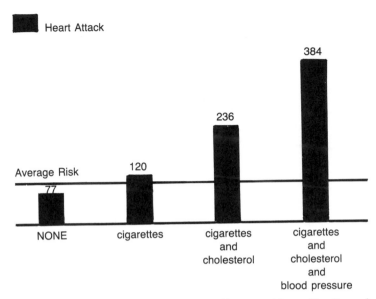

Figure 11-7. *Combining the risk factors. Persons with combinations of risk factors have experienced even more problems with coronary artery disease than those with fewer numbers. How risk factors are combined is a very important consideration. (From Heart Facts 1979, Dallas, Texas, by permission of American Heart Association, Inc. #55-005-C, 1978.)*

than they should is nearly 70% higher than those of normal weight, evidence is lacking to support the contention that a modest gain in body fat is harmful. Although excess body fatness has received great notoriety as a CHD risk factor, existing evidence suggests only a modest relationship, or that the relation is codependent with such factors as hypertension, diabetes mellitus, and cigarette smoking. Angiograms, which provide a picture of the internal dimensions of the coronary arteries, and autopsy studies have *not* revealed a strong association between body fatness per se and the degree of atherosclerosis. However, the overfat condition is often associated with multiple risk factors such as hypertension and elevated serum lipids. In addition, an obese person usually consumes a highly atherogenic diet, that is, one that is high in saturated fats and cholesterol. It certainly appears that extra pounds can mean a greater chance of developing high blood pressure as well as hyperlipidema, impaired glucose tolerance, and abnormal uric acid values. In the presence of these factors, obesity assumes a much stronger role as a health risk.

Weight loss and accompanying fat reduction generally normalize cholesterol and triglyceride levels and have a beneficial effect on blood pressure. In fact, the normally observed relationship between age and blood pressure is partially explained by the fact that as we grow older we have a tendency to put on weight. Although being too fat may not be a primary CHD risk factor, its role as a secondary and contributing factor in heart disease cannot be denied.

PERSONALITY AND BEHAVIOR PATTERNS

There appears to be a distinct type of personality that is susceptible to heart disease. The *coronary-prone* behaviors that typify what psychologists call the Type A personality reflect a lifestyle characterized as hard-driving, ambitious, impatient, short-tempered, hostile, and restless. Unrelenting pressures, drives, deadlines, anxieties, depression, and a constant struggle against the limitations of time are all part of this *stress syndrome*—with its accompanying recurrent and excessive stimulation of the body's "fight or flight" hormonal response that may be detrimental to the health of the heart. The opposite style of behavior, exemplified by the equally-capable, easy going, coronary-resistant Type B personality, is under no time pressure. This personality type is essentially categorized by the absence of Type A behaviors. Generally, one is neither all Type A nor all Type B, but rather a blend of both types of behavior patterns.

The precise manner in which personality traits and behaviors influence the development of CHD is unknown, let alone whether one's basic personality "type" can be significantly altered to influence a disease process. However, it does seem desirable to recognize, manage, and effectively channel excess stress in one's daily life. To this end, exercise blended with the techniques of behavior modification is a positive step in channeling potentially harmful behaviors into ones that will have positive "spin off." Regular exercise is an excellent way to vent tension and reduce stress.

PHYSICAL INACTIVITY

Information on the role of physical activity in protecting one from CHD is sometimes contradictory but generally encouraging. As shown in Table 11-1, physically active people generally have fewer clinical symptoms of heart disease. When a heart attack does strike, their chances for survival are much greater than those of

Table 11-1. *Age-adjusted first myocardial infarction (MI) among middle-aged men: incidence and early mortality in relation to physical activity.*

	MI's PER 1000 MEN AT RISK PER YEAR	PERCENT OF MEN DYING WITH FIRST MI	DEATHS PER 1000 MEN AT RISK PER YEAR
Least Active	6.26	52.6	3.29
Intermediate Active	3.78	26.7	1.01
Most Active	3.81	19.6	0.75

From Frank, D.W., et al.: Myocardial infarction in men: role of physical activity and smoking in incidence and mortality. Journal American Medical Association, *198*:1241, 1966, Copyright © American Medical Association.

their inactive counterparts. In a 9-year study of Californians, sedentary men and women were more than twice as likely to die prematurely compared to those who exercised frequently. In terms of health status, those who reported even mild exercise were better off than completely sedentary people.

Such findings are circumstantial and must be viewed with caution, however, for several reasons. For one thing, comparisons are often made between active and sedentary people with the assumption that other factors (blood lipids, hypertension, cigarette smoking, occupational status, body fatness) are essentially equal. This assumption is frequently not met. It is also possible that people with strong constitutions who are "destined" to live longer select active occupations or leisure-time pursuits. Likewise, as people detect certain symptoms of CHD, they move into a sedentary job or life-style. Thus at the time of death, they are rated as being inactive.

In studies where attempts have been made to account for the limitations of self-selection in research with humans, physical activity still stands out as a protector against heart disease. In two well-controlled studies, large numbers of physically active and less active San Francisco longshoremen and Harvard alumni were paired and matched on known coronary risk variables such as cigarette smoking, blood pressure, and body weight. The results were clear for both the longshoremen and the alumni; those men who were physically active (about 2000 kcal/week of exercise), be it on the job or in recreational pursuits, had a greatly reduced vulnerability to heart attack.

While the results from such studies strongly argue for regular physical activity, "critical or absolute proof" of the protective role of exercise against premature cardiovascular disease in humans is still lacking. Recent experiments made over 3½ years with non-human primates, however, provide some direct evidence for the benefits of exercise. In these studies, monkeys were randomly assigned to a moderate, treadmill exercise program of running, 1 hour three times a week, or no exercise. Both groups were fed a relatively high fat diet. The exercised animals had significantly higher levels of HDL and much lower LDL levels than their sedentary counterparts. Most importantly, they showed *no signs* of the coronary artery narrowing observed in the non-exercised group, and sudden death was observed *only* in the sedentary animals. Upon autopsy of all animals, the researchers noted that exercise was associated with substantially reduced overall atherosclerotic involvement. Exercise produced much larger and heavier hearts that were supplied with larger, healthy-appearing coronary arteries with less atherosclerosis. The conclusion was that moderate exercise may prevent or retard heart disease in primates.

While sufficient direct proof is lacking, the major weight of research on animals and humans indicates that regular exercise may operate against CHD in a variety of beneficial ways to:

1. Improve myocardial circulation and metabolism, which may protect the heart from hypoxic stress; this includes enhanced vascularization, as well as modest increases in cardiac glycogen stores and glycolytic capacity that could be beneficial when the heart's oxygen supply is compromised.

2. Enhance the mechanical or contractile properties of the myocardium; this may enable the conditioned heart to maintain or increase contractility during a specific challenge.

3. Establish more favorable blood clotting characteristics and other hemostatic mechanisms.

Table 11-2. *RISKO—Cardiac risk profile*

(Courtesy of Michigan Heart Association)

Listed below are those risk factors generally associated with an increased danger of heart attack. Study each risk factor and its row, finding the box which applies to yourself. Note the points given in the lower righthand corner of the box. After checking all the risk factors, total your score.

If your score is: 6–11—risk well below average   25–31—risk moderate
12–17—risk below average   32–40—risk dangerous
18–24—risk generally average   41–62—danger urgent! See your physician.

AGE	10 to 20 1	21 to 30 2	31 to 40 3	41 to 50 4	51 to 60 6	61 to 70 and over 8
[a]HEREDITY	No known history of heart disease 1	1 relative with cardiovascular disease Over 60 2	2 relatives with cardiovascular disease Over 60 3	1 relative with cardiovascular disease Under 60 4	2 relatives with cardiovascular disease Under 60 6	3 relatives with cardiovascular disease Under 60 7
WEIGHT	More than 5 lbs. below standard weight 0	−5 to +5 lb. standard weight 1	6–20 lbs. over weight 2	21–35 lbs. over weight 3	36–50 lbs. over weight 5	51–65 lbs. over weight 7
TOBACCO SMOKING	Non-user 0	Cigar and/or pipe 1	10 cigarettes or less a day 2	20 cigarettes a day 4	30 cigarettes a day 6	40 cigarettes a day or more 10
[b]EXERCISE	Intensive occupational and recreational exertion 1	Moderate occupational and recreational exertion 2	Sedentary work and intense recreational exertion 3	Sedentary work and moderate recreational exertion 5	Sedentary work and light recreational exertion 6	Complete lack of all exertion 8
[c]CHOLESTEROL OR FAT % IN DIET	Cholesterol below 180 mg.% Diet Contains no animal or solid fats 1	Cholesterol 181–205 mg.% Diet Contains 10% animal or solid fats 2	Cholesterol 206–230 mg.% Diet Contains 20% animal or solid fats 3	Cholesterol 231–255 mg.% Diet Contains 30% animal or solid fats 4	Cholesterol 256–280 mg.% Diet Contains 40% animal or solid fats 5	Cholesterol 281–300 mg.% Diet Contains 50% animal or solid fats 7
[d]BLOOD PRESSURE	100 upper reading 1	120 upper reading 2	140 upper reading 3	160 upper reading 4	180 upper reading 6	200 or over upper reading 8
SEX	Female under 40 1	Female 40–50 2	Female over 50 3	Male 5	Stocky male 6	Bald stocky male 7

[a]Count parents, grandparents, brothers and sisters who have had a heart attack or stroke.
[b]Lower your score one point if you exercise regularly and frequently.
[c]If you do not know your cholesterol level, the average U.S. diet contains 40% fat.
[d]If you have no recent reading but have passed an insurance or industrial examination, the chances are you have an upper reading of 140 or less.

4. Normalize the blood lipid profile, especially via an increase in HDL and lowering of LDL.

5. Favorably alter heart rate and blood pressure so the work of the myocardium is significantly reduced at rest and during exercise.

6. Achieve a more desirable body composition (higher lean to fat ratio).

7. Establish a more favorable neural-hormonal balance that may conserve oxygen for the myocardium.

8. Provide a favorable outlet for psychologic stress and tensions.

9. Increase the body's ability to dissolve blood clots that could block a blood vessel to cause a stroke (brain) or myocardial infarction (heart).

In light of these findings, most physicians and exercise specialists prescribe exercise as a preventive and rehabilitative health measure.

ASSESS YOUR HEART DISEASE RISK—"RISKO"

Table 11-2 is a chart of risk factors that gives some idea of a person's chances for developing heart disease. This chart is a modified form of a more elaborate version generated from the more than 30 years of research on the natural history of heart disease in the community of Framingham, Massachusetts. The assessment is for adult men and women of all ages. While this is certainly not a substitute for regular medical checkups, the information obtained will be helpful in giving insight as to potential areas for concern. Many of these telltale characteristics are habits or the result of habits that can be controlled.

To play RISKO, assign the appropriate numerical value that represents your present status for each category. Add up the scores in each category to determine your relative risk. Keep in mind that while there is nothing you can do as to your age, sex, and heredity risks, other factors such as blood pressure, tension, cigarette smoking, serum cholesterol, diet, exercise, and obesity can be modified. For example, the Framingham study shows that abstinence from smoking for 2 years reduces heart disease risk by one-half.

12

Questions and Answers About Nutrition, Weight Control, and Exercise

T his chapter contains many of the questions we are often asked about nutrition, weight control, and exercise. We have answered the questions in a conversational manner, omitting supplementary material for the sake of brevity. More in depth coverage can be found in textbooks that specifically deal with exercise physiology or nutrition.

Does the average American have good nutrition?   No. The typical American diet falls far short of what is recommended by the American Heart Association for meeting optimal standards of nutrition, being too high in total fat content, too low in starch, and containing too much salt and too many calories.

Are vitamin and mineral supplements necessary in order to obtain the optimal daily requirements?   For the most part, no. If you eat proper foods from the basic Four Food Groups you should easily obtain all of the necessary vitamins and minerals. Notable exceptions include pregnant women and women who lose large amounts of iron during their menstrual periods. Individuals unable to eat well-balanced meals may require vitamin and mineral supplements in the daily diet.

Are complex carbohydrate food sources better than simple carbohydrate foods?
The simple carbohydrates, the sugars, provide calories but little else in the way of nutrients. In essence, they are "empty calories." On the other hand, the complex carbohydrate foods such as beans, peas, nuts, seeds, vegetables, and whole grain breads and cereal products contain many essential nutrients in addition to calories. Increasing the consumption of certain complex carbohydrates can also increase the proportion of dietary fiber. You can obtain enough fiber in your diet if you eat fruits and vegetables and whole grain breads and cereals. In this case, there is no reason to add fiber to foods that do not already contain it.

Do athletes require different foods for energy?   Careful research has shown that athletes do *not* require any special foods to improve sports performance. Balanced meals containing the necessary vegetables, milk, meat, breads and cereals, and fruit are sufficient to supply the essential vitamins, minerals, amino acids, and calories for athletes as well as non-athletes. For the most part, a person with an increased energy expenditure will increase nutrient intake sufficiently to meet all nutritional demands. Contrary to popular belief, athletes do not require added supplementation of any kind. This includes runners, football players, gymnasts, weight lifters, body builders, skiers, tennis players, hockey, basketball, and baseball players, golfers, bowlers, race car drivers, jockeys, and wrestlers.

How does food preparation affect caloric value? Normal preparation of foods by cooking, freezing, cutting and blending does not appreciably change the caloric content of foods. However, adding rich sauces to meals or frying foods does increase the total number of calories consumed by an amount equal to the added food resources. All foods contain calories—the more you eat, the more calories you consume. Blending foods together doesn't "hide" the calories.

Can I eat all my food at one meal instead of spreading it out over three, four, or five meals? No. This may upset the body's metabolism and cause potentially harmful changes in blood fats. Eating all your calories in one meal may stimulate the body to store more of the calories as fat. For example, a one-meal a day schedule will increase appetite, one of the major causes for breaking a diet.

Are organic or natural grown foods more nutritious than conventionally grown foods? The nutritional value of both is the same. Unfortunately, advocates of health, organic, and natural foods frequently proclaim their products are safer and more nutritious than conventionally grown and marketed foods. Most of these claims, however, have no basis in scientific fact! They do have one thing—they cost much more—often twice as much—without added health benefits or better nutritional quality. Scientific experiments conducted for over 25 years have established no differences between the nutritive value of organic and health foods and foods grown with chemical fertilizers. Vitamins from natural sources have no known nutritional superiority over synthetic vitamins. There's no need to distrust or be fearful of the regular food supply. Remember, the health food business is big business—3 billion dollars worth in 1980, up from 50 million in 1972. Money buys advertising. Lots of it. As one prominent scientist has said of the health food craze, "Americans love hogwash." In short, save your money. Use common sense by eating a balanced diet that incorporates a wide variety of nutritious foods and by practicing moderation in eating any single food.

Will lowering cholesterol intake help to prevent heart disease? Cholesterol is a complex fat-like substance produced by animals. It is a necessary part of the structure of cell membranes and plays an important role in the production of sex and adrenal hormones and of vitamin D. Cholesterol is also essential in the process of repair of the body's tissues. Because of its importance for maintaining health, most cholesterol is made in the body rather than taken in from the foods we eat. While cholesterol is found in all tissues, only the cholesterol found in the blood has been associated with the development of coronary disease. One of the major hotly debated unknowns is whether the cholesterol one consumes has any effect on the total amount of cholesterol in the body.

Recent research has indicated that there are two main carriers of cholesterol in the blood, high density lipoproteins (HDL) and low density lipoproteins (LDL). Cholesterol transported by HDL appears to be a healthy form of cholesterol. It is believed that HDL actually picks up or scavenges cholesterol from the wall of the artery and transports it to the liver where it is broken down and excreted. This should lower the risk of coronary heart disease. Cholesterol carried by LDL is believed to have the opposite effect. LDL appears to carry cholesterol to the arterial wall and deposit it there, thus contributing to the clogging process and the risk of developing coronary disease. Regular aerobic exercise has been shown to significantly raise the HDL and lower the LDL in men and women.

What exercise burns the most calories? Exercises that engage the large muscles of the trunk and extremities produce the highest energy requirements if continued for prolonged periods of time. Cross-country skiing, running, bicycling, swimming, and rowing a boat are excellent examples, but other activities such as skin diving and certain racquet sports can also provide high caloric outputs depending on exercise intensity and duration. From an energy standpoint, it is much better to continue in an activity for a prolonged period of time at a reasonable pace than to perform in the same activity for a short time period. For example, a 150-pound person expends about 110 kcal while jogging a mile in 12 minutes. If continued for 3 miles, the total calorie output would equal 330 kcal. If the same person runs 1 mile at a fast pace of 5 minutes and 30 seconds per mile, then only about 130 kcal are expended.

Is it advisable to lose weight gradually? Most nutrition experts agree that a loss in body fat of up to 2 pounds (0.91 kg) each week is within acceptable medical limits. This guideline is partially based on the fact that those who have been successful in achieving and maintaining a desirable body weight lost no more than 1.5 pounds (0.68 kg) per week during the period of caloric deficit. A more conservative approach would establish a target loss of only 1 pound (0.45 kg) per week. Then even under the best circumstances, the dieter would require 20 weeks to lose 20 pounds (9.1 kg) of fat.

What is the optimal duration of a successful diet plan? This depends on the goals of the program. It must be remembered that the caloric equivalent of each kilogram of weight loss increases substantially as the duration of caloric restriction increases. This is the major reason why it is so important to maintain a calorie deficit for extended time periods; shorter periods of calorie restriction result in a larger percentage of water and carbohydrate loss per unit of weight reduction with only a minimal decrease in body fat. While the calorie equivalent of 1 kg of weight approaches only 3000 kcal during the first 4 or 5 days on a reduced intake, the calorie equivalent reaches 7000 kcal after 2 months of maintaining a caloric deficit.

If I'm trying to lose weight, should I check my weight daily? People react differently to repeated weighings. For those who prefer a daily weigh-in, this provides a "check" to see how they're doing. It's really a stimulus-response situation. If the stimulus (daily weigh-in) provides a "good" response (weight loss), then positive reinforcement occurs and the person will remain motivated to try to maintain the weight loss. In this case, the daily weigh-in serves as the award and provides an accurate appraisal of progress.

Some people abhor daily weighings out of fear of failure—not wishing to be reminded if there is no reward. Even a slight decrease in weight is not enough as people expect large changes quickly. When this doesn't happen, it's easy to become discouraged. If you want to weigh-in daily, do so at a set time each day. Be sure to wear the same clothing and keep all conditions constant prior to your weigh-in, such as exercise, food consumption, and bowel habits.

Can intestinal surgery or wiring the mouth shut correct obesity? Not consistently. These procedures have not proven successful for the majority of people who have tried them, and some of the surgical ones have proved fatal. They are not generally successful because they do not teach people to alter and successfully control their eating and exercise habits. Last resort methods should be reserved for life-threatening situations.

When I was younger it seemed that I could eat as much as I wanted without gaining weight. Why does everything I eat now seem to turn to fat? You have what has been termed "middle age, creeping obesity." As people get older they tend to gain weight for several reasons. They become less active, so they burn less calories than when they were younger. But their food intake often stays the same or even increases slightly. This is coupled to the fact that as you age your metabolism slows down and your body requires fewer calories. It has been estimated that for every decade after age 20, there is a 10% reduction in resting calorie requirement. If eating habits don't change, the additional foods eaten convert to fat. Eating only 10 extra kilocalories a day will add 1 pound (0.45 kg) of fat in a year. At this rate, you would gain 25 pounds (11.3 kg) of fat from age 20 to age 45. The moral is that as you become older, you should eat less and exercise more.

What about isometrics and weight resistance training for weight loss? Exercise that lasts for only a few seconds such as isometrics or weight lifting that involves maximum effort of isolated muscle groups produces a minimal expenditure of calories. These activities are primarily for obtaining and maintaining muscular strength. One form of weight training called circuit weight training, may be helpful in weight reduction. This system involves the performance of many repetititons at a moderate intensity for different exercises within a specified time period. With this system, it is possible to exercise continuously for 30 to 45 minutes; this will burn sufficient calories in the range of 5 to 9 kcal/min to aid in weight loss.

Will I lose more weight if I sweat heavily while exercising? You will weigh less after exercising because of fluid loss, not a diminution of fat tissue. It is not uncommon to lose 2 to 3 pounds due to the sweating that accompanies vigorous exercise. This fluid will and should be replaced shortly after exercise by normal thirst, so don't be fooled by a sudden but brief drop in your weight. Be sure to drink water prior to, during, and after vigorous exercise to prevent dehydration. You should consume fluids whenever you're thirsty. A good rule of thumb is to drink until your thirst is satisfied, and then a little more.

261
*Questions and
Answers About
Nutrition,
Weight Control,
and Exercise*

Will excess carbohydrates make me fat?   Absolutely. Once the carbohydrate reserves of the liver and muscles are filled any excess carbohydrate is converted to fat. Excessive calories be they in the form of protein, fat, or carbohydrate, will make you fat.

Can I change muscle into fat?   Muscle does not change into fat nor fat into muscle. This is a widespread misconception. If you eat too much and exercise too little, any calories beyond those you need to fuel your body will be stored as fat, regardless of whether these excess calories are from carbohydrates, fats, or proteins. If muscles are not used, they will weaken and diminish in size, but they won't change into fat.

How much exercise should an obese person undertake?   As much as possible. Walking at least 1 hour a day, 7 days a week, is highly desirable. Two workouts a day are even better. Depending on the severity of the obesity (and assuming no other medical complications), the initial workouts will depend on individual tolerance to exercise. For the first week or two, sessions should consist of stretching and limbering exercises (5 minutes) and a minimum of 15 minutes of walking at a brisk pace. This 2 week starter program is a "break-in" period where the body adjusts to the new activity level. In the absence of lower leg and ankle pain, the duration should be systematically increased to the 1-hour time period. Coupled with moderate restraint of food intake, such a program will generally produce excellent results in terms of fat loss and a restructuring of daily activity and eating patterns. The obese should not be pampered. Until goals are achieved, there must be a significant increase in exercise output if long-term results are to be maintained.

Is any form of passive exercise effective?   No. This includes rolling machines (they do not remove or redistribute fat), vibrating belts (they do not "break down" fat), vibrating tables (they do not improve posture), massage (absolutely useless for fat reduction), electric stimulators (can be lethal), and figure wrapping (quackery in terms of fat loss or muscle development). Unscrupulous promoters play upon the hopes of millions who are desperate to shed excess fat. There's simply no excuse for the public's apparent support of miraculous weight loss schemes and gimmicks. Hopefully, an educated public can help to stem the tide of erroneous, misleading, and questionable practices.

What's the best diet for weight loss?   Diets are not the key—correct habits are. This means that people who follow sound nutritional practices by eating well-balanced meals, and participate in an exercise program designed to promote improvements in cardiovascular function, have an excellent chance of achieving personal objectives. For people in good health, there is no one "best" diet for promoting long-term results. Weight loss through dieting per se is, for the most part, only temporary. Perhaps the best diet is exercise!

Is there such a thing as cellulite?   Cellulite is best described as fat that bulges out to produce a characteristic waffly, orange peel appearance, usually on the hip, thigh, and buttocks. Cellulite theorists argue that women are more affected than men because of their different hormonal and physical makeup. The advocates of gadgets, gimmicks, and creams to remove cellulite maintain that it is a form of fat gone wrong—a combination of connective tissue, fat, water, and toxic wastes that should be eliminated from the body. Supposedly, this mixture hardens to form the characteristic pockets of the gel-like substance, cellulite.

From a scientific viewpoint, the whole concept of cellulite is irrational and unscientific. Double-blind biopsy studies were made by pathologists of fat from people with dimply, lumpy fatty tissue and those with normal appearing fat tissue. There was no difference in the chemical composition of the fat cells. The difference in appearance of fat is probably caused by an increase in fat cell size (women tend to deposit fat in the hips, buttocks, and thighs) which may cause fat compartments to bulge and produce a waffled appearance of the skin. There simply is no basis in fact for "cellulite." It's Madison Avenue advertising—nothing more!

What is the influence of carbohydrates in exercise? Carbohydrates serve important functions in exercise. They provide rapid energy without oxygen being used. This helps you engage in all-out or sprint-type total exercise. Also, without carbohydrates, the body has difficulty generating energy from fats for sustained moderate exercise. This is what happens when the marathon runner hits "the wall." They have plenty of fat to continue, but the liver and muscle carbohydrate reserves are almost empty. Similarly, people who go on low-carbohydrate diets often suffer chronic fatigue due to the depletion of carbohydrate reserves. It is important that 50 to 60% of your total caloric intake consist of carbohydrates, especially in the complex form of starch—for example, grains, rice, potatoes, vegetables, and spaghetti.

How important is protein as an energy source for exercise? Protein is not a prime energy nutrient for the body as it only provides about 5 to 15% of the body's energy needs. In long-distance exercise and with semi-starvation diets the body relies more and more on protein for energy at the expense of the lean tissue. As a general rule, however, the quantity of protein in a well-balanced diet is more than adequate to supply the needs of vigorous training. If you eat excessive protein, the body simply converts it to fat and stores it as fat.

What about iron loss during a woman's menstrual cycle? Women need about twice the daily iron requirement as men because of the small blood loss during menstruation. The best way to compensate is to take an iron supplement or rely on foods rich in iron, such as beans, chickpeas, prune juice, or liver. If iron insufficiency persists, iron deficiency anemia may develop. Anemia reduces the blood's ability to carry oxygen and, consequently, has an adverse affect on the body's capacity for aerobic exercise.

Is it safe to exercise during pregnancy? Generally, a woman who is enjoying a normal pregnancy should exercise on a regular basis. The additional requirements of exercise during pregnancy are essentially those imposed by the extra weight of the developing fetus. The exercise can consist of large muscle, aerobic activities (walking, cycling, jogging, swimming), as well as light resistive strength building, stretching, and toning exercises. However, we stress the importance of doing this in consultation with a physician. In a normal pregnancy, the exercise is beneficial for the mother, the developing fetus, and for her supply of milk for nursing. Many physicians report significantly less post-delivery complications in women who have maintained a regular exercise program throughout the pregnancy. Strengthening exercises for the abdomen and lower back also help with the quick recovery of muscle tone in those areas in the weeks following delivery. When in doubt, check with a physician.

What exercises can you recommend for use at home? Passive devices, such as belts, shakers, rollers, and other mechanically driven instruments are absolutely worthless. Electrical stimulators are useless for weight control and conditioning. Don't buy them; don't use them; don't waste your money. You are much better off doing just about anything physical that uses your muscle power. Invest in a jump rope, strengthening equipment, a good pair of running shoes, or in a stationary bicycle. But avoid the bicycles with moving handlebars and moving seats. Buy one that weighs at least 50 pounds because it will stand up under heavy use. Such a bicycle is convenient and simple to use but can be expensive; prices range from about $225 to several thousand dollars.

Can extra protein help in muscular development? We need roughly 1 gram of protein per day for each 2.2 pounds of body weight, about 2 to 3 ounces for an average-size adult. While careful research on the protein requirements of weight lifters and body builders has not been done, it is generally believed that the normal protein intake is sufficient to supply the increased protein needs of a developing musculature. In all likelihood, extra protein is of no benefit. Excessive protein intake can be harmful, in fact, because it places a strain on the liver and kidneys. Protein obtained from animal sources (meats, eggs, dairy products) is usually accompanied by relatively large quantities of fat, which is not healthful and besides is high in calories. This problem can be alleviated by consuming protein from diversified plant sources. Additional protein consumed in powder supplements will not transform small muscles to larger ones—despite the overzealous and unsubstantiated claims of manufacturers.

Is it better to exercise harder for a short time or to take it easier but continue longer? For cardiovascular benefits, one should exercise at a training intensity of at least 60% of maximum pulse rate. If it can be tolerated, 70 to 85% is even better. If you exercise intensely, obviously fatigue occurs more quickly. To run a mile "all-out" in 6 minutes may certainly be exhausting, but a slower pace to cover the same distance will also stimulate the development of aerobic fitness and will burn about the same number of calories per mile! And of course, the exercise duration can be continued and several miles covered with few debilitating side-effects compared to the sprint-type exercise. We recommend that people exercise at heart rates within their "training sensitive zone" for a minimum of 30 minutes per session, 3 to 4 times a week.

Is aerobic dancing a good form of exercise? Yes. Not only is it a lot of fun, but the intensity of the workouts (performed within the training sensitive zone), duration

(30- to 45-minute sessions), and frequency (2 to 3 days a week), are sufficient to promote mild to moderate improvements in cardiovascular function and overall toning and muscular endurance.

What is the best type of strength training?   No one really knows! Every manufacturer of strength equipment makes claims about the benefits of their particular products. There is no question that strength does indeed increase when a systematic program of progressive overload is applied. But there is really no good evidence that one brand of machine or device is any more effective than another. A person's perception of what is "best" is probably directly related to the amount of advertising and promotional budget for a particular product.

What kind of clothing is best to wear when exercising in cold weather?   The emphasis should be on lightweight, easy-to-open clothes that allow for evaporation of sweat. Wet, sweat-laden clothing literally sucks heat from the body. Garments made of Gore-tex or similar fabrics help cut the wind and repel water, and at the same time "breathe," so moisture (sweat) isn't trapped inside. When doing exercise with the arms or legs, a large amount of blood flows through these areas as their metabolism increases; this helps ensure adequate warmth. A pair of sweat pants or nylon pants, and in cold weather (below freezing), thermal underwear, will add additional protection. Additional groin protection for men is also called for to avoid frostbite in that area. Also, wear mittens, not gloves because mittens keep the fingers together to provide more warmth. When worn, a wool cap can reduce as much as 40% of the body's heat loss during moderate to intense exercise. In extreme cold or with severe wind chill, a scarf will help reduce the chance of frostbite around the face and ears. The important consideration is to keep warm initially during exercise, but then to remove layers of clothing as the body warms up. Parkas are fine for ice fishing or sitting in a football stadium, but they can be a problem when jogging, ice skating, or cross-country skiing.

What is the ideal dress for exercise in warm weather?   Warm weather clothing should be lightweight and loose fitting to permit the free circulation of air between the skin and environment. This promotes evaporation and subsequent body cooling. Cottons and linens absorb moisture readily, whereas heavy "sweat shirts" and clothing made of rubber or plastic retard the vaporization of moisture from the skin surface; this significantly inhibits or even prevents evaporative cooling. Color is also important because dark colors absorb heat, whereas light colors reflect heat rays.

Can frigid air cause lung damage during exercise?   No. All the evidence shows that even the coldest air warms up in the nose and throat before it enters the lungs. Lung tissue can't freeze while you exercise. Cold weather exercise may produce an uncomfortable dryness in the throat because the incoming cold air is dry and absorbs considerable moisture from the respiratory passages. This may aggravate an existing respiratory or asthmatic condition.

Can air pollution affect exercise performance?   Yes. There are considerable individual differences, especially among asthmatics and others who suffer from allergies or pulmonary problems. Many new medications are available that provide relief, and people should consult with their physician about their use prior to and during exercise. If outdoor air irritates whatever condition you have, exercise should be confined to an air-conditioned gym, or the confines of one's home. People should be especially cautious during an air pollution alert or when the air quality is "unacceptable."

Should I wear an exercise suit made of rubber or vinyl? Absolutely not! This kind of garment is harmful because it heats the body while preventing its normal refrigeration system from working properly. No cooling can take place because evaporation is thwarted. The body continues to sweat, forcing the body temperature up and fluid reserves down. No benefits result and dangerous dehydration can occur. In extreme cases this will cause death from heat stroke!

What are the effects of cigarette smoking on regular exercise and performance? The regular smoker tends to show a decrease in the lung's functional capacity. Fifteen inhalations on a cigarette during a 5-minute period can triple resistance to breathing, whether or not a person is a chronic smoker. While long-term smoking may have only a minor effect during light exercise, it can be a handicap during more vigorous exercise because the total oxygen available for muscular exercise is reduced. The good news is that when a smoker abstains for just 1 day, exercise response improves noticeably.

Are salt tablets useful during or immediately following exercise? All the experts in the field (with whom we heartily agree) believe that the easiest and best way to replace the salt lost by sweating is to sprinkle a little extra on your food. Too much salt can aggravate high blood pressure, irritate the stomach, and actually create an unfavorable water distribution in the body. Under no circumstances should you routinely take salt tablets. If you've been exercising strenuously for several days in hot weather, mix one-third teaspoon of salt with each quart of water consumed.

Is it helpful to drink a sugary solution, such as Gatorade, during exercise? Research indicates that the best way to get fluids back into your body is to drink cool water. Any addition of glucose (sugar) to the water actually retards water absorption. Thus, if the weather is hot, the primary concern should be to replace water loss by drinking cool water. If you engage in prolonged exercise during cold weather, water loss is not as significant, and some sugar in the water can help replenish the body's depleted supply of carbohydrates.

Are potassium supplements useful? Research suggests that potassium loss during exercise generally is not significant, so taking potassium tablets would not really help. Potassium excretion during excessive sweating can be replaced by eating a banana or drinking a glass of orange juice.

Is it true that there are certain stimulants that enhance performance? The best advice we can offer is to avoid all drugs. While stimulants like amphetamines ("uppers" or pep pills) arouse the nervous system, they have never been shown to have a consistently positive effect on exercise capacity. More important, the dangers of addictive and harmful side effects greatly outweigh the chances of any small performance improvement.

An exception to this general rule may be caffeine. It has been shown that consuming the amount of caffeine commonly found in 2.5 cups of coffee 60 minutes before exercising significantly enhances long-term endurance in moderately strenuous exercise. The caffeine also makes the work feel easier, probably via effects on the nervous system and by increasing the use of fat for energy instead of depleting the body's limited carbohydrate reserves. Generally, this would only be of value in prolonged exercise of an hour or longer.

What is a stress test and should I take one before starting an exercise program? Stress tests involve exercising on a motor driven treadmill or bicycle ergometer while the heart is monitored by an electrocardiogram or ECG. Many people who have a normal heart response during rest may have abnormal response patterns during exercise stress. Such abnormal responses may be an indication of some form of coronary disease. The validity of some of the responses encountered during such diagnostic stress tests is still being questioned by the medical community. However, individuals over the age of 40 who have not exercised for many years and who have a pattern of risk factors such as high blood pressure, family history of heart disease, obesity, high blood fat levels, or who have chest pains probably should have a stress test before undertaking a comprehensive exercise program. For everyone, medical clearance for exercise is advised before such programs are begun.

Will weight lifting exercises slow you down and make you less flexible? Absolutely not. There is no research evidence to indicate that weight lifting makes you inflexible or slows down your speed of movement. In fact many weight lifting exercises require that a particular body part be moved through its full range of motion, thus enhancing joint flexibility.

What's the best way to recover following vigorous exercise? Recovery is fastest if you keep moving at a moderate pace just as soon as you complete your particular exercise program. The lactic acid built up as a result of the vigorous anaerobic exercise is actually used by the muscles and heart as you continue to exercise at a slow pace. For example, after you run a mile, select a comfortable walking or jogging pace for 5 to 10 minutes until you feel "recovered," or until your pulse is in the range of 100 to 120 beats per minute.

How important are flexibility exercises in a daily fitness program? Flexibility seems to be a product of heredity as well as exercise. It is also rather specific. You can have good flexibility in your ankle but not in your shoulder. Chronic lower back pain seems to be related directly to poor flexibility in the legs' hamstring muscles and to weakened abdominal muscles. Although there is no conclusive proof, most specialists in sports medicine agree that good flexibility seems to help prevent or at least lessen the occurrence of certain types of injuries. Any flexibility exercise should be done *slowly* with the stretch position held for about 15 to 30 seconds.

Should a woman exercise during her menstrual period? Yes. A woman should exercise whenever she feels like exercising. Sport events are not scheduled with any regard for the menstrual cycles of the participating female athletes, and many women have achieved world records while menstruating. Researchers have been unable to detect any significant diminution in physical performance during menstruation among healthy women with normal menstrual flow.

Is there any biologic basis to the phenomenon called the "runner's high"? The runner's high has been described by those experiencing it as a type of altered state manifested by feelings of euphoria and well-being during prolonged exercise. Recent evidence has indicated that vigorous exercise like running stimulates the body's production of natural opiate-like, mood-influencing compounds. These compounds, called endorphins and enkelphins, act as natural pain killers in much the same way as morphine. This may help the exerciser tolerate high levels of physical activity with minimal discomfort.

This form of high may have positive attributes. These natural opiates do not distort or impair mental function; they may even increase alertness. In fact, their production may help explain the claim that exercise aids to reduce depression, to improve one's ability to deal with stress, to increase relaxation and create a more positive state of mental well-being. It is quite possible that regular and vigorous exercise is truly a positive addiction!

Is it true that regular participation in a vigorous exercise program will place an extra demand on the body's iron stores and lead to an anemic condition? While the answers as to the effects of exercise on the body's mineral requirements are far from complete, the general belief is that regular physical activity places no additional demand on the body's need for iron. Some research shows a change in the blood characteristics of exercising men and women with the hemoglobin and hematocrit levels moving slightly lower during the early phase of training. However, these values return to normal and continue at this level for the duration of the program. Generally speaking, highly active people are no more or no less anemic than their sedentary counterparts. Clearly, however, those desiring to exercise must pay careful attention to their iron intake (10 mg/day men; 18 mg/day women) because any negative effects of dietary iron insufficiency will be magnified during the stress of vigorous aerobic exercise.

I am a swimmer and would like to further develop my aerobic capabilities to improve my endurance for swimming. Can I use running, cycling, and swimming interchangeably with equal effectiveness? Recall from our discussion of aerobic training in Chapter 10 that effective training results from the overloading of two systems, the central circulation and the peripheral musculature. In essence, we must train the heart to pump blood and the specific muscles to develop their ability to both deliver oxygen and process it in the reactions of aerobic energy metabolism. While running and cycling may provide an appropriate aerobic overload for enhancing heart function, these leg exercises would have only minimal effect in improving metabolic function in the muscles of the upper body which are used primarily in swimming. Although swimming, running, and cycling can each work the heart and burn significant calories, only swimming per se can engage the musculature in precisely the manner required by the swimming movement. As a rule, the best way to enhance performance in a specific sport is to train with the movements of that sport. Consequently, swimmers should swim, runners should run, and cyclists should train with bicycle exercise.

Do manufacturers of sports equipment conduct research on their products? The answer depends on the definition of research. Few manufacturers conduct a rigorous and thorough laboratory testing program typically carried out by scientists. For example, many machines used in weight training are the brain child of one or two individuals who have the resources to design, construct, distribute, and advertise their products. Some products are sold based on testimonial or personal opinion, without any formal research done to evaluate the effectiveness of the particular product. The key question to pose to salesmen or others involved in the distribution of fitness related products is, "Have the results of experiments to evaluate your claims been published in a scientific journal?". Such journals have a policy of peer review, which means other scientists have reviewed carefully the results of the experiments and have found the experimental design, methodology, statistical analysis, and inferences about the results to meet the rigors of a proper scientific experiment. In a way, this is an effective means to separate emotion from fact. Scientific research is published in appropriate scientific journals; personal points of view, interviews in the lay press, hand-outs from sales representatives, quotes from a popular coaching or quasi-fitness magazine, or TV blurbs, do not constitute research. The burden of responsibility rests with the manufacturer to provide facts, usually gathered by an independent team of scientists following appropriate procedures of the scientific method of inquiry. You can be sure of one thing; an equipment manufacturer who provides the "facts" without solid evidence, or who pontificates about the virtues of a given piece of equipment, probably does so for one of at least three reasons—ego, ignorance, or economic gain. As one eminent scholar phrased it, "Get the facts and the truth shall emerge."

What are some of the life-style modifications I can make to increase my chances of keeping my blood cholesterol at a desirable level? In many instances the blood lipids can be favorably affected by factors which we can control or at least modify. For one thing, diet can affect the lipid profile in both a positive and negative factor. Diets rich in saturated fat and cholesterol tend to raise blood cholesterol, while a low fat intake with a predominance of unsaturated fatty acids has the opposite effect. Also, diets rich in fiber, the non-digestible structural components and coverings of fruits, grains, and vegetables may also exert a lowering effect by binding cholesterol in the digestive tract and removing it from the body. Regular and vigorous aerobic exercise not only reduces total blood cholesterol, but also tends to elevate the high density lipoproteins (HDL) which favorably protect against the process of atherosclerosis. And, of course, adequate control of body weight is an important step in normalizing blood lipids. In summary, the "big three" life-style factors are: nutrition, weight control, and exercise!

General References

Åstrand, P.O., and K. Rodahl: Textbook of Work Physiology, 2nd ed. New York, McGraw-Hill Book Co., 1977.

Cioffi, L.A., W.P.T. Jones, and T.B. Van Itallie: The Body Weight Regulatory System: Normal and Disturbed Mechanisms. New York, Raven Press, 1981.

Consolazio, F.C., R.E. Johnson, and L.J. Pecora: Physiological Measurements of Metabolic Functions in Man. New York, McGraw-Hill Book Co., 1963.

Durnin, J.V.G.A., and R. Passmore: Energy, Work and Leisure. London, Hueneman Educational Books, 1967.

Food and Nutrition Board: Recommended Dietary Allowances. Washington, D.C., National Academy of Sciences, revised, 1980.

Hamilton, E.M. and E. Whitney: Nutrition. Concepts and Controversies. St. Paul, West Publishing Company, 1979.

Haskell, W., J. Scala, and J. Whittam (Eds.): Nutrition and Athletic Performance. Palo Alto, Bull Publishing Co., 1982.

Komi, P.V.: Exercise and Sport Biology. Champaign, Illinois, Human Kinetics Publishers, 1982.

Krause, M.V., and M.A. Hunscher: Food, Nutrition and Diet Therapy. Philadelphia, W.B. Saunders Co., 1972.

Lehninger, A.L.: Bioenergetics, 2d ed. Menlo Park, Calif., W.A. Benjamin, 1971.

McArdle, W.D., F.I. Katch, and V.L. Katch: Exercise Physiology. Energy, Nutrition, and Human Performance. Philadelphia, Lea & Febiger, 1981.

Pollock, M.L., J.H. Wilmore, and S.M. Fox III: Health and Fitness Through Physical Activity. New York, John Wiley & Sons, 1978.

Shephard, R.J.: Physical Activity and Aging. Chicago, Year Book Medical Publishers, Inc., 1978.

Smith, E. and R.C. Serfass: Exercise and Aging. Hillside, N.J., Enslow Publishers, 1981.

Smith, N.J.: Food for Sport. Bull Publishing Co., Palo Alto, Calif., 1976.

Vander, A.J. et al.: Human Physiology: The Mechanisms of Body Function. New York, McGraw-Hill Book Co., 1975.

Watt, B.K., and A.L. Merrill: Composition of Foods—Raw, Processed and Prepared. Handbook no. 8, Washington, D.C., U.S. Department of Agriculture, 1963.

Williams, M.H.: Nutritional Aspects of Human Physical and Athletic Performance. Springfield, Charles C Thomas, 1976.

Worthington-Roberts, B.S.: Contemporary Developments in Nutrition. St. Louis, C.V. Mosby Co., 1981.

269

References

CHAPTER 1   NUTRIENTS IN FOOD

American College of Sports Medicine: Position statement on prevention of heat injuries during distance running. *Medicine and Science in Sports.* 7:VII, 1975.

Bogert, L.J. et al.: Nutrition and Physical Fitness. Philadelphia, W.B. Saunders Co., 1979.

Costill, D.L. et al.: Dietary potassium and heavy exercise: effects on muscle, water and electrolytes. *American Journal of Clinical Nutrition.* 36:266, 1982.

Deutsch, R.M.: Realities of Nutrition. Palo Alto, Bull Publishing Co., 1976.

Dwyer, J.: Vegetarianism. *Contemporary Nutrition.* 4, no. 6, 1979.

Gardner, G.W. et al.: Cardiorespiratory, hematological and physical performance responses of anemic subjects to iron treatment. *American Journal of Clinical Nutrition.* 28:982, 1975.

Goodhart, R.S., and M.E. Shils (Eds.): Modern Nutrition in Health and Disease, 6th ed., Philadelphia, Lea & Febiger, 1980.

McArdle, W.D. et al.: Body composition and temperature regulation during rest and exercise in air and water. *Medicine and Science in Sports and Exercise.* 14:127, 1982.

Nutrition For Athletes: A Handbook For Coaches. Washington, D.C., American Association for Health, Physical Education, and Recreation, 1971.

Palumbo, J.D. and G.L. Blackburn: Human protein requirements. *Contemporary Nutrition.* 5, no. 1, 1980.

Parizkova, J., and V.A. Rogozkin: Nutrition, Physical Fitness and Health. Baltimore, University Park Press, 1978.

Percy, E.C.: Ergogenic aids in athletes. *Medicine and Science in Sports.* 10:298, 1978.

Reed, P.B.: Nutrition: An Applied Science. St. Paul, West Publishing Company, 1980.

Reiser, R.: A critique of universal diet recommendations for prevention of coronary heart disease. *Contemporary Nutrition.* 6(10), 1981.

Scott, M.L.: Advances in our understanding of vitamin E. *Federation Proceedings.* 39:2736, 1980.

Scrimshaw, N.S. and V.R. Young: The requirements of human nutrition. *Scientific American.* 235:50, 1976.

Shekelle, R.B. et al.: Dietary vitamin A and risk of cancer in the Western Electric study. *Lancet.* 2:1186, November 28, 1981.

Sims, L.: Dietary status of lactating women. *Journal of the American Dietetic Association.* 73:139, 1978.

Vitovsek, S.H.: Is more better? *Nutrition Today.* 14:10, 1979.

Wilcox, A.R.: The effects of caffeine and exercise on body weight, fat-pad weight, and fat cell size. *Medicine and Science in Sports and Exercise. 14:*317, 1982.

Williams, M.H.: Nutritional aspects of human physical and athletic performance. Springfield, Charles C Thomas, 1976.

Williams, R.J.: Nutrition in a Nutshell. New York, Dolphin Books, 1962.

Winston, M.: Diet and coronary heart disease. *Contemporary Nutrition. 6*(9), 1981.

CHAPTER 2   OPTIMAL NUTRITION FOR EXERCISE AND SPORT

Bentivegna, A. et al.: Diet, fitness and athletic performance. *The Physician and Sports Medicine. 7:*99, 1979.

Blair, S.N. et al.: Comparison of nutrient intake in middle-aged men and women runners and controls. *Medicine and Science in Sports and Exercise. 13:*310–315, 1981.

Buskirk, E.R.: Some nutritional considerations in the conditioning of athletes. *Annual Review of Nutrition. 1:*319, 1981.

Connor, W.E. et al.: The plasma lipids, lipoproteins, and diet of the Tarahumara Indians of Mexico. *American Journal of Clinical Nutrition. 31:*1131, 1978.

Costill, D.L.: Nutritional requirements for endurance athletes, In: Toward an Understanding of Human Performance. Edited by E.J. Burke, Ithaca, N.Y., Mouvement Publications, 1977.

Girandola, R.N. et al.: Effects of pangamic acid (B-15) ingestion on metabolic response to exercise. *Biochemical Medicine. 24:*218, 1980.

Higdon, H.: The Complete Diet. Mountain View, Calif., World Publication, 1978.

Lemon, P.W.R. and F.J. Nagle: Effects of exercise on protein and amino acid metabolism. *Medicine and Science in Sports and Exercise. 13:*141, 1981.

Lewis, S. and B. Gutin: Nutrition and endurance. *American Journal of Clinical Nutrition. 26:*1011, 1973.

Nelson, R.A.: What athletes should eat. Unmixing folly and facts. *The Physician and Sportsmedicine. 3:*67, 1975.

Nutrition and Athletic Performance. *Dairy Council Digest. 46:*7, 1975.

Serfas, R.C.: Nutrition for the athlete. *Contemporary Nutrition. 2,* No. 5, 1977.

Stare, F.J.: Nutrition-sense and nonsense. *Postgraduate Medicine. 67:*147, 1980.

Van Dam, B.: Vitamins and Sports. *British Journal of Sports Medicine. 12:*74, 1978.

CHAPTER 3   ENERGY SYSTEMS FOR EXERCISE

Appenzeller, O. and R. Atkinson (Eds.): Sports Medicine. Baltimore, Urban & Schwarzenberg, 1981.

Bergh, V. et al.: Maximal oxygen uptake and muscle fiber types in trained and untrained humans. *Medicine and Science in Sports. 10:*151, 1978.

Chapman, C.B. and J.H. Mitchell: The physiology of exercise. *Scientific American. 212:*88, 1965.

Gollnick, P.: Energy release in the muscle cell. *Medicine and Science in Sports. 1:*23, 1969.

Goodman, M.N. and N.B. Ruderman: Influence of muscle use on amino acid metabolism. In: Exercise and Sport Science Reviews. Vol. 10. Edited by R.L. Terjung. Philadelphia, Franklin Institute Press, 1982.

Grimby, G.: Respiration in exercise. *Medicine and Science in Sports. 1:*9, 1969.

Holloszy, J.O.: Biochemical adaptation to exercise: Aerobic metabolism. In Exercise and Sport Science Reviews. Vol. I. J. Wilmore (Ed.). New York, Academic Press, 1973.

Rowell, L.B.: Human cardiovascular adjustments to exercise and thermal stress. *Physiological Reviews. 4:*75, 1974.

Rushmer, R.F.: Cardiovascular Dynamics. Philadelphia, W.B. Saunders Co., 1976.

Saltin, B.: Metabolic fundamentals in exercise. *Medicine and Science in Sports.* 5:137, 1973.

Saltin, B.: Physiological effects of physical conditioning. *Medicine and Science in Sports.* 1:50, 1969.

Saltin, B. et al.: Fiber types and metabolic potentials of skeletal muscles in sedentary man and endurance runners. *Annals of the New York Academy of Science. 301:*3, 1977.

Stanisby, W.N. and J.K. Barclay: Exercise metabolism: O_2 deficit, steady level O_2 uptake and O_2 in recovery. *Medicine and Science in Sports. 2:*177, 1970.

CHAPTER 4   ENERGY VALUE OF FOOD AND PHYSICAL ACTIVITY

Behnke, A.R.: The relation of lean body weight to metabolism and some consequent systematizations. *Annals of the New York Academy of Sciences.* 56:1095, 1953.

Brobeck, J.R.: Energy balance and food intake. In: Medical Physiology, V.B. Mountcastle (Ed.), 12th ed., Vol. I. St. Louis, C.V. Mosby Co., 1968.

Calloway, D. H. and E. Zanni: Energy requirements and energy expenditure of elderly men. *American Journal of Clinical Nutrition. 33:*2088, 1980.

Cohen, J.L. et al.: Cardiorespiratory responses to ballet exercise and the $\dot{V}O_{2max}$ of elite ballet dancers. *Medicine and Science in Sports and Exercise. 14:*212, 1982.

Consolazio, C.F., R.E. Johnson, and L.J. Pecora: Physiological Measurements of Metabolic Functions in Man. New York, McGraw-Hill Book Co., 1963.

Cunningham, J.J.: A reanalysis of the factors influencing basal metabolic rate in normal adults. *American Journal of Clinical Nutrition. 33:*2372, 1980.

Garry, R.C., et al.: Expenditure of energy and the consumption of food by miners and clerks. *Medical Research Council,* Report No. 289. Fife, Scotland, Her Majesty's Stationery Office, 1955.

Girandola, R.N., and F.I. Katch: Effects of physical training on ventilatory equivalent and respiratory exchange ratio during weight supported, steady-state exercise. *European Journal of Applied Physiology. 35:*119, 1976.

Glaser, R.M., and W.D. McArdle: A radiotelemetry transmitter for monitoring heart rate of humans engaged in physical activity. *Research Quarterly. 40:*640, 1969.

Knuttgen, H.G., and K. Emerson, Jr.: Physiological response to pregnancy at rest and during exercise. *Journal of Applied Physiology. 36:*549, 1974.

McArdle, W.D. et al.: Metabolic and cardiovascular adjustment to work in air and water at 18, 25, 33°C. *Journal of Applied Physiology. 40:*85, 1976.

McArdle, W.D., et al.: Aerobic capacity, heart rate, and estimated energy cost during women's competitive basketball. *Research Quarterly. 42:*178, 1971.

McArdle, W.D., et al.: Reliability and interrelationships between maximal oxygen intake, physical work capacity, and step test scores in college women. *Medicine and Science in Sports. 4:*182, 1972.

Passmore, R., and M.H. Draper. The chemical anatomy of the human body. In Biochemical Disorders in Human Disease, R.H.S. Thompson and E.J. King (Eds.), 2d ed. London, Churchill, 1964.

President's Council on Physical Fitness and Sports: National Adult Physical Fitness Survey. Washington, D.C., May, 1973.

Rothwell, N.J. and M.J. Stock: Regulation of energy balance. *Annual Review of Nutrition. 1:*235, 1981.

Town, G.P. et al.: The effect of rope skipping rate on energy expenditure of males and females. *Medicine and Science in Sports and Exercise. 12:*295, 1980.

CHAPTER 5   EVALUATION OF BODY COMPOSITION

Behnke, A.R., and J.H. Wilmore: Evaluation and Regulation of Body Build and Composition. Englewood Cliffs, N.J. Prentice-Hall, 1974.

Behnke, A.R., F.I. Katch, and V.L. Katch: Routine anthropometry and arm radiography in assessment of nutritional status: Its potential. *Journal of Parenteral and Enteral Nutrition. 2:*532, 1978.

Borkan, G.A. et al.: Assessment of abdominal fat content by computed tomography. *American Journal of Clinical Nutrition. 36:*172, 1982.

Freedson, P.F. et al.: Physique, body composition and psychological characteristics of competitive female body builders. *Physician and Sportsmedicine. 11:*85–93, 1983.

Garrett, W.N.: Experiences in the use of body density as an estimator of body composition of animals. In: Body Composition in Animals and Man. Washington, D.C., National Academy of Sciences, Publication 1598, 1968.

Katch, F.I., E.D. Michael, and S.M. Horvath: Estimation of body volume by underwater weighing: Description of a simple method. *Journal of Applied Physiology. 23:*811, 1967.

Katch, F.I., and W.D. McArdle: Validity of body composition prediction equations for college men and women. *American Journal of Clinical Nutrition. 28:*105, 1975.

Katch, F.I., A.R. Behnke, and V.L. Katch: Estimation of body fat from skinfolds and surface area. *Human Biology. 51:*411, 1979.

Katch, F.I., V.L. Katch and A.R. Behnke: The underweight female. *Physician and Sportsmedicine. 8:*55, 1980.

Katch, F.I. and V.L. Katch: Measurement and prediction errors in body composition assessment and the search for the perfect prediction equation. *Research Quarterly for Exercise and Sport. 51:*249, 1980.

Katch, V.L. et al.: Muscular development and lean body weight in body builders and weight lifters. *Medicine and Science in Sports and Exercise. 12:*340, 1980.

Kissebah, A.H. et al.: Relation of body fat distribution to metabolic complications of obesity. *Journal of Clinical Endocrinology and Metabolism. 54:*254, 1981.

Lukaski, H.C. et al.: A comparison of methods of assessment of body composition including neutron activation analysis of total body nitrogen. *Metabolism. 30:*777, 1981.

Pitts, G.C.: Studies of body composition by direct dissection. *Annals of the New York Academy of Sciences. 110:*11, 1963.

Siri, W.E.: Gross composition of the body. In: Advances in Biological and Medical Physics, J.H. Lawrence and C.A. Tobias (Eds.) vol. IV. New York, Academic Press, 1956.

CHAPTER 6 OBESITY

Ashwell, M. and C.J. Meade: Obesity: Can some fat cells enlarge while others are shrinking? *Lipids. 16:*475, 1981.

Bray, G.A., and J.E. Bethune, (Eds.): Treatment and Management of Obesity. New York, Harper & Row, 1974.

Bukowiecki, L. et al.: Mechanism of enhanced lipolysis in adipose tissue of exercise-trained rats. *American Journal of Physiology. 239:*422, 1980.

Chumlea, W.C. et al.: Adipocytes and adiposity in adults. *American Journal of Clinical Nutrition. 34:*1798, 1981.

Chumlea, W.C. et al.: Size and number of adipocytes and measures of body fat in boys and girls 10 to 18 years of age. *American Journal of Nutrition. 34:*1791, 1981.

Drenick, E.J.: Risk of obesity and surgical indications. *International Journal of Obesity. 5:*387, 1980.

Faust, I.M., P.R. Johnson, and J. Hirsch: Long-term effects of early nutritional experience on the development of obesity in the rat. *Journal of Nutrition. 110:*2027, 1980.

Garn, S.M. and P.E. Cole: Do the obese remain obese and the lean remain lean? *American Journal of Public Health. 70:*351, 1980.

Ginsberg-Fellner, F. et al.: Overweight and obesity in preschool children in New York City. *American Journal of Clinical Nutrition. 34:*2236, 1981.

Ginsberg-Fellner, F. and J.L. Knittle: Weight reduction in young obese children. 1. Effects on adipose tissue cellularity and metabolism. *Pediatric Research. 15:*1381, 1981.

Hirsch, J., and P.W. Han: Cellularity of rat adipose tissue: Effects of growth, starvation and obesity. *Journal of Lipid Research. 10:*77, 1969.

Hirsch, J., and J. Knittle: Cellularity of obese and nonobese human adipose tissue. *Federation Proceedings. 28:*1516, 1970.

Knittle, J., and J. Hirsch: Effect of early nutrition on the development of rat epididymal fat pads: Cellularity and metabolism. *Journal of Clinical Investigation. 47:*2091, 1968.

Oscai, L., et al.: Effects of exercise and of food restriction on adipose tissue cellularity. *Journal of Lipid Research. 13:*588, 1972.

Oscai, L., et al.: Exercise or food restriction: Effect on adipose tissue cellularity. *American Journal of Physiology. 227:*901, 1974.

Roche, A.F.: The adipocyte-number hypothesis. *Child Development. 52:*31, 1981.

Salans, L.B., et al.: Studies of human adipose tissue: Adipose cell size and number in nonobese and obese patients. *Journal of Clinical Investigation. 52:*929, 1973.

Sims, E.A.H., and E.S. Horton: Endocrine and metabolic adaptation to obesity and starvation. *American Journal of Clinical Nutrition. 21:*1455, 1968.

Stern, J. and M.R.C. Greenwood: A review of development of adipose cellularity in man and animals. *Federation Proceedings. 33:*1952, 1974.

Thompson, J.K. et al.: Exercise and obesity: Etiology, physiology, and intervention. *Psychological Bulletin. 91:*55, 1982.

Ylitalo, V.: Treatment of obese school children. *Acta Paediactrica Scandinavica.* Suppl. 290, 1981.

CHAPTER 7   WEIGHT CONTROL

American Medical Association Council on Food and Nutrition: *Journal of the American Medical Association. 224:*1418, 1973.

Bennett, W. and J. Gurin: The Dieter's Dilemma. New York, Basic Books, Inc., 1982.

Bjorntorp, P., et al.: Effect of an energy reduced dietary regimen in relation to adipose tissue cellularity in obese women. *American Journal of Clinical Nutrition. 28:*445, 1975.

Bray, G.: Effect of caloric restriction on energy expenditure in obese subjects. *Lancet. 2:*397, 1969.

Brownell, K.D. and F.S. Kaye: A school-based behavior modification, nutrition education, and physical activity program for obese children. *American Journal of Clinical Nutrition. 35:*277, 1982.

Craighead, L.W., et al.: Behavior therapy and pharmacotherapy for obesity. *Archives of General Psychiatry. 38:*763, 1981.

Frank, A., et al.: Fatalities on the liquid-protein diet: An analysis of possible causes. *International Journal of Obesity. 5:*243, 1981.

Glucksman, M.L. and J. Hirsch: The response of obese patients to weight reduction. *Psychosomatic Medicine. 30:*1, 1968.

Grande, F.: Nutrition and energy balance in body composition studies. In: Techniques for Measuring Body Composition. Washington, D.C., National Academy of Sciences-National Research Council, 1961.

Karvonen, M.J., et al.: Consumption and selection of food in competitive lumber work. *Journal of Applied Physiology. 6:*603, 1954.

Katch, F.I., et al.: Effects of physical training on the body composition and diet of females. *Research Quarterly. 40:*99, 1969.

Kinsell, L.W., et al.: Calories do count. *Metabolism. 3:*195, 1964.

Nisbett, R.E.: Eating behavior and obesity in men and animals. *Advances in Psychosomatic Medicine. 7:*173, 1972.

Schachter, S.: Obesity and eating: Internal and external cues differentially affect the eating behavior of obese and normal subjects. *Science. 161:*751, 1968.

Schachter, S.: Some extraordinary facts about obese humans and rats. *American Psychologist. 26:*129, 1971.

Sours, H.E., et al.: Sudden death associated with very low caloric weight reduction regimens. *American Journal of Clinical Nutrition. 34:*453, 1981.

Stunkard, A.J., and M. McLaren-Hume: The results of treatment for obesity. *Archives of Internal Medicine. 103:*79, 1959.

CHAPTER 8   MODIFICATION OF EATING AND EXERCISE BEHAVIORS

Brownell, K.D. and F.S. Kaye: A school-based behavior modification, nutrition education, and physical activity program for obese children. *The American Journal of Clinical Nutrition. 35:*277, 1982.

Foreyt, J.P., and W.A. Kennedy: Treatment of overweight by aversion therapy. *Behaviour Research and Therapy. 9:*29, 1971.

Johnson, M.L., et al.: Relative importance of inactivity and overeating in the energy balance of obese high school girls. *American Journal of Clinical Nutrition. 4:*37, 1956.

Jordan, H.A., and L.S. Levitz: Behavior modification in a self-help group. *Journal of the American Dietetic Association. 62:*27, 1973.

Leon, G.R.: The behavior modification approach to weight reduction. *Contemporary Nutrition. 4*(8): 1979.

Penick, S.B., et al.: Behaviour modifications in the treatment of obesity. *Psychosomatic Medicine. 33:*49, 1971.

Stuart, R.B., and B. Davis: Slim Chance in a Fat World: Behavioral Control of Obesity, Champaign, Ill., Research Press, 1971.

Stunkard, A.J.: Environment and obesity: Recent advances in our understanding of regulation of food intake in man. *Federation Proceedings.* 1367, 1968.

Stunkard, A.J.: New therapies for the eating disorders: Behavior modification of obesity and anorexia nervosa. *Archives of General Psychiatry. 26:*391, 1972.

Stunkard, A.J., et al.: The management of obesity: Patient self help and medical treatment. *Archives of Internal Medicine. 125:*1067, 1970.

Stunkard, A.J. and S.B. Penick: Behavior modification in the treatment of obesity: The problem of maintaining weight loss. *Archives of General Psychiatry. 36:*801, 1979.

Wilson, G.T., et al.: Behavior therapy for obesity: Including family members in the treatment process. *Behavior Therapy. 9:*943, 1978.

Wollersheim, J.P.: The effectiveness of group therapy based upon learning principles in the treatment of overweight women. *Journal of Abnormal Psychology. 76:*462, 1970.

CHAPTER 9   CONDITIONING FOR MUSCULAR STRENGTH

Caiozzo, V.J., J.J. Perrine, and V.R. Edgerton: Training-induced alterations of the in vivo force-velocity relationship of human muscle. *Journal of Applied Physiology: Respiration, Environmental, Exercise Physiology. 51:*750, 1981.

Costill, D.L., et al.: Adaptations in skeletal muscle following strength training. *Journal of Applied Physiology: Respiration, Environmental, Exercise Physiology. 46:*96, 1979.

Davies, K.J.A., et al.: Biochemical adaptation of mitochondria, muscle, and whole-animal respiration to endurance training. *Archives of Biochemistry and Biophysics. 209:*539, 1981.

Gettman, L.R. and M.L. Pollock: Circuit weight training: a critical review of its physiological benefits. *Physician and Sportsmedicine.9:*44, 1980.

Gettman, L.R., P. Ward, and R.D. Hagan: A comparison of combined running and weight training with circuit weight training. *Medicine and Science in Sports and Exercise. 14:*229–234, 1982.

Goldberg, A.L., et al.: Mechanism of work induced hypertrophy. *Medicine and Science in Sports. 7:*185, 1975.

Gregor, R.J., et al.: Skeletal muscle properties and performance in elite female track athletes. *European Journal of Applied Physiology. 47:*355, 1981.

Ikai, M., and A.H. Steinhaus: Some factors modifying the expression of human strength. *Journal of Applied Physiology. 16:*157, 1961.

Katch, F.I., et al.: Relationship of maximal leg force and leg composition to treadmill and bicycle ergometer maximum oxygen uptake. *Medicine and Science in Sports. 6:*38, 1974.

Katch, F.I., and G. Danielson: Bicycle ergometer endurance in women related to maximal force, leg volume, and body composition. *Research Quarterly. 47:*366, 1976.

Larsson, L.: Physical training effects on muscle morphology in sedentary males at different ages. *Medicine and Science in Sports and Exercise. 14:*203, 1982.

MacDougall, J.D. et al.: Muscle ultrastructural characteristics of elite powerlifters and bodybuilders. *European Journal of Applied Physiology. 48:*117, 1982.

McArdle, W.D., and G.F. Foglia: Energy cost and cardiorespiratory stress of isometric and weight training exercise. *Journal of Sports Medicine and Physical Fitness. 9:*23, 1969.

Saltin, B. et al.: Fiber types and metabolic potentials of skeletal muscles in sedentary man and endurance runners. *Annals of New York Academy of Sciences. 301:*3, 1977.

Wilmore, J.H.: Alterations in strength, body composition, and anthropometric measurements consequent to a 10-week weight training program. *Medicine and Science in Sports. 6:*133, 1974.

Winter, D.A. et al.: Errors in the use of isokinetic dynamometers. *European Journal of Applied Physiology. 46:*397, 1981.

CHAPTER 10   CONDITIONING FOR ANAEROBIC AND AEROBIC POWER

American College of Sports Medicine: The recommended quantity and quality of exercise for developing and maintaining fitness in healthy adults. *Medicine and Science in Sports. 10:*7, 1978.

Costill, D.L.: Physiology of marathon running. *Journal of the American Medical Association. 221:*1024, 1972.

Greer, N.L. and F.I. Katch: Validity of palpation recovery pulse rate following four intensities of bench step exercise. *Research Quarterly for Exercise and Sport. 53:*340, 1982.

Katch, V.L. et al.: Biological variability in maximum aerobic power. *Medicine and Science in Sports and Exercise. 14:*21, 1982.

Magel, J.R. et al.: Specificity of swim training on maximum oxygen uptake. *Journal of Applied Physiology. 38:*151, 1975.

McArdle, W.D. et al.: Specificity of run training on $\dot{V}O_2$ max and heart rate changes during running and swimming. *Medicine and Science in Sports. 10:*16, 1978.

Pollock, M.L.: The quantification of endurance training programs. In: Exercise and Sport Sciences Reviews. Vol. 1. J. Wilmore (Ed.). New York, Academic Press, 1973.

Ready, A.E., and H.A. Quinney: Alterations in anaerobic threshold as the result of endurance training and detraining. *Medicine and Science in Sports and Exercise. 14:*292, 1982.

Sawka, M.N. et al.: Alactic capacity and power. *European Journal of Applied Physiology. 45:*109, 1980.

Scheuer, J. and C.M. Tipton: Cardiovascular adaptations to training. *Annual Review of Physiology. 39:*221, 1977.

Stamford, B.A. et al.: Exercise recovery above and below anaerobic threshold following maximal work. *Journal of Applied Physiology. 51:*840, 1981.

Withers, R.T. et al.: Specificity of the anaerobic threshold in endurance trained cyclists and runners. *European Journal of Applied Physiology. 47:*93, 1981.

CHAPTER 11   AGING, EXERCISE, AND CARDIOVASCULAR HEALTH

Amsterdam, E.A., J.H. Wilmore, and A.N. DeMaria, (Eds.): Exercise in Cardiovascular Health and Disease. New York, Yorke Medical Books, 1977.

Brunner, D. (Ed.): Physical Activity and Aging. Baltimore, University Park Press, 1970.

Ehsani, A.A. et al.: Effects of 12 months of intense exercise training on ischemic ST-segment depression in patients with coronary artery disease. *Circulation. 64:*1116, 1981.

Fisher, A.: The Healthy Heart. Virginia, Time-Life Books, 1981.

Friedman, M. and R. Rosenman: Type A Behavior and Your Heart. New York, Alfred A. Knopf, 1974.

Froelicher, V.: Exercise and health. *The American Journal of Medicine. 70:*987, 1981.

Hartung, G.H.: Jogging—The potential for prevention of heart disease. *Comprehensive Therapy. 6:*28, 1980.

Hartung, G.H. et al.: Effects of marathon running, jogging and diet on coronary risk factors in middle-aged men. *Preventive Medicine. 10:*316, 1981.

Keys, A.: Is overweight a risk factor for coronary heart disease? *Cardiovascular Medicine. 4:*1233, 1979.

Kramsch, D.M. et al.: Reduction of coronary atherosclerosis by moderate conditioning exercise in monkeys on an atherogenic diet. *New England Journal of Medicine. 305:*1483, 1981.

Leon, A.S. et al.: Effects of a vigorous walking program on body composition, and carbohydrate and lipid metabolism of obese young men. *American Journal of Clinical Nutrition. 32:*1776, 1979.

Miller, G.J.: High density lipoproteins and atherosclerosis. *Annual Review of Medicine. 31:*97, 1980.

Montoye, H.J.: Physical Activity and Health: An Epidemiologic Study of an Entire Community. Englewood Cliffs, N.J., Prentice-Hall, 1975.

Morris, J.N. et al.: Vigorous exercise in leisure time: protection against coronary heart disease. *Lancet. 2:*1207, 1980.

Paffenbarger, R.S. et al.: Physical activity as an index of heart disease risk in college alumni. *American Journal of Epidemiology. 108:*161, 1975.

Paffenbarger, R.S. et al.: Energy expenditure, cigarette smoking, and blood pressure level as related to death from specific diseases. *American Journal of Epidemiology. 108:*12, 1978.

Pollock, M.L. and D.H. Schmidt, (Eds.): Heart Disease and Rehabilitation. Boston, Houghton-Mifflin, 1979.

Ransford, C.P.: A role for amines in the antidepressant effects of exercise: a review. *Medicine and Science in Sports and Exercise. 14:*1, 1982.

Shephard, R.J.: Ischaemic Heart Disease and Exercise. Chicago, Year Book Medical Publishers Inc., 1981.

Smith, E.L.: Exercise for prevention of osteoporosis: A review. *The Physician and Sportsmedicine. 3:*72, 1982.

Spirduso, W.W.: Physical fitness, aging, and psychomotor speed: A review. *Journal of Gerontology. 35:*850, 1980.

Stamler, J.: Diet and coronary heart disease. *Biometrics. 38:*95, 1982.

Toll, A. and Small, D.M.: Current Concepts: Plasma high density lipoproteins. *New England Journal of Medicine. 229:*1232, 1978.

A*

Nutritive Value of Commonly Used Foods

Explanation of the Table

The foods have been arranged in alphabetical order. The weight of the food is given in grams (g) as well as in ounces (oz), followed by the approximate measure of the food and its description. The next columns present the caloric value of the food (kcal); the number of grams of protein, fat, and carbohydrates; and the number of milligrams of calcium, iron, ascorbic acid, thiamin, riboflavin, and vitamin-A activity expressed in international units (IU). Page 304 lists the caloric value of alcoholic beverages, and pages 304 to 307 list the caloric value of specialty items purchased at selected fast-food chain stores. The abbreviation *tr* indicates that only a trace of a food nutrient is present.

Equivalents by Weight

1 pound (16 ounces)	= 454 grams
1 ounce	= 28.4 grams
$3\frac{1}{2}$ ounces	= 100 grams

Equivalents by Volume

1 quart	= 4 cups
1 cup	= 8 fluid ounces
	= $\frac{1}{2}$ pint
	= 16 tablespoons
2 tablespoons	= 1 fluid ounce
1 tablespoon	= 3 teaspoons
1 pound regular margarine or butter	= 4 sticks
	= 2 cups
1 pound whipped butter or margarine	= 6 sticks
	= two 8-ounce containers

---

*Data from B. K. Watt and A. L. Merrill, *Composition of Foods—Raw, Processed and Prepared*, U.S. Department of Agriculture, Washington, D.C., 1963; *Nutritive Value of Foods*, Home and Garden Bulletin no. 72, rev, U.S. Department of Agriculture, Washington, D.C., 1971.

FOOD	WEIGHT G	WEIGHT OZ	APPROXIMATE MEASURE AND DESCRIPTION	KCAL
Alcoholic beverages (*see* page 474)				
Apples, raw	150	5.3	1 apple, about 3 per lb.	70
Apple, baked	130	4.6	1 medium apple, 2½ in. dia.	120
Apple brown betty	115	4.0	½ cup	175
Apple juice (sweet cider)	124	4.3	½ cup, bottled or canned	60
Apple pie (*see* pies)				
Applesauce, canned sweetened	128	4.5	½ cup	115
Apricots, fresh raw (as purchased)	114	4.0	3 apricots, about 12 per lb.	55
Apricots, canned	130	4.6	½ cup or 4 medium halves, 2 tbsp. juice (syrup pack)	110
Apricots, dried, stewed	108	3.8	½ cup (scant) or 8 halves, 2 tbsp. juice, sweetened	135
Apricot nectar (peach and pear nectar have similar values)	125	4.4	½ cup	70
Asparagus, cooked, green	73	2.6	½ cup, 1½- to 2-in. lengths	15
Avocado, raw (as purchased)	142	5.0	½ avocado, 3⅛ in. dia., pitted and peeled	185
Bacon, broiled or fried	15	0.5	2 slices, cooked crisp (20 slices per lb., raw)	90
Bacon, Canadian, cooked	43	1.5	3 slices, cooked crisp	100
Bananas, raw (as purchased)	175	6.1	1 medium banana	100
Bavarian cream, orange	99	3.5	½ cup	210
Bean sprouts, mung, cooked	63	2.2	½ cup, drained	18
Beans, green snap, cooked	63	2.2	½ cup	15
Beans, dry, green lima, cooked	144	5.0	¾ cup	195
Beans, immature, green lima, cooked	85	2.8	½ cup	95
Beans, dry, red kidney, canned	191	6.7	¾ cup	173
Beans, dry, white, canned with tomato sauce, without pork	196	6.9	¾ cup	233
Beans, dry, white, canned with tomato sauce and pork	191	6.7	¾ cup	233
Beef, corned, canned	85	3.0	3 slices, 3 × 2 × ¼ in.	185
Beef, corned hash, canned	85	3.0	½ cup (approx.)	155
Beef, dried or chipped	57	2.0	4 thin slices, 4 × 5 in.	115
Beef, hamburger, broiled	85	3.0	1 patty, 3 in. dia. (regular ground beef)	245
Beef, heart, braised	85	3.0	2 round slices, 2½ in. dia., ½ in. thick	160

PROTEIN G	FAT G	CARBOHYDRATE G	CALCIUM MG	IRON MG	VITAMIN-A ACTIVITY IU	ASCORBIC ACID MG	THIAMIN MG	RIBOFLAVIN MG
tr	tr	18	8	0.4	50	3	0.04	0.02
tr	tr	30	8	0.4	50	3	0.04	0.02
2	4	34	21	0.7	115	2	0.07	0.05
tr	tr	15	8	0.8	—	1	0.01	0.03
tr	tr	31	5	0.7	50	2	0.03	0.02
1	tr	14	18	0.5	2890	10	0.03	0.04
1	tr	29	14	0.4	2255	5	0.03	0.03
2	tr	34	26	1.5	2287	3	tr	0.04
1	tr	19	12	0.3	1190	4	0.02	0.02
2	tr	3	15	0.5	655	19	0.12	0.13
3	19	7	11	0.7	315	15	0.12	0.22
5	8	1	2	0.5	0	—	0.08	0.05
18	12	tr	13	2.2	0	0	0.62	0.12
1	tr	26	10	0.8	230	12	0.06	0.07
2	10	30	27	0.1	627	54	0.10	0.05
2	tr	4	11	0.6	15	4	0.06	0.07
1	tr	4	32	0.4	340	8	0.05	0.06
12	1	37	41	4.2	—	—	0.19	0.08
7	1	17	40	2.2	240	15	0.16	0.09
11	1	32	56	3.5	8	—	0.10	0.08
12	1	45	133	3.9	120	4	0.14	0.07
12	5	37	104	3.5	248	4	0.15	0.06
22	10	0	17	3.7	20	—	0.01	0.20
7	10	9	11	1.7	—	—	0.01	0.08
9	4	0	11	2.9	—	—	0.04	0.18
21	17	0	9	2.7	30	—	0.07	0.18
27	5	1	5	5.0	20	1	0.21	1.04

FOOD	WEIGHT		APPROXIMATE MEASURE AND DESCRIPTION	KCAL
	G	OZ		
Beef liver (*see* liver)				
Beef loaf (*see* meat loaf)				
Beef potpie, baked	227	7.9	1 pie, $4\frac{1}{4}$ in. dia.	560
Beef, pot roast, cooked	85	3.0	1 piece, $4 \times 3\frac{3}{4} \times \frac{1}{2}$ in.	245
Beef roast, oven-cooked	85	3.0	2 slices, $6 \times 3\frac{1}{4} \times \frac{1}{8}$ in., relatively lean	165
Beef steak, broiled	85	3.0	1 piece, $3\frac{1}{2} \times 2 \times \frac{3}{4}$ in., relatively fat, no bone	330
Beef stroganoff, cooked	130	4.6	$\frac{1}{2}$ cup	250
Beef tongue, braised	85	3.0	7 slices, $2\frac{1}{4} \times 2\frac{1}{4} \times \frac{1}{8}$ in.	210
Beets, cooked	85	3.0	$\frac{1}{2}$ cup, diced	28
Beverages, alcoholic (*see* page 304)				
Beverages, cola-type	185	6.5	about $\frac{3}{4}$ cup	75
Beverages, ginger ale	240	8.4	1 cup	75
Biscuits, baking powder	28	1.0	1 biscuit, 2 in. dia. (enriched flour)	105
Blackberries, raw	72	2.5	$\frac{1}{2}$ cup	45
Blueberries, raw	70	2.5	$\frac{1}{2}$ cup	45
Bluefish, cooked	85	3.0	1 piece, $3\frac{1}{2} \times 2 \times \frac{1}{2}$ in.	135
Bologna (*see* sausage)				
Bouillon cubes	4	0.1	1 cube, $\frac{5}{8}$ in.	5
Bran flakes	26	0.9	$\frac{3}{4}$ cup, 40% bran, (thiamin and iron added)	80
Bread, Boston brown	48	1.7	1 slice, $3 \times \frac{3}{4}$ in.	100
Bread, cracked wheat	25	0.9	1 slice, 18 slices per lb. loaf	65
Bread, French or Vienna	20	0.7	1 slice, $3\frac{1}{4} \times 2 \times 1$ in. (enriched flour)	60
Bread, Italian	20	0.7	1 slice, $3\frac{1}{4} \times 2 \times 1$ in. (enriched flour)	5
Bread, light rye	25	0.9	1 slice, 18 slices per lb. loaf ($\frac{1}{3}$ rye, $\frac{2}{3}$ wheat)	6
Bread, pumpernickel	34	1.2	1 slice, $3\frac{1}{4} \times 2 \times 1$ in. (dark rye flour)	8
Bread, raisin	25	0.9	1 slice, 18 slices per lb. loaf	6
Bread, white firm crumb (enriched)	23	0.8	1 slice, 20 slices per lb. loaf	6
Bread, white soft crumb (enriched)	25	0.9	1 slice, 18 slices per lb loaf	7
Bread, white soft crumb (enriched), toasted	22	0.8	1 slice, 18 slices per lb loaf	7
Bread, white soft crumb (unenriched)	25	0.9	1 slice, 18 slices per lb loaf	7
Bread, whole wheat firm crumb	25	0.9	1 slice, 18 slices per lb loaf	6
Bread crumbs	25	0.9	$\frac{1}{4}$ cup, dry grated	9

PROTEIN G	FAT G	CARBOHYDRATE G	CALCIUM MG	IRON MG	VITAMIN-A ACTIVITY IU	ASCORBIC ACID MG	THIAMIN MG	RIBOFLAVIN MG
23	33	43	32	4.1	1860	7	0.25	0.27
23	16	0	10	2.9	30	—	0.04	0.18
25	7	0	11	3.2	10	—	0.06	0.19
20	27	0	9	2.5	50	—	0.05	0.16
17	18	6	41	2.6	395	2	0.12	0.29
18	14	tr	6	1.9	—	—	0.04	0.25
1	tr	6	12	0.5	15	5	0.03	0.04
0	0	19	—	—	0	0	0	0
0	0	19	—	—	0	0	0	0
2	5	13	34	0.4	tr	tr	0.06	0.06
1	1	10	23	0.7	145	15	0.03	0.03
1	1	11	11	0.7	70	10	0.02	0.04
22	4	0	25	0.6	40	—	0.09	0.08
1	tr	tr	—	—	—	—	—	—
3	1	21	19	9.3	0	0	0.11	0.05
3	1	22	43	0.9	0	0	0.05	0.03
2	1	13	22	0.3	tr	tr	0.03	0.02
2	1	11	9	0.4	tr	tr	0.06	0.04
2	tr	11	3	0.4	0	0	0.06	0.04
2	tr	13	19	0.4	0	0	0.05	0.02
3	0	19	30	0.8	0	0	0.08	0.05
2	1	13	18	0.3	tr	tr	0.01	0.02
2	1	12	22	0.6	tr	tr	0.06	0.05
2	1	13	21	0.6	tr	tr	0.06	0.05
2	1	13	21	0.6	tr	tr	0.05	0.05
2	1	13	21	0.2	tr	tr	0.02	0.02
3	1	12	25	0.8	tr	tr	0.06	0.03
3	1	18	31	0.9	tr	tr	0.06	0.08

FOOD	WEIGHT G	WEIGHT OZ	APPROXIMATE MEASURE AND DESCRIPTION	KCAL
Broccoli, cooked	78	2.7	$\frac{1}{2}$ cup, stalks cut into $\frac{1}{2}$-in. pieces	20
Brussels sprouts, cooked	78	2.7	$\frac{1}{2}$ cup or 5 medium sprouts	28
Buns (see rolls)				
Butter	14	0.5	1 tbsp or $\frac{1}{8}$ stick	100
Cabbage, cooked	73	2.6	$\frac{1}{2}$ cup, cooked short time in little water	15
Cabbage, raw	45	1.6	$\frac{1}{2}$ cup, finely shredded	10
Cabbage, raw, Chinese	38	1.3	$\frac{1}{2}$ cup, 1-in. pieces	5
Cake, angel food (from mix)	53	1.9	1 piece, $\frac{1}{12}$ of 10-in.-dia. cake	135
Cake, Boston cream pie	69	2.4	1 piece, $\frac{1}{12}$ of 8-in.-dia. pie (unenriched flour)	210
Cake, plain chocolate-iced cupcake (from mix)	36	1.3	1 cupcake, $2\frac{1}{2}$ in. dia.	130
Cake, plain uniced cupcakes (from mix)	25	0.9	1 cupcake, $2\frac{1}{2}$ in. dia.	90
Cake, 2-layer devil's food with chocolate icing (from mix)	69	2.4	1 piece (mix), $\frac{1}{16}$ of 9-in.-dia. cake	235
Cake, fruit, dark	15	0.5	1 slice, $\frac{1}{30}$ of 8-in.-long loaf (enriched flour)	55
Cake, pound	30	1.1	1 slice, $2\frac{3}{4} \times 3 \times \frac{5}{8}$ in. (unenriched flour)	140
Cake, sponge	66	1.4	1 piece, $\frac{1}{12}$ of 10-in.-dia. cake (unenriched)	195
Cake, 2-layer white with chocolate icing	71	2.5	1 piece, $\frac{1}{16}$ of 9-in.-dia. cake	250
Candy, caramels	28	1.0	4 small	115
Candy, plain chocolate	28	1.0	1 bar, $3\frac{3}{4} \times 1\frac{1}{2} \times \frac{1}{4}$ in.	145
Candy, chocolate with almonds	51	1.8	1 bar, $5\frac{1}{3} \times 1\frac{7}{8} \times \frac{1}{3}$ in.	265
Candy, chocolate creams	28	1.0	2 pieces, $1\frac{1}{4}$ in. dia. (base), $\frac{5}{8}$ in. thick	110
Candy, chocolate fudge	28	1.0	1 piece, $1\frac{1}{4} \times 1\frac{1}{4} \times 1$ in.	115
Candy, hard	28	1.0	6 pieces, 1 in. dia., $\frac{1}{4}$ in. thick	110
Candy, peanut brittle	28	1.0	1 piece, $3\frac{1}{4} \times 2\frac{1}{2} \times \frac{1}{4}$ in.	125
Cantaloupes	385	13.5	$\frac{1}{2}$ melon, 5 in. dia.	60
Carrots, raw grated	55	1.9	$\frac{1}{2}$ cup grated	23
Carrots, raw whole or strips	50	1.8	1 carrot, $5\frac{1}{2}$ in. long, or 25 thin strips	20
Carrots, cooked	73	2.6	$\frac{1}{2}$ cup diced	23
Catsup, tomato (see tomato)				
Cauliflower, cooked	60	2.1	$\frac{1}{2}$ cup flowerets	13
Celery, raw diced	50	1.8	$\frac{1}{2}$ cup	8
Celery, raw whole	40	1.4	1 stalk, large outer, 8 in. long	5
Cheese, blue (Roquefort type)	28	1.0	$\frac{3}{4}$-in. sector or 3 tbsp	105

PROTEIN G	FAT G	CARBOHYDRATE G	CALCIUM MG	IRON MG	VITAMIN-A ACTIVITY IU	ASCORBIC ACID MG	THIAMIN MG	RIBOFLAVIN MG
3	1	4	68	0.6	1940	70	0.07	0.16
4	1	5	25	0.9	405	68	0.06	0.11
tr	12	tr	3	0	470	0	—	—
1	tr	3	32	0.2	95	24	0.03	0.03
1	tr	3	22	0.2	60	21	0.03	0.03
1	tr	1	16	0.3	55	10	0.02	0.02
3	tr	32	50	0.2	0	0	tr	0.06
4	6	34	46	0.3	140	tr	0.02	0.08
2	5	21	47	0.3	60	tr	0.01	0.04
1	3	14	40	0.1	40	tr	0.01	0.03
3	9	40	41	0.6	100	tr	0.02	0.06
1	2	9	11	0.4	20	tr	0.02	0.02
2	9	14	6	0.2	80	0	0.01	0.03
5	4	36	20	0.8	300	tr	0.03	0.09
3	8	45	70	0.4	40	tr	0.01	0.06
1	3	22	42	0.4	tr	tr	0.01	0.05
2	9	16	65	0.3	80	tr	0.02	0.10
4	19	25	102	1.4	70	0	0.07	0.25
1	4	20	—	—	—	0	—	—
1	4	21	22	0.3	tr	tr	0.01	0.03
0	tr	28	6	0.5	0	0	0	0
2	4	21	11	0.6	10	0	0.03	0.01
1	tr	14	27	0.8	6540	63	0.08	0.06
1	tr	6	21	0.4	6050	5	0.03	0.03
1	tr	5	18	0.4	5500	4	0.03	0.03
1	tr	5	24	0.5	7610	5	0.04	0.04
2	tr	3	13	0.4	35	33	0.06	0.05
1	tr	2	20	0.2	120	5	0.02	0.02
tr	tr	2	16	0.1	100	4	0.01	0.01
6	9	1	89	0.1	350	0	0.01	0.17

FOOD	WEIGHT G	WEIGHT OZ	APPROXIMATE MEASURE AND DESCRIPTION	KCAL
Cheese, cheddar (American), cubed	28	1.0	1 cube, $1\frac{1}{8}$ in.	115
Cheese, cheddar (American), grated	7	0.3	1 tbsp	30
Cheese, creamed cottage	61	2.1	$\frac{1}{4}$ cup (made from skim milk)	65
Cheese, uncreamed cottage	28	1.0	2 tbsp (made from skim milk)	25
Cheese, cream	16	0.5	1 tbsp	60
Cheese, Swiss (domestic)	28	1.0	1 slice, $7 \times 4 \times \frac{1}{8}$ in.	105
Cheese foods, cheddar	28	1.0	2 round slices, $1\frac{5}{8}$ in. dia., $\frac{1}{4}$ in. thick or 2 tbsp	90
Cheese sauce	60	2.1	$\frac{1}{4}$ cup	110
Cheese soufflé	79	2.8	$\frac{3}{4}$ cup	200
Cheesecake	162	5.7	$\frac{1}{10}$ of 9-in.-dia. cake	400
Cherries, raw sweet	130	4.6	1 cup with stems	80
Cherries, raw West Indian (acerola)	11	0.4	2 medium cherries	3
Chick peas, dry raw (garbanzos)	105	3.7	$\frac{1}{2}$ cup	380
Chicken, broiled	85	3.0	3 slices, flesh only	115
Chicken, canned	85	3.0	$\frac{1}{3}$ cup boned meat	170
Chicken, creamed	99	3.5	$\frac{1}{2}$ cup	222
Chicken breast, fried	94	3.3	$\frac{1}{2}$ breast with bone	155
Chicken drumstick, fried	59	2.1	1 drumstick with bone	90
Chicken pie (see poultry potpie)				
Chili con carne with beans, canned	188	6.5	$\frac{3}{4}$ cup	250
Chili con carne without beans, canned	191	6.7	$\frac{3}{4}$ cup	383
Chili powder	15	0.5	1 tbsp hot red peppers, dried and ground	50
Chili sauce	17	0.6	1 tbsp, mainly tomatoes	20
Chocolate, bitter (baking chocolate)	28	1.0	1 square	145
Chocolate candy (see candy)				
Chocolate-flavored milk drink	250	8.8	1 cup (made with skim milk)	190
Chocolate morsels	15	0.5	30 morsels or $1\frac{1}{2}$ tbsp	80
Chocolate syrup	40	1.4	2 tbsp	80
Chop suey, cooked	122	4.3	$\frac{3}{4}$ cup	325
Clams, canned	85	3.0	$\frac{1}{2}$ cup or 3 medium clams	45
Cocoa, beverage	182	6.3	$\frac{3}{4}$ cup (made with milk)	176
Coconut, dried shredded, sweetened	16	0.6	$\frac{1}{4}$ cup	85
Coconut, fresh shredded	33	1.2	$\frac{1}{4}$ cup	113
Codfish, dried	51	1.8	$\frac{1}{2}$ cup	190
Coffee cake, frosted	79	2.8	1 piece, $3 \times 3 \times 1\frac{1}{4}$ in.	260
Cole slaw	60	2.1	$\frac{1}{2}$ cup	50
Cookies, brownies	26	0.9	1 piece, $1\frac{7}{8} \times 1\frac{7}{8} \times \frac{5}{8}$ in.	145
Cookies, chocolate chip	11	0.4	1 cookie, $2\frac{1}{4}$ in. diameter	60
Cookies, coconut bar chews	11	0.4	1 cookie, $3 \times \frac{7}{8} \times \frac{1}{3}$ in.	55
Cookies, oatmeal with raisins and nuts	11	0.4	1 cookie, $2\frac{1}{8}$ in. diameter	65

PROTEIN G	FAT G	CARBOHYDRATE G	CALCIUM MG	IRON MG	VITAMIN-A ACTIVITY IU	ASCORBIC ACID MG	THIAMIN MG	RIBOFLAVIN MG
6	10	2	206	0.3	368	0	0.02	0.13
2	2	tr	52	0.1	90	0	tr	0.03
8	3	2	58	0.2	105	0	0.02	0.15
5	tr	1	26	0.1	tr	0	0.01	0.08
1	6	tr	10	tr	250	0	tr	0.04
8	8	1	262	0.3	320	0	tr	0.11
6	6	2	160	0.2	280	0	tr	0.16
5	9	4	156	0.1	337	1	0.02	0.14
10	16	7	210	1.0	826	1	0.08	0.23
15	23	35	128	0.8	958	1	0.08	0.33
2	tr	20	26	0.5	130	12	0.06	0.07
—	—	1	1	—	—	100	—	0.01
22	5	64	97	7.5	tr	2	0.58	0.19
20	2	0	8	1.4	80	—	0.05	0.16
18	10	0	18	1.3	200	3	0.03	0.11
20	12	6	84	1.1	445	1	0.04	0.20
25	5	1	9	1.3	70	—	0.04	0.17
12	4	tr	6	0.9	50	—	0.03	0.15
14	11	23	60	3.2	113	—	0.06	0.14
20	29	11	73	2.7	285	—	0.04	0.23
2	2	8	40	2.3	9750	2	0.03	0.17
tr	tr	4	3	0.1	240	3	0.02	0.01
3	15	8	22	1.9	20	0	0.01	0.07
8	6	27	270	0.5	210	3	0.10	0.40
1	4	10	5	0.3	tr	0	tr	tr
tr	tr	22	6	0.6	—	—	—	—
19	20	16	43	2.9	85	17	0.11	0.13
7	1	2	47	3.5	—	—	0.01	0.09
7	8	20	215	0.7	293	2	0.07	0.34
1	6	8	3	0.3	0	0	0.01	0.01
1	12	3	4	0.6	0	1	0.02	0.01
41	2	0	25	1.8	0	0	0.04	0.23
4	11	37	25	1.0	477	0	0.12	0.13
1	4	5	24	0.3	40	25	0.03	0.03
2	9	17	12	0.5	231	—	0.03	0.04
1	3	7	4	0.2	81	—	0.01	0.01
tr	2	9	7	0.3	76	0	0.01	0.01
1	4	6	5	0.3	18	tr	0.04	0.02

FOOD	WEIGHT		APPROXIMATE MEASURE AND DESCRIPTION	KCAL
	G	OZ		
Cookies, sugar, plain	9	0.3	1 cookie, $2\frac{1}{2}$ in. diameter	40
Corn, sweet, cooked	140	4.9	1 ear, 5 in. long	70
Corn, sweet, canned	128	4.5	$\frac{1}{2}$ cup, solids and liquid	85
Corn grits, cooked	163	5.7	$\frac{2}{3}$ cup, enriched and degermed	85
Corn muffins	40	1.4	1 muffin, $2\frac{3}{8}$ in. dia., enriched flour and enriched degermed meal	125
Corned beef (see beef)				
Corned beef hash (see beef)				
Cornflakes	33	1.2	$1\frac{1}{3}$ cup (added nutrients)	133
Cornmeal, dry	138	4.8	1 cup, white or yellow, enriched and degermed	500
Cow peas (see peas)				
Crabmeat, canned	85	3.0	$\frac{1}{2}$ cup flakes	85
Crackers, graham, plain	14	0.6	2 medium or 4 small	55
Crackers, saltines	8	0.3	2 crackers, 2 in. square	35
Cranberry juice, canned	125	4.4	$\frac{1}{2}$ cup or 1 small glass, ascorbic acid added	85
Cranberry sauce, canned	69	2.4	$\frac{1}{4}$ cup, strained and sweetened	85
Cream, coffee (light cream)	15	0.5	1 tbsp	30
Cream, half-and-half	15	0.5	1 tbsp	20
Cream, heavy, whipping	15	0.5	1 tbsp, unwhipped (volume doubled when whipped)	55
Creamer, coffee (imitation cream)	2	—	1 tsp powder	10
Cucumber, raw	50	1.8	6 slices, pared, $\frac{1}{8}$ in. thick	5
Custard, baked	124	4.3	$\frac{1}{2}$ cup	143
Dates, pitted	45	1.6	$\frac{1}{4}$ cup or 8 dates	123
Dessert topping, whipped	11	0.4	2 tbsp (low-calorie, with nonfat dry milk)	17
Doughnuts, cake-type	32	1.1	1 (enriched flour)	125
Egg, raw, boiled, or poached	50	1.8	1 whole egg	80
Egg white, raw	33	1.2	1 egg white	15
Egg yolk, raw	17	0.6	1 egg yolk	60
Eggs, creamed	113	4.0	$\frac{1}{2}$ cup (1 egg in $\frac{1}{4}$ cup white sauce)	190
Eggs, fried	54	1.9	1 egg, cooked in 1 tsp fat	115
Eggs, scrambled	64	2.2	1 egg, with milk and fat	110
Endive, curly, raw	57	2.0	3 leaves (includes escarole)	10
Farina, cooked	163	5.7	$\frac{2}{3}$ cup (quick, enriched)	70
Fats, cooking, lard	13	0.5	1 tbsp solid fat	115
Fats, cooking, vegetable	13	0.5	1 tbsp solid fat	110
Figs, dried	21	0.7	1 large fig, 1 × 2 in.	60
Figs, fresh raw	114	4.0	3 small, $1\frac{1}{2}$ in. dia.,	90
Fish (see various kinds of fish)				

PROTEIN G	FAT G	CARBOHYDRATE G	CALCIUM MG	IRON MG	VITAMIN-A ACTIVITY IU	ASCORBIC ACID MG	THIAMIN MG	RIBOFLAVIN MG
1	2	6	2	0.1	64	0	0.02	0.01
3	1	16	2	0.5	310	7	0.09	0.08
3	1	20	5	0.5	345	7	0.04	0.06
2	tr	18	1	0.5	100	0	0.07	0.05
3	4	19	42	0.7	120	tr	0.08	0.09
3	tr	28	5	0.5	0	0	0.15	0.03
11	2	108	8	4.0	610	0	0.61	0.36
15	2	1	38	0.7	—	—	0.07	0.07
1	1	10	6	0.2	0	0	0.01	0.03
1	1	6	2	0.1	0	0	tr	tr
tr	tr	21	7	0.4	tr	20	0.02	0.02
tr	tr	21	4	0.1	13	1	0.01	0.01
1	3	1	15	tr	130	tr	tr	0.02
1	2	1	16	tr	70	tr	tr	0.02
tr	6	1	11	tr	230	tr	tr	0.02
tr	1	1	1	tr	tr	—	—	—
tr	tr	2	8	0.2	tr	6	0.02	0.02
7	7	14	139	0.5	435	1	0.05	0.24
1	tr	33	26	1.3	23	0	0.04	0.04
1	—	3	29	—	1	1	0.01	0.04
1	6	16	13	0.4	30	tr	0.05	0.05
6	6	tr	27	1.1	590	0	0.05	0.15
4	tr	tr	3	tr	0	0	tr	0.09
3	5	tr	24	0.9	580	0	0.04	0.07
9	14	7	103	1.2	928	tr	0.07	0.25
6	10	tr	28	1.1	590	0	0.05	0.15
7	8	1	51	1.1	690	0	0.05	0.18
1	tr	2	46	1.0	1870	6	0.04	0.08
2	tr	14	98	0.5	0	0	0.08	0.05
0	13	0	0	0	0	0	0	0
0	13	0	0	0	—	0	0	0
1	tr	15	26	0.6	20	0	0.02	0.02
1	tr	23	40	0.7	90	2	0.07	0.06

FOOD	WEIGHT G	WEIGHT OZ	APPROXIMATE MEASURE AND DESCRIPTION	KCAL
Fish, creamed (tuna, salmon, or other, in white sauce)	136	4.8	½ cup	220
Fish sticks, breaded, cooked	114	4.0	5 sticks, each 3.8 × 1.0 × 0.5 in.	200
Frankfurter, heated	56	2.0	1 frankfurter	170
French toast, fried	79	2.8	1 slice (enriched bread)	180
Fruit balls, raw (dried apricots, dates, nuts)	11	0.4	1 ball, 1 in. dia.	45
Fruit cocktail, canned	128	4.5	½ cup, with heavy syrup	98
Gelatin, plain, dry	7	0.3	1 tbsp (1 envelope)	25
Gelatin dessert, plain	120	4.2	½ cup, ready to eat	70
Gingerbread	63	2.2	1 piece (mix), ⅑ of 8-in.-square cake	175
Grapefruit, white, raw (as purchased)	241	8.4	½ medium, 3¾ in. dia.	45
Grapefruit, white, canned	125	4.4	½ cup, syrup pack	88
Grapefruit juice, canned	124	4.3	½ cup, unsweetened	50
Grapefruit juice, dehydrated crystals	124	4.3	½ cup or 1 small glass, prepared, ready to serve	50
Grapes, raw American-type	153	5.4	1 cup or 1 medium bunch (slip skin, as Concord)	65
Grapes, raw European-type	160	5.6	1 cup or 40 grapes (adherent skin, as Tokay)	95
Grape juice, canned	127	4.4	½ cup	83
Greens, collards, cooked	95	3.3	½ cup	28
Greens, dandelion, cooked	90	3.2	½ cup	30
Greens, kale, cooked	55	1.9	½ cup, leaves and stems	15
Greens, mustard, cooked	70	2.5	½ cup	18
Greens, spinach, cooked	90	3.2	½ cup	20
Greens, turnip, cooked	73	2.6	½ cup	15
Guavas, raw	82	2.8	1 guava	50
Haddock, fried	85	3.0	1 fillet, 4 × 2½ × ½ in.	140
Ham, boiled	57	2.0	1 slice, 6¼ × 3¾ × ⅛ in.	135
Ham, cured, roasted	85	3.0	2 slices, 5½ × 3¾ × ⅛ in.	245
Ham, luncheon, canned	57	2.0	2 tbsp, spiced or unspiced	165
Hamburger (see beef, hamburger)				
Honey, strained	21	0.7	1 tbsp.	65
Hot dog (see frankfurter)				
Ice cream, plain	50	1.8	1 container, 3 fluid oz (factory packed)	9?
Ice cream, plain brick	71	2.5	1 slice, ⅛ of qt brick	14?
Ice milk	66	2.3	½ cup	10?

PROTEIN G	FAT G	CARBOHYDRATE G	CALCIUM MG	IRON MG	VITAMIN-A ACTIVITY IU	ASCORBIC ACID MG	THIAMIN MG	RIBOFLAVIN MG
20	13	8	81	0.9	385	tr	0.05	0.18
19	10	8	13	0.5	—	—	0.05	0.08
7	15	1	3	0.8	—	—	0.08	0.11
6	12	14	78	1.0	568	tr	0.09	0.17
1	1	8	10	0.4	285	tr	0.02	0.02
1	tr	25	12	0.5	180	3	0.03	0.02
6	tr	0	—	—	—	—	—	—
2	0	17	—	—	—	—	—	—
2	4	32	57	1.0	tr	tr	0.02	0.06
1	tr	12	19	0.5	10	44	0.05	0.02
1	tr	22	16	0.4	10	38	0.04	0.02
1	tr	12	10	0.5	10	42	0.04	0.02
1	tr	12	11	0.1	10	46	0.05	0.03
1	1	15	15	0.4	100	3	0.05	0.03
1	tr	25	17	0.6	140	6	0.07	0.04
1	tr	21	14	0.4	—	tr	0.05	0.03
3	1	5	145	0.6	5130	44	0.14	0.19
2	1	6	126	1.6	10,530	16	0.12	0.15
2	1	2	74	0.7	4070	34	—	—
2	1	3	97	1.3	4060	34	0.06	0.10
3	1	3	84	2.0	7290	25	0.07	0.13
2	tr	3	126	0.8	4135	34	0.08	0.17
1	tr	12	21	0.5	180	212	0.05	0.03
17	5	5	34	1.0	—	2	0.03	0.06
11	10	0	6	1.6	0	—	0.25	0.09
18	19	0	8	2.2	0	—	0.40	0.16
8	14	1	5	1.2	0	—	0.18	0.12
tr	0	17	1	0.1	0	tr	tr	0.01
2	5	10	73	0.2	220	1	0.02	0.11
3	9	15	87	0.1	370	1	0.03	0.13
3	4	15	102	0.1	140	1	0.04	0.15

FOOD	WEIGHT		APPROXIMATE MEASURE AND DESCRIPTION	KCAL
	G	OZ		
Jams, jellies, preserves	20	0.7	1 tbsp	55
Kale (*see* greens)				
Lamb chop, cooked	137	4.8	1 thick chop with bone	400
Lamb, leg, roasted	85	3.0	2 slices, $3 \times 3\frac{1}{4} \times \frac{1}{8}$ in., lean and fat, no bone	235
Lard (*see* fats, cooking)				
Lemon juice, fresh	15	0.5	1 tbsp	5
Lemonade	248	8.7	1 cup (made from frozen, sweetened concentrate)	110
Lentils, dry, cooked	100	3.5	$\frac{1}{2}$ cup	120
Lettuce, headed, raw	454	16.0	1 head (compact, as iceberg), $4\frac{3}{4}$ in. dia.	60
Lettuce, loose leaf, raw	50	1.8	2 large leaves or 4 small leaves	10
Lime juice, canned	62	2.2	$\frac{1}{4}$ cup	15
Liver, beef, fried	57	2.0	1 slice, $5 \times 2 \times \frac{1}{3}$ in.	130
Liver, calf, fried	74	2.6	1 slice, $5 \times 2 \times \frac{1}{2}$ in.	230
Liver, chicken, fried	85	3.0	3 medium livers	235
Liver, pork, fried	70	2.5	1 slice, $3\frac{3}{4} \times 1\frac{3}{4} \times \frac{1}{2}$ in.	225
Macaroni, cooked	105	3.7	$\frac{3}{4}$ cup (enriched)	115
Macaroni and cheese, baked	150	5.3	$\frac{3}{4}$ cup (enriched macaroni)	325
Mackerel, broiled	85	3.0	1 piece	200
Mangoes, raw	198	7.0	1 medium mango	90
Margarine	14	0.5	1 tbsp or $\frac{1}{8}$ stick (fortified with vitamin A)	100
Marshmallows	9	0.3	1, $1\frac{1}{4}$ in. dia.	25
Meat loaf, beef, baked	77	2.7	1 slice, $3\frac{3}{4} \times 2\frac{1}{4} \times \frac{3}{4}$ in.	240
Milk, dry skim (nonfat)	17	0.6	$\frac{1}{4}$ cup powder, instant	61
Milk, dry whole	26	0.9	$\frac{1}{4}$ cup powder	129
Milk, evaporated, canned	126	4.4	$\frac{1}{2}$ cup, undiluted and unsweetened	173
Milk, fluid, skim or buttermilk	245	8.6	1 cup ($\frac{1}{2}$ pt)	90
Milk, fluid, whole	244	8.5	1 cup ($\frac{1}{2}$ pt), 3.5% fat	160
Milk, malted, plain	353	12.4	1 fountain size glass (about $1\frac{1}{2}$ cup)	368
Milkshake, chocolate	342	12.0	1 fountain size glass	420
Molasses, cane, black-strap	20	0.7	1 tbsp, 3rd extraction	45
Molasses, cane, light	20	0.7	1 tbsp, 1st extraction	50
Muffins, plain	40	1.4	1 muffin, $2\frac{3}{4}$ in. dia. (enriched white flour)	120
Mushrooms, canned	122	4.3	$\frac{1}{2}$ cup, solids and liquid	20
Noodles, egg, cooked	120	4.2	$\frac{3}{4}$ cup (enriched)	150
Nuts, almonds	36	1.3	$\frac{1}{4}$ cup shelled	213
Nuts, cashew, rosted	35	1.2	$\frac{1}{4}$ cup	196
Nuts, peanuts (*see* peanuts, roasted)				
Nuts, pecan halves	27	0.9	$\frac{1}{4}$ cup	185
Nuts, walnut halves	25	0.9	$\frac{1}{4}$ cup, English or Persian	163

PROTEIN G	FAT G	CARBOHYDRATE G	CALCIUM MG	IRON MG	VITAMIN-A ACTIVITY IU	ASCORBIC ACID MG	THIAMIN MG	RIBOFLAVIN MG
tr	tr	14	4	0.2	tr	tr	tr	0.01
25	33	0	10	1.5	—	—	0.14	0.25
22	16	0	9	1.4	—	—	0.13	0.23
tr	tr	1	1	tr	tr	7	tr	tr
tr	tr	28	2	tr	tr	17	tr	0.02
9	tr	22	12	2.5	200	0	0.20	0.09
4	tr	13	91	2.3	1500	29	0.29	0.27
1	tr	2	34	0.7	950	9	0.03	0.04
tr	tr	6	6	0.1	5	13	0.01	0.01
15	6	3	6	5.0	30,280	15	0.15	2.37
15	15	4	5	9.0	19,130	30	0.18	2.65
20	15	5	15	6.4	27,370	17	0.19	2.11
17	15	3	8	15.3	12,070	19	0.34	2.53
4	1	24	6	1.0	0	0	0.15	0.08
13	17	30	272	1.4	645	tr	0.15	0.30
19	13	0	5	1.0	450	—	0.13	0.23
1	—	23	12	0.3	8380	55	0.08	0.07
tr	12	tr	3	0	470	0	—	—
tr	0	8	2	0.2	0	0	0	tr
19	17	3	34	2.9	138	—	0.10	0.21
6	tr	9	220	0.1	5	1	0.06	0.30
7	7	10	234	0.1	290	2	0.08	0.38
9	10	12	318	0.2	405	2	0.05	0.43
9	tr	12	296	0.1	10	2	0.09	0.44
9	9	12	288	0.1	350	2	0.07	0.41
17	15	42	476	1.1	885	3	0.21	0.74
11	18	58	363	0.9	687	4	0.12	0.55
—	—	11	137	3.2	—	—	0.02	0.04
—	—	13	33	0.9	—	—	0.01	0.01
3	4	17	42	0.6	40	tr	0.07	0.09
3	tr	3	8	0.6	tr	2	0.02	0.30
5	2	28	12	1.1	83	0	0.17	0.11
7	19	7	83	1.7	0	tr	0.09	0.33
6	16	10	13	1.3	35	—	0.15	0.09
3	19	4	20	0.7	35	1	0.23	0.04
4	16	4	25	0.8	8	1	0.08	0.03

293

FOOD	WEIGHT		APPROXIMATE MEASURE	KCAL
	G	OZ	AND DESCRIPTION	
Oatmeal or rolled oats, cooked	160	5.6	$\frac{2}{3}$ cup (regular or quick-cooking)	87
Oils, salad or cooking	14	0.5	1 tbsp	125
Okra, cooked	43	1.5	4 pods, $3 \times \frac{5}{8}$ in.	13
Olives, green	16	0.6	4 medium or 3 large	15
Olives, ripe	10	0.4	3 small or 2 large	15
Onions, raw	110	3.9	1 onion, $2\frac{1}{2}$ in. dia.	40
Onions, cooked	105	3.7	$\frac{1}{2}$ cup or 5 onions, $1\frac{1}{4}$ in. dia.	30
Onions, young green	50	1.8	6 small, without tops	20
Oranges	180	6.3	1 orange, $2\frac{5}{8}$ in. dia. (all commercial varieties)	65
Orange juice, fresh	124	4.3	$\frac{1}{2}$ cup or 1 small glass (all varieties)	55
Orange juice, canned unsweetened	125	4.4	$\frac{1}{2}$ cup or 1 small glass	60
Orange juice, frozen concentrate	125	4.4	$\frac{1}{2}$ cup or 1 small glass, diluted, ready to serve	60
Orange juice, dehydrated crystals	124	4.3	$\frac{1}{2}$ cup or 1 small glass, prepared, ready to serve	60
Oysters, raw	120	4.2	$\frac{1}{2}$ cup or 8–10 oysters	80
Oyster stew, milk	230	8.1	1 cup with 3–4 oysters	200
Pancakes, wheat	27	0.9	1 griddle cake, 4 in. dia. (enriched flour)	60
Papayas, raw	91	3.2	$\frac{1}{2}$ cup in $\frac{1}{2}$-in. cubes	35
Parsley, raw	4	0.1	1 tbsp chopped	tr
Parsnips, cooked	77	2.7	$\frac{1}{2}$ cup	50
Peaches, canned halves or slices	129	4.5	$\frac{1}{2}$ cup, solids and liquid, syrup-pack	100
Peaches, canned whole	123	4.3	$\frac{1}{2}$ cup, solids liquid (water pack)	38
Peaches, raw sliced	84	2.9	$\frac{1}{2}$ cup fresh or frozen	33
Peaches, raw whole	114	4.0	1 peach, 2 in. dia.	35
Peanuts, roasted	36	1.3	$\frac{1}{4}$ cup halves, salted	210
Peanut butter	32	1.1	2 tbsp	190
Pears, canned	117	4.1	2 medium halves with 2 tbsp juice (syrup pack)	90
Pears, raw (as purchased)	182	6.3	1 pear, $3 \times 2\frac{1}{2}$ in. dia.	100
Peas, cowpeas, dry, cooked (blackeye peas or frijoles)	124	4.3	$\frac{1}{2}$ cup	95
Peas, green, cooked	80	2.8	$\frac{1}{2}$ cup	58
Peas, pigeon, dry raw (gandules)	99	3.5	6 tbsp	310
Peas, split, dry cooked	125	4.4	$\frac{1}{2}$ cup	145
Peppers, green, stuffed	113	4.0	1 medium pepper, cooked with meat stuffing	200
Peppers, hot red (see chili powder)				
Peppers, pimientos, canned	38	1.3	1 medium pod	10
Peppers, raw sweet green	74	2.6	1 medium pod without stem and seeds, 5 pods per lb	15

PROTEIN G	FAT G	CARBOHYDRATE G	CALCIUM MG	IRON MG	VITAMIN-A ACTIVITY IU	ASCORBIC ACID MG	THIAMIN MG	RIBOFLAVIN MG
3	1	15	15	0.9	0	0	0.13	0.03
0	14	0	0	0	—	0	0	0
1	tr	3	39	0.2	210	9	0.06	0.08
tr	2	tr	8	0.2	40	—	—	—
tr	2	tr	9	0.1	10	—	tr	tr
2	tr	10	30	0.6	40	11	0.04	0.04
2	tr	7	25	0.4	40	7	0.03	0.03
1	tr	5	20	0.3	tr	12	0.02	0.02
1	tr	16	54	0.5	260	66	0.13	0.05
1	1	13	14	0.3	250	62	0.11	0.04
1	tr	14	13	0.5	250	50	0.09	0.03
1	tr	15	13	0.1	275	60	0.11	0.01
l	tr	14	13	0.3	250	55	0.10	0.04
10	2	4	113	6.6	370	—	0.17	0.22
11	12	11	269	3.3	640	—	0.13	0.41
2	2	9	27	0.4	30	tr	0.05	0.06
1	tr	9	18	0.3	1595	51	0.04	0.04
tr	tr	tr	8	0.2	340	7	tr	0.01
1	1	12	35	0.5	25	8	0.06	0.07
1	tr	26	5	0.4	550	4	0.01	0.03
1	tr	10	5	0.4	550	4	0.01	0.03
1	tr	8	8	0.4	1115	6	0.02	0.04
1	tr	10	9	0.5	1320	7	0.02	0.05
9	18	7	27	0.8	—	0	0.12	0.05
8	16	6	18	0.6	—	0	0.04	0.04
tr	tr	23	6	0.2	tr	2	0.01	0.02
1	1	25	13	0.5	30	7	0.04	0.07
7	1	17	21	1.6	10	tr	0.21	0.06
5	1	10	19	1.5	430	17	0.22	0.09
22	2	50	140	4.0	169	0	0.45	0.34
10	1	26	14	2.1	50	—	0.19	0.11
12	14	12	31	1.9	637	64	0.09	0.14
tr	tr	2	3	0.6	870	36	0.01	0.02
1	tr	4	7	0.5	310	94	0.06	0.06

FOOD	WEIGHT G	WEIGHT OZ	APPROXIMATE MEASURE AND DESCRIPTION	KCAL
Peppers, raw sweet red	60	2.1	1 medium pod without stem and seeds	20
Perch, ocean, fried	85	3.0	1 piece, $4 \times 3 \times \frac{1}{2}$ in.	195
Persimmons, raw (Japanese)	125	4.4	1 fruit, $2\frac{1}{2}$ in. dia.	75
Pickle relish	15	0.5	1 tbsp	20
Pickles, cucumber, bread and butter	42	1.5	6 slices, $\frac{1}{4} \times 1\frac{1}{2}$ in. diameter	30
Pickles, cucumber, dill	65	2.3	1 large pickel, $3\frac{3}{4} \times 1\frac{1}{4}$ in.	10
Pickles, cucumber, sweet	15	0.5	1 pickle, $2\frac{1}{2} \times \frac{3}{4}$ in. diameter	20
Pie, apple	135	4.7	4-in. sector or $\frac{1}{7}$ of 9-in.-dia. pie (unenriched flour)	350
Pie, cherry	135	4.7	4-in. sector or $\frac{1}{7}$ of 9-in.-dia. pie (unenriched flour)	350
Pie, custard	130	4.6	4-in. sector or $\frac{1}{7}$ of 9-in.-dia. pie (unenriched flour)	285
Pie, lemon meringue	120	4.2	4-in. sector or $\frac{1}{7}$ of 9-in.-dia. pie (unenriched flour)	305
Pie, mince	135	4.7	4-in. sector or $\frac{1}{7}$ of 9-in.-dia. pie (unenriched flour)	365
Pie, pumpkin	130	4.6	4-in. sector or $\frac{1}{7}$ of 9-in.-dia. pie (unenriched flour)	275
Pineapple, canned crushed	130	4.6	$\frac{1}{2}$ cup (syrup pack)	100
Pineapple, canned slices	122	4.3	1 large or 2 small slices, 2 tbsp juice (syrup pack)	90
Pineapple, raw	70	2.5	$\frac{1}{2}$ cup, diced	38
Pineapple juice, canned	125	4.4	$\frac{1}{2}$ cup or 1 small glass	68
Pizza (cheese)	75	2.6	$5\frac{1}{2}$-in. sector or $\frac{1}{8}$ of 14-in.-dia. pie	185
Plantain, raw, green	100	3.5	1 baking banana, 6 in.	135
Plums, canned	128	4.5	$\frac{1}{2}$ cup or 3 plums with 2 tbsp juice (syrup pack)	100
Plums, raw	60	2.1	1 plum, 2 in. diameter	25
Popcorn, popped	9	0.3	1 cup (oil and salt) added	40
Pork chop, cooked	99	3.5	1 thick chop, trimmed, with bone	260
Pork roast, cooked	85	3.0	2 slices, $5 \times 4 \times \frac{1}{8}$ in.	310
Potato chips	20	0.7	10 medium chips, 2 in. diameter	115
Potatoes, baked	99	3.5	1 medium potato, about 3 per pound raw	90
Potatoes, boiled	122	4.3	1 potato, peeled before boiling	80
Potatoes, French fried	57	2.0	10 pieces, $2 \times \frac{1}{2} \times \frac{1}{2}$ in., cooked in deep fat	155
Potatoes, mashed	98	3.4	$\frac{1}{2}$ cup (milk and butter added)	95
Poultry (chicken or turkey) potpie	227	7.9	1 indiv. pie, $4\frac{1}{4}$ in. diameter	535
Pretzels	3	0.1	5, $3\frac{1}{8}$-in. sticks	10
Prunes, dried, cooked	105	3.7	5 medium prunes with 2 tbsp juice, sweetened	160
Prune juice, canned	128	4.5	$\frac{1}{2}$ cup or 1 small glass	100
Pudding, chocolate blanc mange	130	4.6	$\frac{1}{2}$ cup	190

PROTEIN G	FAT G	CARBOHYDRATE G	CALCIUM MG	IRON MG	VITAMIN-A ACTIVITY IU	ASCORBIC ACID MG	THIAMIN MG	RIBOFLAVIN MG
1	tr	4	8	0.4	2670	122	0.05	0.05
16	11	6	1.1	1.1	—	—	0.08	0.09
1	tr	20	6	0.4	2740	11	0.03	0.02
tr	tr	5	3	0.1	—	—	—	—
tr	tr	7	13	0.8	80	4	0.01	0.02
1	tr	1	17	0.7	70	4	tr	0.01
tr	tr	6	2	0.2	10	1	tr	tr
3	15	51	11	0.4	40	1	0.03	0.03
4	15	52	19	0.4	590	tr	0.03	0.03
8	14	30	125	0.8	300	0	0.07	0.21
4	12	45	17	0.6	200	4	0.04	0.10
3	16	56	38	1.4	tr	1	0.09	0.05
5	15	32	66	0.7	3210	tr	0.04	0.13
1	tr	25	15	0.4	60	9	0.10	0.03
tr	tr	24	13	0.4	50	8	0.09	0.03
1	tr	10	12	0.4	50	12	0.06	0.02
1	tr	17	19	0.4	60	11	0.06	0.02
7	6	27	107	0.7	290	4	0.04	0.12
1	—	32	8	0.8	380	28	0.07	0.04
1	tr	27	11	1.1	1485	2	0.03	0.03
tr	tr	7	7	0.3	140	3	0.02	0.02
1	2	5	1	0.2	—	0	—	0.01
16	21	0	8	2.2	0	—	0.63	0.18
21	24	0	9	2.7	0	—	0.78	0.22
1	8	10	8	0.4	tr	3	0.04	0.01
3	tr	21	9	0.7	tr	20	0.10	0.04
2	tr	18	7	0.6	tr	20	0.11	0.04
2	7	20	9	0.7	tr	12	0.07	0.04
2	4	12	24	0.4	165	9	0.08	0.05
23	31	42	68	3.0	3020	5	0.25	0.26
tr	tr	2	1	tr	0	0	tr	tr
1	tr	42	21	1.5	733	1	0.03	0.06
1	tr	25	18	5.3	—	3	0.02	0.02
6	8	26	158	0.9	211	1	0.06	0.27

FOOD	WEIGHT G	WEIGHT OZ	APPROXIMATE MEASURE AND DESCRIPTION	KCAL
Pudding, cornstarch (plain blanc mange)	124	4.3	½ cup	140
Pudding, rice with raisins (old-fashioned)	136	4.8	½ cup	300
Pudding, tapioca	74	2.6	½ cup	140
Radishes, raw	40	1.4	4 small	5
Raisins, seedless	10	0.4	1 tbsp pressed down	30
Raspberries, raw, red	62	2.2	½ cup	35
Rhubarb, cooked	136	4.8	½ cup (sugar added)	190
Rice, parboiled, cooked	131	4.6	¾ cup (enriched)	140
Rice, puffed	15	0.5	1 cup (nutrients added)	60
Rice flakes	30	1.1	1 cup (nutrients added)	115
Rolls, bagel (egg)	55	1.9	1 roll, 3 in. diameter	165
Rolls, barbecue bun	40	1.3	1 bun, 3½ in. diameter (enriched)	120
Rolls, hard	52	1.8	1 round roll	160
Rolls, plain, white	28	1.0	1 commercial pan roll (enriched flour)	85
Rolls, sweet, pan	43	1.5	1 roll	135
Rutabagas, cooked	77	2.7	½ cup	25
Salad, chicken	125	4.4	½ cup, with mayonnaise	280
Salad, egg	128	4.5	½ cup, with mayonnaise	190
Salad, fresh fruit (orange, apple, banana, grapes)	125	4.4	½ cup, with French dressing	130
Salad, jellied, vegetable	122	4.3	½ cup, no dressing	70
Salad, lettuce	130	4.6	¼ solid head, with French dressing	80
Salad, potato	139	4.9	½ cup, with mayonnaise	185
Salad, tomato aspic	119	4.2	½ cup, no dressing	45
Salad, tuna fish	102	3.6	½ cup, with mayonnaise	250
Salad dressing, blue cheese	15	0.5	1 tbsp	75
Salad dressing, boiled	16	0.6	1 tbsp, home-made	25
Salad dressing, commercial	15	0.5	1 tbsp, mayonnaise-type	65
Salad dressing, French	16	0.6	1 tbsp	65
Salad dressing, low-calorie	26	0.9	2 tbsp (cottage cheese, nonfat dry milk, no oil)	17
Salad dressing, mayonnaise	14	0.5	1 tbsp	100
Salad dressing, Thousand Island	16	0.6	1 tbsp	80
Salmon, boiled or baked	119	4.2	1 steak, 4 × 3 × ½ in.	200
Salmon, pink, canned	85	3.0	½ cup	120
Salmon loaf	113	4.0	½ cup or 1 slice, 4 × 1¼ × 1¼ in.	235
Sardines, canned oil	57	2.0	5 small fish, 3 × 1 × ¼ in.	120
Sauce, chocolate	40	1.4	2 tbsp	75
Sauce, custard	31	1.1	2 tbsp (low calorie, with nonfat dry milk)	45
Sauce, hard	17	0.6	1 tbsp	90

PROTEIN G	FAT G	CARBOHYDRATE G	CALCIUM MG	IRON MG	VITAMIN-A ACTIVITY IU	ASCORBIC ACID MG	THIAMIN MG	RIBOFLAVIN MG
5	5	20	145	0.1	195	1	0.04	0.20
8	8	52	243	0.8	313	3	0.10	0.35
5	5	12	104	0.4	327	1	0.04	0.19
tr	tr	1	12	0.4	tr	10	0.01	0.01
tr	tr	8	7	0.4	2	tr	0.01	0.01
1	1	9	14	0.6	80	16	0.02	0.06
1	tr	50	106	0.8	110	9	0.03	0.08
3	tr	31	25	1.1	0	0	0.14	0.02
1	tr	13	3	0.3	0	0	0.07	0.01
2	tr	26	9	0.5	0	0	0.10	0.02
6	2	28	9	1.2	30	0	0.14	0.10
3	2	21	30	0.8	tr	tr	0.11	0.07
5	2	31	24	0.4	tr	tr	0.03	0.05
2	2	15	21	0.5	tr	tr	0.08	0.05
4	4	21	37	0.3	30	tr	0.03	0.06
1	tr	6	43	0.3	270	18	0.04	0.06
25	19	1	20	1.7	200	1	0.04	0.15
6	18	1	35	1.3	630	1	0.06	0.16
—	6	21	25	0.6	154	22	0.06	0.05
3	—	16	14	0.2	25	20	0.03	0.02
1	6	5	28	0.7	618	9	0.05	0.10
2	12	17	21	0.8	40	17	0.11	0.05
5	0	7	12	0.5	1441	22	0.07	0.05
21	18	1	14	1.2	98	1	0.04	0.09
1	8	1	12	tr	30	tr	tr	0.02
1	2	2	14	0.1	80	tr	0.01	0.03
tr	6	2	2	tr	30	—	tr	tr
tr	6	3	2	0.1	—	—	—	—
2	0	2	31	0	18	1	0.01	0.06
tr	11	tr	3	0.1	40	—	tr	0.01
tr	8	3	2	0.1	50	tr	tr	tr
34	7	tr	—	1.4	—	—	0.12	0.33
17	5	0	167	0.7	60	—	0.03	0.16
29	10	5	43	1.8	332	2	0.08	0.20
13	6	0	248	1.7	127	—	0.01	0.11
1	4	9	32	0.2	87	—	0.01	0.05
2	1	7	56	0.2	89	—	0.02	0.09
—	6	11	1	0	231	0	0	0

FOOD	WEIGHT G	WEIGHT OZ	APPROXIMATE MEASURE AND DESCRIPTION	KCAL
Sauce, hollandaise (mock)	26	0.9	2 tbsp	75
Sauce, lemon	28	1.0	2 tbsp	40
Sauerkraut, canned	118	4.1	$\frac{1}{2}$ cup, solids and liquid	25
Sausage, bologna	57	2.0	2 slices, 4.1 × 0.1 in.	173
Sausage, frankfurters (see frankfurters)				
Sausage, liverwurst	57	2.0	3 slices, 2$\frac{1}{2}$ in. diameter $\frac{1}{4}$ in. thick	150
Sausage, pork, cooked	26	0.9	2 small patties or links	125
Sausage, Vienna	16	0.6	1 canned sausage, about 2 in. long	40
Shad, baked	85	3.0	1 piece, 4 × 3 × $\frac{1}{2}$ in.	170
Sherbet, orange	97	3.4	$\frac{1}{2}$ cup	130
Shrimp, canned	85	3.0	$\frac{1}{2}$ cup, meat only	100
Syrup, table blends	21	0.7	1 tbsp, light and dark	60
Soup, bean with pork, canned	250	8.8	1 cup, ready to serve	170
Soup, beef broth, bouillon, consommé, canned	240	8.4	1 cup, ready to serve	30
Soup, chicken noodle, canned	250	8.8	1 cup, ready to serve	65
Soup, clam chowder, canned	255	8.9	1 cup, ready to serve	85
Soup, cream of vegetable (e.g., tomato, mushroom), canned	240	8.4	1 cup, ready to serve	135
Soup, minestrone, canned	245	8.6	1 cup, ready to serve	105
Soup, tomato, canned	245	8.6	1 cup, ready to serve	90
Soup, vegetable, canned	250	8.8	1 cup, ready to serve	80
Spaghetti, cooked	105	3.7	$\frac{3}{4}$ cup (enriched)	115
Spaghetti, in tomato sauce, with cheese	188	6.5	$\frac{3}{4}$ cup	200
Spaghetti, in tomato sauce, with meat balls	186	6.5	$\frac{3}{4}$ cup	250
Spinach (see greens)				
Squash, summer, cooked	105	3.7	$\frac{1}{2}$ cup, diced	15
Squash, winter, baked	103	3.6	$\frac{1}{2}$ cup, mashed	65
Stew, beef and vegetable	176	6.2	$\frac{3}{4}$ cup	160
Strawberries, raw	75	2.6	$\frac{1}{2}$ cup, capped	30
Sugar, brown	14	0.5	1 tbsp firmly packed	50
Sugar, granulated	11	0.4	1 tbsp (beet or cane)	40
Sugar, lump	6	0.2	1 domino, 1$\frac{1}{8}$ × $\frac{3}{4}$ × $\frac{3}{8}$ in.	25
Sugar, powdered	8	0.3	1 tbsp	30
Sweet potatoes, baked	110	3.9	1 medium potato, about 6 oz raw	155
Sweet potatoes, candied	175	6.1	1 potato, 3$\frac{1}{2}$ × 2$\frac{1}{4}$ in.	295
Tangerine	116	4.1	1 medium tangerine, 2$\frac{3}{8}$ in. diameter	40

PROTEIN G	FAT G	CARBOHYDRATE G	CALCIUM MG	IRON MG	VITAMIN-A ACTIVITY IU	ASCORBIC ACID MG	THIAMIN MG	RIBOFLAVIN MG
2	7	3	36	0.2	353	1	0.02	0.06
0	1	8	—	—	34	2	—	—
1	tr	5	43	0.6	60	17	0.04	0.05
7	16	1	4	1.0	—	—	0.09	0.12
10	12	1	5	3.1	3260	0	0.10	0.63
5	11	tr	2	0.6	0	—	0.21	0.09
2	3	tr	1	0.3	—	—	0.01	0.02
20	10	0	20	0.5	20	—	0.11	0.22
1	1	30	16	tr	60	2	0.01	0.03
21	1	1	98	2.6	50	—	0.01	0.03
0	0	15	9	0.8	0	0	0	0
8	6	22	63	2.3	650	3	0.13	0.08
5	0	3	tr	0.5	tr	—	tr	0.02
4	2	8	10	0.5	50	tr	0.02	0.02
2	3	13	36	1.0	920	—	0.03	0.03
2	10	10	41	0.5	70	tr	0.02	0.12
5	3	14	37	1.0	2350	—	0.07	0.05
2	3	16	15	0.7	1000	12	0.05	0.05
3	2	14	20	0.8	3250	—	0.05	0.02
4	1	24	8	1.0	0	0	0.15	0.08
7	7	28	60	1.7	810	10	0.18	0.14
15	9	30	93	2.8	1193	17	0.20	0.23
1	tr	4	26	0.4	410	11	0.05	0.08
2	1	16	29	0.8	4305	14	0.05	0.14
11	8	11	21	2.1	1733	11	0.10	0.13
1	1	7	16	0.8	45	44	0.02	0.05
0	0	13	12	0.5	0	0	tr	tr
0	0	11	0	tr	0	0	0	0
0	0	6	0	tr	0	0	0	0
0	0	8	0	tr	0	0	0	0
2	1	36	44	1.0	8910	24	0.10	0.07
2	6	60	65	1.6	11,030	17	0.10	0.08
1	tr	10	34	0.3	360	27	0.05	0.02

FOOD	WEIGHT G	WEIGHT OZ	APPROXIMATE MEASURE AND DESCRIPTION	KCAL
Tartar sauce (see salad dressing, mayonnaise)				
Toast, melba	6	0.2	1 slice, $3\frac{3}{4} \times 1\frac{3}{4}$ in.	20
Tomato catsup	15	0.5	1 tbsp	15
Tomato juice, canned	122	4.3	$\frac{1}{2}$ cup or 1 small glass	23
Tomatoes, canned	121	4.2	$\frac{1}{2}$ cup	25
Tomatoes, raw	200	7.0	1 tomato, about 3 in. diameter, $2\frac{1}{8}$ in. high	40
Topping, whipped	4	0.1	1 tbsp, pressurized	10
Tortillas	20	0.7	1 tortilla, 5 in. diameter	50
Tuna fish, canned in oil	85	3.0	$\frac{1}{2}$ cup, drained solids	170
Tuna salad (see salad, tuna fish)				
Turnip greens (see greens)				
Turnips, cooked	78	2.7	$\frac{1}{2}$ cup, diced	18
Veal cutlet, breaded (wiener schnitzel)	136	4.8	2 slices, $2\frac{1}{2} \times 2\frac{1}{2} \times \frac{3}{4}$ in.	315
Veal cutlet, broiled	85	3.0	1 cutlet, $3\frac{3}{4} \times 3 \times \frac{1}{2}$ in.	185
Veal roast, cooked	85	3.0	2 slices, $3 \times 2\frac{1}{2} \times \frac{1}{4}$ in.	230
Vinegar	15	0.5	1 tbsp	2
Waffles	75	2.6	1 waffle, 7 in. diameter (enriched flour)	210
Watermelon, raw	925	32.4	1 wedge, 4×8 in., with rind	115
Welsh rarebit	125	4.4	$\frac{1}{2}$ cup	330
Wheat flour, white enriched	115	4.0	1 cup, sifted	420
Wheat flour, white unenriched	110	3.9	1 cup, sifted	400
Wheat flour, whole wheat	120	4.2	1 cup, hard wheat	400
Wheat germ	9	0.3	2 tbsp	30
Wheat flakes	30	1.1	1 cup (nutrients added)	105
Wheat, shredded	25	0.9	1 biscuit, $4 \times 2\frac{1}{4}$ in.	90
White sauce (medium)	65	2.3	$\frac{1}{4}$ cup	110
Yeast, brewers, dry	8	0.3	1 tbsp	25
Yeast, compressed	28	1.0	one 1-oz cake	25
Yeast, dry active	28	1.0	four $\frac{1}{4}$-oz packages	80
Yogurt, plain	245	8.6	1 cup (made from partially skimmed milk)	125

PROTEIN G	FAT G	CARBOHYDRATE G	CALCIUM MG	IRON MG	VITAMIN-A ACTIVITY IU	ASCORBIC ACID MG	THIAMIN MG	RIBOFLAVIN MG
1	tr	4	5	0.1	0	0	0.01	0.01
tr	tr	4	3	0.1	210	2	0.01	0.01
1	tr	5	9	1.1	970	20	0.06	0.04
1	1	5	7	0.6	1085	21	0.06	0.04
2	4	9	24	0.9	1640	42	0.11	0.07
tr	1	tr	tr	—	20	—	—	0
1	1	10	22	0.4	40	—	0.04	0.01
24	7	0	7	1.6	70	—	0.04	0.10
1	tr	4	27	0.3	tr	17	0.03	0.04
26	21	5	37	4.2	295	—	0.22	0.41
23	9	—	9	2.7	—	—	0.06	0.21
23	14	0	10	2.9	—	—	0.11	0.26
0	—	1	1	0.1	—	—	—	—
7	7	28	85	1.3	250	tr	0.13	0.19
2	1	27	30	2.1	2510	30	0.13	0.13
19	26	6	534	0.7	1118	—	0.04	0.40
12	1	88	18	3.3	0	0	0.51	0.30
12	1	84	18	0.9	0	0	0.07	0.05
16	2	85	49	4.0	0	0	0.66	0.14
2	1	4	6	0.8	0	0	0.17	0.06
3	tr	24	12	1.3	0	0	0.19	0.04
2	1	20	11	0.9	0	0	0.06	0.03
3	8	6	76	0.1	305	tr	0.03	0.11
3	tr	3	17	1.4	tr	tr	1.25	0.34
3	tr	3	4	1.4	tr	tr	0.20	0.47
12	tr	12	12	4.4	tr	tr	0.69	1.52
8	4	13	294	0.1	170	2	0.10	0.44

303

Alcoholic Beverages

BEVERAGE	AMOUNT	NUMBER OF CALORIES
Beer	8-oz glass	100
Eggnog, holiday variety, made with whiskey and rum	$\frac{1}{2}$ cup	225
Whiskey, gin, rum, vodka		
100 proof	1 jigger ($1\frac{1}{2}$ oz)	125
90 proof	1 jigger ($1\frac{1}{2}$ oz)	110
86 proof	1 jigger ($1\frac{1}{2}$ oz)	105
80 proof	1 jigger ($1\frac{1}{2}$ oz)	100
70 proof	1 jigger ($1\frac{1}{2}$ oz)	85
Wines		
table wines (such as chablis, claret, Rine wine and sauterne)	1 wine glass (about 3 oz)	75
dessert wines (such as muscatel, port, sherry, or Tokay)	1 wine glass (about 3 oz)	125

Specialty and Fast Food Items (Dashes indicate information not provided by sources.)

	WT (G)	KCAL	PRO-TEIN (G)	FAT (G)	CAR-BOHY-DRATE (G)	CAL-CIUM (MG)	IRON (MG)	VITAMIN A ACTIVITY (IU)	ASCORBIC ACID (MG)	THIA-MIN (MG)	RIBO-FLAVIN (MG)
BURGER CHEF											
Big Shef	186	542	23	34	35	189	3.4	282	2	0.34	0.35
Cheeseburger	104	304	14	17	24	156	2.0	266	1	0.22	0.23
Double Cheeseburger	145	434	24	26	24	246	3.1	430	1	0.25	0.34
French Fries	68	187	3	9	25	10	0.9	tr	14	0.09	0.05
Hamburger, Regular	91	258	11	13	24	69	1.9	114	1	0.22	0.18
Mariner Platter	373	680	32	24	85	137	4.7	448	24	0.37	0.40
Rancher Platter	316	640	30	38	44	57	5.1	367	24	0.30	0.37
Shake	305	326	11	11	47	411	0.2	10	2	0.11	0.57
Skipper's Treat	179	604	21	37	47	201	2.5	303	1	0.29	0.30
Super Shef	252	600	29	37	39	240	4.2	763	9	0.37	0.43
Source: Burger Chef Systems, Inc., Indianapolis, Ind. 1978 (analyses obtained from USDA Handbook No. 8).											
BURGER KING											
Cheeseburger	—	305	17	13	29	141	2.0	195	0.5	0.01	0.02
Hamburger	—	252	14	9	29	45	2.0	21	0.5	0.01	0.01
Whopper	—	606	29	32	51	37	6.0	641	13.0	0.02	0.03
French Fries	—	214	3	10	28	12	1.0	0	16.0	0.01	0.01
Vanilla Shake	—	332	11	11	50	390	0.2	9	tr	0.01	0.05
Whaler	—	486	18	46	64	70	1.0	141	1.3	0.01	0.01
Hot Dog	—	291	11	17	23	40	2.0	0	0	0.04	0.02
Source: Chart House, Inc., Oak Brook, Ill., 1978.											
DAIRY QUEEN											
Big Brazier Deluxe	213	470	28	24	36	111	5.2	—	<2.5	0.34	0.37
Big Brazier Regular	184	184	27	23	37	113	5.2	—	<2.0	0.37	0.39
Big Brazier W/Cheese	213	553	32	30	38	268	5.2	495	<2.3	0.34	0.53
Brazier W/Cheese	121	318	18	14	30	163	3.5	—	<1.2	0.29	0.29
Brazier Cheese Dog	113	330	15	19	24	168	1.6	—	—	—	0.18
Brazier Chili Dog	128	330	13	20	25	86	2.0	—	11.0	0.15	0.23
Brazier Dog	99	273	11	15	23	75	1.5	—	11.0	0.12	0.15
Brazier French Fries, 2.5 oz.	71	200	2	10	25	tr	0.4	tr	3.6	0.06	tr
Brazier French Fries, 4.0 oz.	113	320	3	16	40	tr	0.4	tr	4.8	0.09	0.03
Brazier Onion Rings	85	300	6	17	33	20	0.4	tr	2.4	0.09	tr

	WT (G)	KCAL	PRO-TEIN (G)	FAT (G)	CAR-BOHY-DRATE (G)	CAL-CIUM (MG)	IRON (MG)	VITAMIN A ACTIVITY (IU)	ASCORBIC ACID (MG)	THIA-MIN (MG)	RIBO-FLAVIN (MG)
DAIRY QUEEN (*cont.*)											
Brazier Regular	106	260	13	9	28	70	3.5	—	<1.0	0.28	0.26
Fish Sandwich	170	400	20	17	41	60	1.1	tr	tr	0.15	0.26
Fish Sandwich W/Cheese	177	440	24	21	39	150	0.4	100	tr	0.15	0.26
Super Brazier	298	783	53	48	35	282	7.3	—	<3.2	0.39	0.69
Super Brazier Dog	182	518	20	30	41	158	4.3	tr	14.0	0.42	0.44
Super Brazier Dog W/Cheese	203	593	26	36	43	297	4.4	—	14.0	0.43	0.48
Super Brazier Chili Dog	210	555	23	33	42	158	4.0	—	18.0	0.42	0.48
Banana Split	383	540	10	15	91	350	1.8	750	18.0	0.60	0.60
Buster Bar	149	390	10	22	37	200	0.7	300	tr	0.09	0.34
DQ Chocolate Dipped Cone, sm.	78	150	3	7	20	100	tr	100	tr	0.03	0.17
DQ Chocolate Dipped Cone, med.	156	300	7	13	40	200	0.4	300	tr	0.09	0.34
DQ Chocolate Dipped Cone, lg.	234	450	10	20	58	300	0.4	400	tr	0.12	0.51
DQ Chocolate Malt, sm.	241	340	10	11	51	300	1.8	400	2.4	0.06	0.34
DQ Chocolate Malt, med.	418	600	15	20	89	500	3.6	750	3.6	0.12	0.60
DQ Chocolate Malt, lg.	588	840	22	28	125	600	5.4	750	6.0	0.15	0.85
DQ Chocolate Sundae, sm.	106	170	4	4	30	100	0.7	100	tr	0.03	0.17
DQ Chocolate Sundae, med.	184	300	6	7	53	200	1.1	300	tr	0.06	0.26
DQ Chocolate Sundae, lg.	248	400	9	9	71	300	1.8	400	tr	0.09	0.43
DQ Cone, sm.	71	110	3	3	18	100	tr	100	tr	0.03	0.14
DQ Cone, med.	142	230	6	7	35	200	tr	300	tr	0.09	0.26
DQ Cone, lg.	213	340	10	10	52	300	tr	400	tr	0.15	0.43
Dairy Queen Parfait	284	460	10	11	81	300	1.8	400	tr	0.12	0.43
Dilly Bar	85	240	4	15	22	100	0.4	100	tr	0.06	0.17
DQ Float	397	330	6	8	59	200	tr	100	tr	0.12	0.17
DQ Freeze	397	520	11	13	89	300	tr	200	tr	0.15	0.34
DQ Sandwich	60	140	3	4	24	60	0.4	100	tr	0.03	0.14
Fiesta Sundae	269	570	9	22	84	200	tr	200	tr	0.23	0.26
Hot Fudge Brownie Delight	266	570	11	22	83	300	1.1	500	tr	0.45	0.43
Mr. Misty Float	404	440	6	8	85	200	tr	120	tr	0.12	0.17
Mr. Misty Freeze	411	500	10	12	87	300	tr	200	tr	0.15	0.34

Source: International Dairy Queen, Inc., Minneapolis, Minn. 1978. Dairy Queen stores in the State of Texas do not conform to Dairy Queen-approved products. Any nutritional information shown does not necessarily pertain to their products.

KENTUCKY FRIED CHICKEN											
Original Recipe Dinner*	425	830	52	46	56	150‡	4.5‡	750‡	27.0‡	0.38‡	0.56‡
Extra Crispy Dinner*	437	950	52	54	63	150‡	3.6‡	750‡	27.0‡	0.38‡	0.56‡
Individual Pieces†											
(Original Recipe)											
Drumstick	54	136	14	8	2	20	0.9	30	0.6	0.04	0.12
Keel	96	283	25	13	6	—	0.9	50	1.2	0.07	0.13
Rib	82	241	19	15	8	55	1.0	58	<1.0	0.06	0.14
Thigh	97	276	20	19	12	39	1.4	74	<1.0	0.08	0.24
Wing	45	151	11	10	4	—	0.6	—	<1.0	0.03	0.07
9 Pieces	652	1892	152	116	59	—	8.8	—	—	0.49	1.27

Source: Nutritional Content of Average Serving, Heublein Food Service and Franchising Group, June 1976.
* Dinner comprises mashed potatoes and gravy, cole slaw, roll, and three pieces of chicken, either 1) wing, rib, and thigh; 2) wing, drumstick, and thigh; or 3) wing, drumstick, and keel.
† Edible portion of chicken.
‡ Calculated from percentage of US RDA.

TACO BELL											
Bean Burrito	166	343	11	12	48	98	2.8	1657	15.2	0.37	0.22
Beef Burrito	184	466	30	21	37	83	4.6	1675	15.2	0.30	0.39
Beefy Tostada	184	291	19	15	21	208	3.4	3450	12.7	0.16	0.27
Bellbeefer	123	221	15	7	23	40	2.6	2961	10.0	0.15	0.20
Bellbeefer W/Cheese	137	278	19	12	23	147	2.7	3146	10.0	0.16	0.27
Burrito Supreme	225	457	21	22	43	121	3.8	3462	16.0	0.33	0.35
Combination Burrito	175	404	21	16	43	91	3.7	1666	15.2	0.34	0.31
Enchirito	207	454	25	21	42	259	3.8	1178	9.5	0.31	0.37
Pintos 'N' Cheese	158	168	11	5	21	150	2.3	3123	9.3	0.26	0.16

	WT (G)	KCAL	PRO-TEIN (G)	FAT (G)	CAR-BOHY-DRATE (G)	CAL-CIUM (MG)	IRON (MG)	VITAMIN A ACTIVITY (IU)	ASCORBIC ACID (MG)	THIA-MIN (MG)	RIBO-FLAVIN (MG)
TACO BELL (cont.)											
Taco	83	186	15	8	14	120	2.5	120	0.2	0.09	0.16
Tostada	138	179	9	6	25	191	2.3	3152	9.7	0.18	0.15

Sources: Menu Item Portions, July 1976. Taco Bell Co., San Antonio, Tex.
Adams CF: *Nutritive Value of American Foods in Common Units.* USDA Agricultural Research Service, Agricultural Handbook No. 456, November 1975.
Church CF, Church HN: *Food Values of Portions Commonly Used,* ed 12. Philadelphia, J. B. Lippincott Co., 1975.
Valley Baptist Medical Center, Food Service Department: Descriptions of Mexican-American Foods, NASCO, Fort Atkinson, Wisc.

	WT (G)	KCAL	PRO-TEIN (G)	FAT (G)	CAR-BOHY-DRATE (G)	CAL-CIUM (MG)	IRON (MG)	VITAMIN A ACTIVITY (IU)	ASCORBIC ACID (MG)	THIA-MIN (MG)	RIBO-FLAVIN (MG)
BEVERAGES											
Coffee, 6 oz.	180	2	tr	tr	tr	4	0.2	0	0	0	tr
Tea, 6 oz.	180	2	tr	tr	—	5	0.2	0	1	0	0.04
Orange Juice, 6 oz.	183	82	1	tr	20	17	0.2	366	82.4	0.17	0.02
Chocolate Milk, 8 oz.	250	213	9	9	28	278	0.5	330	3.0	0.08	0.40
Skim Milk, 8 oz.	245	88	9	tr	13	296	0.1	10	2.0	0.09	0.44
Whole Milk, 8 oz.	244	159	9	9	12	188	tr	342	2.4	0.07	0.41
Coca-Cola, 8 oz.	246	96	0	0	24	—	—	—	—	—	—
Fanta Ginger Ale, 8 oz.	244	84	0	0	21	—	—	—	—	—	—
Fanta Grape, 8 oz.	247	114	0	0	29	—	—	—	—	—	—
Fanta Orange, 8 oz.	248	117	0	0	30	—	—	—	—	—	—
Fanta Root Beer, 8 oz.	246	103	0	0	27	—	—	—	—	—	—
Mr. Pibb, 8 oz.	245	93	0	0	25	—	—	—	—	—	—
Mr. Pibb Without Sugar, 8 oz.	237	1	0	0	tr	—	—	—	—	—	—
Sprite, 8 oz.	245	95	0	0	24	—	—	—	—	—	—
Sprite Without Sugar, 8 oz.	237	3	0	0	0	—	—	—	—	—	—
Tab, 8 oz.	237	tr	0	0	tr	—	—	—	—	—	—
Fresca, 8 oz.	237	2	0	0	0	—	—	—	—	—	—

Sources: Adams CF: *Nutritive Value of American Foods in Common Units.* USDA Agricultural Research Service, Agricultural Handbook No. 456, November 1975.
Coca-Cola Company, Atlanta, Ga., January 1977.
American Hospital Formulary Service. Washington, American Society of Hospital Pharmacists, Section 28:20, March 1978.

	WT (G)	KCAL	PRO-TEIN (G)	FAT (G)	CAR-BOHY-DRATE (G)	CAL-CIUM (MG)	IRON (MG)	VITAMIN A ACTIVITY (IU)	ASCORBIC ACID (MG)	THIA-MIN (MG)	RIBO-FLAVIN (MG)
LONG JOHN SILVER'S											
Breaded Oysters, 6 pc.	—	460	14	19	58	—	—	—	—	—	—
Breaded Clams, 5 oz.	—	465	13	25	46	—	—	—	—	—	—
Chicken Planks, 4 pc.	—	458	27	23	35	—	—	—	—	—	—
Cole Slaw, 4 oz.	—	138	1	8	16	—	—	—	—	—	—
Corn on Cob, 1 pc.	—	174	5	4	29	—	—	—	—	—	—
Fish W/Batter, 2 pc.	—	318	19	19	19	—	—	—	—	—	—
Fish W/Batter, 3 pc.	—	477	28	28	28	—	—	—	—	—	—
Fryes, 3 oz.	—	275	4	15	32	—	—	—	—	—	—
Hush Puppies, 3 pc.	—	158	1	7	20	—	—	—	—	—	—
Ocean Scallops, 6 pc.	—	257	10	12	27	—	—	—	—	—	—
Peg Leg W/Batter, 5 pc.	—	514	25	33	30	—	—	—	—	—	—
Shrimp W/Batter, 6 pc.	—	269	9	13	31	—	—	—	—	—	—
Treasure Chest											
2 pc. Fish, 2 Peg Legs	—	467	25	29	27	—	—	—	—	—	—

Source: Long John Silver's Seafood Shoppes, Jan. 8, 1978 (nutritional analysis information furnished in study conducted by the Department of Nutrition and Food Science, University of Kentucky).

	WT (G)	KCAL	PRO-TEIN (G)	FAT (G)	CAR-BOHY-DRATE (G)	CAL-CIUM (MG)	IRON (MG)	VITAMIN A ACTIVITY (IU)	ASCORBIC ACID (MG)	THIA-MIN (MG)	RIBO-FLAVIN (MG)
McDONALD'S											
Egg McMuffin	132	352	18	20	26	187	3.2	361	1.6	0.36	0.60
English Muffin, Buttered	62	186	6	6	28	87	1.6	106	<0.7	0.22	0.14
Hot Cakes, W/Butter & Syrup	206	472	8	9	89	54	2.4	255	<2.1	0.31	0.43
Sausage (Pork)	48	184	9	17	tr	13	0.9	36	<0.5	0.22	0.13
Scrambled Eggs	77	162	12	12	2	49	2.2	514	<0.8	0.07	0.60
Big Mac	187	541	26	31	39	175	4.3	327	2.4	0.35	0.37
Cheeseburger	114	306	16	13	31	158	2.9	372	1.6	0.24	0.30
Filet O Fish	131	402	15	23	34	105	1.8	152	4.2	0.28	0.28
French Fries	69	211	3	11	26	10	0.5	<52	11.0	0.15	0.03

	WT (G)	KCAL	PRO-TEIN (G)	FAT (G)	CAR-BOHY-DRATE (G)	CAL-CIUM (MG)	IRON (MG)	VITAMIN A ACTIVITY (IU)	ASCORBIC ACID (MG)	THIA-MIN (MG)	RIBO-FLAVIN (MG)
McDONALD'S *(cont.)*											
Hamburger	99	257	13	9	30	63	3.0	231	1.8	0.23	0.23
Quarter Pounder	164	418	26	21	33	79	5.1	164	2.3	0.31	0.41
Quarter Pounder W/Cheese	193	518	31	29	34	251	4.6	683	2.9	0.35	0.59
Apple Pie	91	300	2	19	31	12	0.6	<69	2.7	0.02	0.03
Cherry Pie	92	298	2	18	33	12	0.4	213	1.3	0.02	0.03
McDonaldland Cookies	63	294	4	11	45	10	1.4	<48	1.4	0.28	0.23
Chocolate Shake	289	364	11	9	60	338	1.0	318	<2.9	0.12	0.89
Strawberry Shake	293	345	10	9	57	339	0.2	322	<2.9	0.12	0.66
Vanilla Shake	289	323	10	8	52	346	0.2	346	<2.9	0.12	0.66

Source: "Nutritional analysis of food served at McDonald's restaurants." WARF Institute, Inc., Madison, Wisc., June 1977

	WT (G)	KCAL	PRO-TEIN (G)	FAT (G)	CAR-BOHY-DRATE (G)	CAL-CIUM (MG)	IRON (MG)	VITAMIN A ACTIVITY (IU)	ASCORBIC ACID (MG)	THIA-MIN (MG)	RIBO-FLAVIN (MG)
PIZZA HUT＊											
Thin 'N' Crispy											
Beef†	—	490	29	19	51	350	6.3	750	<1.2	0.30	0.60
Pork†	—	520	27	23	51	350	6.3	1000	<1.2	0.38	0.68
Cheese	—	450	25	15	54	450	4.5	750	<1.2	0.30	0.51
Pepperoni	—	430	23	17	45	300	4.5	1000	<1.2	0.30	0.51
Supreme	—	510	27	21	51	350	7.2	1250	2.4	0.38	0.68
Thick 'N' Chewy											
Beef†	—	620	38	20	73	400	7.2	750	<1.2	0.68	0.60
Pork†	—	640	36	23	71	400	7.2	750	1.2	0.90	0.77
Cheese	—	560	34	14	71	500	5.4	1000	<1.2	0.68	0.68
Pepperoni	—	560	31	18	68	400	5.4	1250	3.6	0.68	0.68
Supreme	—	640	36	22	74	400	7.2	1000	9.0	0.75	0.85

Source: Research 900 and Pizza Hut, Inc., Wichita, Kan.
＊Based on a serving size of one half of a 10-inch pizza (3 slices).
†Topping mixture of ingredients.

B*

Energy Expenditure in Household, Recreational, and Sports Activitie
(in kcal · min⁻¹)

ACTIVITY	kcal·min⁻¹·kg⁻¹	kg / lb	50 / 110	53 / 117	56 / 123	59 / 130	62 / 137	65 / 143	68 / 15
Archery	0.065		3.3	3.4	3.6	3.8	4.0	4.2	4.4
Badminton	0.097		4.9	5.1	5.4	5.7	6.0	6.3	6.6
Bakery, general (F)	0.035		1.8	1.9	2.0	2.1	2.2	2.3	2.4
Basketball	0.138		6.9	7.3	7.7	8.1	8.6	9.0	9.4
Billiards	0.042		2.1	2.2	2.4	2.5	2.6	2.7	2.9
Bookbinding	0.038		1.9	2.0	2.1	2.2	2.4	2.5	2.6
Boxing									
in ring	0.222		6.9	7.3	7.7	8.1	8.6	9.0	9.4
sparring	0.138		11.1	11.8	12.4	13.1	13.8	14.4	15.1
Canoeing									
leisure	0.044		2.2	2.3	2.5	2.6	2.7	2.9	3.0
racing	0.103		5.2	5.5	5.8	6.1	6.4	6.7	7.0
Card playing	0.025		1.3	1.3	1.4	1.5	1.6	1.6	1.7
Carpentry, general	0.052		2.6	2.8	2.9	3.1	3.2	3.4	3.5
Carpet sweeping (F)	0.045		2.3	2.4	2.5	2.7	2.8	2.9	3.1
Carpet sweeping (M)	0.048		2.4	2.5	2.7	2.8	3.0	3.1	3.3
Circuit-training	0.185		9.3	9.8	10.4	10.9	11.5	12.0	12.6
Cleaning (F)	0.062		3.1	3.3	3.5	3.7	3.8	4.0	4.2
Cleaning (M)	0.058		2.9	3.1	3.2	3.4	3.6	3.8	3.9
Climbing hills									
with no load	0.121		6.1	6.4	6.8	7.1	7.5	7.9	8.2
with 5-kg load	0.129		6.5	6.8	7.2	7.6	8.0	8.4	8.8
with 10-kg load	0.140		7.0	7.4	7.8	8.3	8.7	9.1	9.5
with 20-kg load	0.147		7.4	7.8	8.2	8.7	9.1	9.6	10.0
Coal mining									
drilling coal, rock	0.094		4.7	5.0	5.3	5.5	5.8	6.1	6.4
erecting supports	0.088		4.4	4.7	4.9	5.2	5.5	5.7	6.0
shoveling coal	0.108		5.4	5.7	6.0	6.4	6.7	7.0	7.3
Cooking (F)	0.045		2.3	2.4	2.5	2.7	2.8	2.9	3.1
Cooking (M)	0.048		2.4	2.5	2.7	2.8	3.0	3.1	3.3
Cricket									
batting	0.083		4.2	4.4	4.6	4.9	5.1	5.4	5.6
bowling	0.090		4.5	4.8	5.0	5.3	5.6	5.9	6.1

* Data from E. W. Bannister and S. R. Brown, The relative energy requirements of physical activity in H. B. Falls, ed., *Exercise Physiology*, Aca
Press, New York, 1968; E. T. Howley and M. E. Glover, The caloric costs of running and walking one mile for men and women, *Medicine and Scien
Sports* 6:235, 1974; R. Passmore and J. V. G. A. Durnin, Human energy expenditure, *Physiological Reviews* 35:801, 1955.
Note: Symbols (M) and (F) denote experiments for males and females, respectively. See page 95 for instructions on how to use this appe

| 71 | 74 | 77 | 80 | 83 | 86 | 89 | 92 | 95 | 98 |
157	163	170	176	183	190	196	203	209	216
4.6	4.8	5.0	5.2	5.4	5.6	5.8	6.0	6.2	6.4
6.9	7.2	7.5	7.8	8.1	8.3	8.6	8.9	9.2	9.5
2.5	2.6	2.7	2.8	2.9	3.0	3.1	3.2	3.3	3.4
9.8	10.2	10.6	11.0	11.5	11.9	12.3	12.7	13.1	13.5
3.0	3.1	3.2	3.4	3.5	3.6	3.7	3.9	4.0	4.1
2.7	2.8	2.9	3 0	3.2	3.3	3.4	3.5	3.6	3.7
9.8	10.2	10.6	11.0	11.5	11.9	12.3	12.7	13.1	13.5
5.8	16.4	17.1	17.8	18.4	19.1	19.8	20.4	21.1	21.8
3.1	3.3	3.4	3.5	3.7	3.8	3.9	4.0	4.2	4.3
7.3	7.6	7.9	8.2	8.5	8.9	9.2	9.5	9.8	10.1
1.8	1.9	1.9	2.0	2.1	2.2	2.2	2.3	2.4	2.5
3.7	3.8	4.0	4.2	4.3	4.5	4.6	4.8	4.9	5.1
3.2	3.3	3.5	3.6	3.7	3.9	4.0	4.1	4.3	4.4
3.4	3.6	3.7	3.8	4.0	4.1	4.3	4.4	4.6	4.7
3.1	13.7	14.2	14.8	15.4	15.9	16.5	17.0	17.6	18.1
4.4	4.6	4.8	5.0	5.1	5.3	5.5	5.7	5.9	6.1
4.1	4.3	4.5	4.6	4.8	5.0	5.2	5.3	5.5	5.7
8.6	9.0	9.3	9.7	10.0	10.4	10.8	11.1	11.5	11.9
9.2	9.5	9.9	10.3	10.7	11.1	11.5	11.9	12.3	12.6
9.9	10.4	10.8	11.2	11.6	12.0	12.5	12.9	13.3	13.7
0.4	10.9	11.3	11.8	12.2	12.6	13.1	13.5	14.0	14.4
6.7	7.0	7.2	7.5	7.8	8.1	8.4	8.6	8.9	9.2
6.2	6.5	6.8	7.0	7.3	7.6	7.8	8.1	8.4	8.6
7.7	8.0	8.3	8.6	9.0	9.3	9.6	9.9	10.3	10.6
3.2	3.3	3.5	3.6	3.7	3.9	4.0	4.1	4.3	4.4
3.4	3.6	3.7	3.8	4.0	4.1	4.3	4.4	4.6	4.7
5.9	6.1	6.4	6.6	6.9	7.1	7.4	7.6	7.9	8.1
6.4	6.7	6.9	7.2	7.5	7.7	8.0	8.3	8.6	8.8

ACTIVITY	kcal·min⁻¹·kg⁻¹	kg / lb	50 / 110	53 / 117	56 / 123	59 / 130	62 / 137	65 / 143	68 / 150
Croquet	0.059		3.0	3.1	3.3	3.5	3.7	3.8	4.
Cycling									
leisure, 5.5 mph	0.064		3.2	3.4	3.6	3.8	4.0	4.2	4.
leisure, 9.4 mph	0.100		5.0	5.3	5.6	5.9	6.2	6.5	6.
racing	0.169		8.5	9.0	9.5	10.0	10.5	11.0	11.
Dancing									
ballroom	0.051		2.6	2.7	2.9	3.0	3.2	3.3	3.
choreographed			8.4	8.9	9.4	9.9	10.4	10.9	11.
"twist," "wiggle"	0.168		5.2	5.5	5.8	6.1	6.4	6.7	7.
Digging trenches	0.145		7.3	7.7	8.1	8.6	9.0	9.4	9.
Drawing (standing)	0.036		1.8	1.9	2.0	2.1	2.2	2.3	2.
Eating (sitting)	0.023		1.2	1.2	1.3	1.4	1.4	1.5	1.
Electrical work	0.058		2.9	3.1	3.2	3.4	3.6	3.8	3.
Farming									
barn cleaning	0.135		6.8	7.2	7.6	8.0	8.4	8.8	9.
driving harvester	0.040		2.0	2.1	2.2	2.4	2.5	2.6	2.
driving tractor	0.037		1.9	2.0	2.1	2.2	2.3	2.4	2
feeding cattle	0.085		4.3	4.5	4.8	5.0	5.3	5.5	5
feeding animals	0.065		3.3	3.4	3.6	3.8	4.0	4.2	4
forking straw bales	0.138		6.9	7.3	7.7	8.1	8.6	9.0	9
milking by hand	0.054		2.7	2.9	3.0	3.2	3.3	3.5	3
milking by machine	0.023		1.2	1.2	1.3	1.4	1.4	1.5	1
shoveling grain	0.085		4.3	4.5	4.8	5.0	5.3	5.5	5
Field hockey	0.134		6.7	7.1	7.5	7.9	8.3	8.7	9
Fishing	0.062		3.1	3.3	3.5	3.7	3.8	4.0	4
Food shopping (F)	0.062		3.1	3.3	3.5	3.7	3.8	4.0	4
Food shopping (M)	0.058		2.9	3.1	3.2	3.4	3.6	3.8	3
Football	0.132		6.6	7.0	7.4	7.8	8.2	8.6	9
Forestry									
ax chopping, fast	0.297		14.9	15.7	16.6	17.5	18.4	19.3	20
ax chopping, slow	0.085		4.3	4.5	4.8	5.0	5.3	5.5	5
barking trees	0.123		6.2	6.5	6.9	7.3	7.6	8.0	8
carrying logs	0.186		9.3	9.9	10.4	11.0	11.5	12.1	12
felling trees	0.132		6.6	7.0	7.4	7.8	8.2	8.6	9
hoeing	0.091		4.6	4.8	5.1	5.4	5.6	5.9	6
planting by hand	0.109		5.5	5.8	6.1	6.4	6.8	7.1	7
sawing by hand	0.122		6.1	6.5	6.8	7.2	7.6	7.9	8
sawing, power	0.075		3.8	4.0	4.2	4.4	4.7	4.9	6
stacking firewood	0.088		4.4	4.7	4.9	5.2	5.5	5.7	6
trimming trees	0.129		6.5	6.8	7.2	7.6	8.0	8.4	8
weeding	0.072		3.6	3.8	4.0	4.2	4.5	4.7	4
Furriery	0.083		4.2	4.4	4.6	4.9	5.1	5.4	5
Gardening									
digging	0.126		6.3	6.7	7.1	7.4	7.8	8.2	8
hedging	0.077		3.9	4.1	4.3	4.5	4.8	5.0	5
mowing	0.112		5.6	5.9	6.3	6.6	6.9	7.3	7
raking	0.054		2.7	2.9	3.0	3.2	3.3	3.5	3
Golf	0.085		4.3	4.5	4.8	5.0	5.3	5.5	5
Gymnastics	0.066		3.3	3.5	3.7	3.9	4.1	4.3	4
Horse-grooming	0.128		6.4	6.8	7.2	7.6	7.9	8.3	8
Horse-racing									
galloping	0.137		6.9	7.3	7.7	8.1	8.5	8.9	9

| 71 | 74 | 77 | 80 | 83 | 86 | 89 | 92 | 95 | 98 |
157	163	170	176	183	190	196	203	209	216
4.2	4.4	4.5	4.7	4.9	5.1	5.3	5.4	5.6	5.8
4.5	4.7	4.9	5.1	5.3	5.5	5.7	5.9	6.1	6.3
7.1	7.4	7.7	8.0	8.3	8.6	8.9	9.2	9.5	9.8
2.0	12.5	13.0	13.5	14.0	14.5	15.0	15.5	16.1	16.6
3.6	3.8	3.9	4.1	4.2	4.4	4.5	4.7	4.8	5.0
1.9	12.4	12.9	13.4	13.9	14.4	15.0	15.5	16.0	16.5
7.3	7.6	7.9	8.2	8.5	8.9	9.2	9.5	9.8	10.1
0.3	10.7	11.2	11.6	12.0	12.5	12.9	13.3	13.8	14.2
2.6	2.7	2.8	2.9	3.0	3.1	3.2	3.3	3.4	3.5
1.6	1.7	1.8	1.8	1.9	2.0	2.0	2.1	2.2	2.3
4.1	4.3	4.5	4.6	4.8	5.0	5.2	5.3	5.5	5.7
9.6	10.0	10.4	10.8	11.2	11.6	12.0	12.4	12.8	13.2
2.8	3.0	3.1	3.2	3.3	3.4	3.6	3.7	3.8	3.9
2.6	2.7	2.8	3.0	3.1	3.2	3.3	3.4	3.5	3.6
6.0	6.3	6.5	6.8	7.1	7.3	7.6	7.8	8.1	8.3
4.6	4.8	5.0	5.2	5.4	5.6	5.8	6.0	6.2	6.4
9.8	10.2	10.6	11.0	11.5	11.9	12.3	12.7	13.1	13.5
3.8	4.0	4.2	4.3	4.5	4.6	4.8	5.0	5.1	5.3
1.6	1.7	1.8	1.8	1.9	2.0	2.0	2.1	2.2	2.3
6.0	6.3	6.5	6.8	7.1	7.3	7.6	7.8	8.1	8.3
9.5	9.9	10.3	10.7	11.1	11.5	11.9	12.3	12.7	13.1
4.4	4.6	4.8	5.0	5.1	5.3	5.5	5.7	5.9	6.1
4.4	4.6	4.8	5.0	5.1	5.3	5.5	5.7	5.9	6.1
4.1	4.3	4.5	4.6	4.8	5.0	5.2	5.3	5.5	5.7
9.4	9.8	10.2	10.6	11.0	11.4	11.7	12.1	12.5	12.9
1.1	22.0	22.9	23.8	24.7	25.5	26.4	27.3	28.2	29.1
6.0	6.3	6.5	6.8	7.1	7.3	7.6	7.8	8.1	8.3
8.7	9.1	9.5	9.8	10.2	10.6	10.9	11.3	11.7	12.1
3.2	13.8	14.3	14.9	15.4	16.0	16.6	17.1	17.7	18.2
9.4	9.8	10.2	10.6	11.0	11.4	11.7	12.1	12.5	12.9
6.5	6.7	7.0	7.3	7.6	7.8	8.1	8.4	8.6	8.9
7.7	8.1	8.4	8.7	9.0	9.4	9.7	10.0	10.4	10.7
8.7	9.0	9.4	9.8	10.1	10.5	10.9	11.2	11.6	12.0
.3	5.6	5.8	6.0	6.2	6.5	6.7	6.9	7.1	7.4
.2	6.5	6.8	7.0	7.3	7.6	7.8	8.1	8.4	8.6
.2	9.5	9.9	10.3	10.7	11.1	11.5	11.9	12.3	12.6
.1	5.3	5.5	5.8	6.0	6.2	6.4	6.6	6.8	7.1
.9	6.1	6.4	6.6	6.9	7.1	7.4	7.6	7.9	8.1
.9	9.3	9.7	10.1	10.5	10.8	11.2	11.6	12.0	12.3
.5	5.7	5.9	6.2	6.4	6.6	6.9	7.1	7.3	7.5
.0	8.3	8.6	9.0	9.3	9.6	10.0	10.3	10.6	11.0
.8	4.0	4.2	4.3	4.5	4.6	4.8	5.0	5.1	5.3
.0	6.3	6.5	6.8	7.1	7.3	7.6	7.8	8.1	8.3
.7	4.9	5.1	5.3	5.5	5.7	5.9	6.1	6.3	6.5
.1	9.5	9.9	10.2	10.6	11.0	11.4	11.8	12.2	12.5
7	10.1	10.6	11.0	11.4	11.8	12.2	12.6	13.0	13.4

ACTIVITY	kcal·min^{-1}·kg^{-1}	kg 50	53	56	59	62	65	68
		lb 110	117	123	130	137	143	15
Horse-racing								
trotting	0.110	5.5	5.8	6.2	6.5	6.8	7.2	7.
walking	0.041	2.1	2.2	2.3	2.4	2.5	2.7	2.
Ironing (F)	0.033	1.7	1.7	1.8	1.9	2.0	2.1	2.
Ironing (M)	0.064	3.2	3.4	3.6	3.8	4.0	4.2	4.
Judo	0.195	9.8	10.3	10.9	11.5	12.1	12.7	13
Knitting, sewing (F)	0.022	1.1	1.2	1.2	1.3	1.4	1.4	1
Knitting, sewing (M)	0.023	1.2	1.2	1.3	1.4	1.4	1.5	1
Locksmith	0.057	2.9	3.0	3.2	3.4	3.5	3.7	3
Lying at ease	0.022	1.1	1.2	1.2	1.3	1.4	1.4	1
Machine-tooling								
machining	0.048	2.4	2.5	2.7	2.8	3.0	3.1	3
operating lathe	0.052	2.6	2.8	2.9	3.1	3.2	3.4	3
operating punch press	0.088	4.4	4.7	4.9	5.2	5.5	5.7	6
tapping and drilling	0.065	3.3	3.4	3.6	3.8	4.0	4.2	4
welding	0.052	2.6	2.8	2.9	3.1	3.2	3.4	3
working sheet metal	0.048	2.4	2.5	2.7	2.8	3.0	3.1	3
Marching, rapid	0.142	7.1	7.5	8.0	8.4	8.8	9.2	9
Mopping floor (F)	0.062	3.1	3.3	3.5	3.7	3.8	4.0	4
Mopping floor (M)	0.058	2.9	3.1	3.2	3.4	3.6	3.8	3
Music playing								
accordion (sitting)	0.032	1.6	1.7	1.8	1.9	2.0	2.1	2
cello (sitting)	0.041	2.1	2.2	2.3	2.4	2.5	2.7	2
conducting	0.039	2.0	2.1	2.2	2.3	2.4	2.5	2
drums (sitting)	0.066	3.3	3.5	3.7	3.9	4.1	4.3	4
flute (sitting)	0.035	1.8	1.9	2.0	2.1	2.2	2.3	2
horn (sitting)	0.029	1.5	1.5	1.6	1.7	1.8	1.9	2
organ (sitting)	0.053	2.7	2.8	3.0	3.1	3.3	3.4	3
piano (sitting)	0.040	2.0	2.1	2.2	2.4	2.5	2.6	2
trumpet (standing)	0.031	1.6	1.6	1.7	1.8	1.9	2.0	2
violin (sitting)	0.045	2.3	2.4	2.5	2.7	2.8	2.9	2
woodwind (sitting)	0.032	1.6	1.7	1.8	1.9	2.0	2.1	2
Painting, inside	0.034	1.7	1.8	1.9	2.0	2.1	2.2	2
Painting, outside	0.077	3.9	4.1	4.3	4.5	4.8	5.0	5
Planting seedlings	0.070	3.5	3.7	3.9	4.1	4.3	4.6	
Plastering	0.078	3.9	4.1	4.4	4.6	4.8	5.1	5
Printing	0.035	1.8	1.9	2.0	2.1	2.2	2.3	
Running, cross-country	0.163	8.2	8.6	9.1	9.6	10.1	10.6	1
Running, horizontal								
11 min, 30 s per mile	0.135	6.8	7.2	7.6	8.0	8.4	8.8	
9 min per mile	0.193	9.7	10.2	10.8	11.4	12.0	12.5	1
8 min per mile	0.208	10.8	11.3	11.9	12.5	13.1	13.6	1
7 min per mile	0.228	12.2	12.7	13.3	13.9	14.5	15.0	1
6 min per mile	0.252	13.9	14.4	15.0	15.6	16.2	16.7	1
5 min, 30 s per mile	0.289	14.5	15.3	16.2	17.1	17.9	18.8	1
Scraping paint	0.063	3.2	3.3	3.5	3.7	3.9	4.1	
Scrubbing floors (F)	0.109	5.5	5.8	6.1	6.4	6.8	7.1	
Scrubbing floors (M)	0.108	5.4	5.7	6.0	6.4	6.7	7.0	
Shoe repair, general	0.045	2.3	2.4	2.5	2.7	2.8	2.9	

71 157	74 163	77 170	80 176	83 183	86 190	89 196	92 203	95 209	98 216
7.8	8.1	8.5	8.8	9.1	9.5	9.8	10.1	10.5	10.8
2.9	3.0	3.2	3.3	3.4	3.5	3.6	3.8	3.9	4.0
2.3	2.4	2.5	2.6	2.7	2.8	2.9	3.0	3.1	3.2
4.5	4.7	4.9	5.1	5.3	5.5	5.7	5.9	6.1	6.3
13.8	14.4	15.0	15.6	16.2	16.8	17.4	17.9	18.5	19.1
1.6	1.6	1.7	1.8	1.8	1.9	2.0	2.0	2.1	2.2
1.6	1.7	1.8	1.8	1.9	2.0	2.0	2.1	2.2	2.3
4.0	4.2	4.4	4.6	4.7	4.9	5.1	5.2	5.4	5.6
1.6	1.6	1.7	1.8	1.8	1.9	2.0	2.0	2.1	2.2
3.4	3.6	3.7	3.8	4.0	4.1	4.3	4.4	4.6	4.7
3.7	3.8	4.0	4.2	4.3	4.5	4.6	4.8	4.9	5.1
6.2	6.5	6.8	7.0	7.3	7.6	7.8	8.1	8.4	8.6
4.6	4.8	5.0	5.2	5.4	5.6	5.8	6.0	6.2	6.4
3.7	3.8	4.0	4.2	4.3	4.5	4.6	4.8	4.9	5.1
3.4	3.6	3.7	3.8	4.0	4.1	4.3	4.4	4.6	4.7
0.1	10.5	10.9	11.4	11.8	12.2	12.6	13.1	13.5	13.9
4.4	4.6	4.8	5.0	5.1	5.3	5.5	5.7	5.9	6.1
4.1	4.3	4.5	4.6	4.8	5.0	5.2	5.	5.5	5.7
2.3	2.4	2.5	2.6	2.7	2.8	2.8	2.9	3.0	3.1
2.9	3.0	3.2	3.3	3.4	3.5	3.6	3.8	3.9	4.0
2.8	2.9	3.0	3.1	3.2	3.4	3.5	3.6	3.7	3.8
4.7	4.9	5.1	5.3	5.5	5.7	5.9	6.1	6.3	6.6
2.5	2.6	2.7	2.8	2.9	3.0	3.1	3.2	3.3	3.4
2.1	2.1	2.2	2.3	2.4	2.5	2.6	2.7	2.8	2.8
3.8	3.9	4.1	4.2	4.4	4.6	4.7	4.9	5.0	5.2
2.8	3.0	3.1	3.2	3.3	3.4	3.6	3.7	3.8	3.9
2.2	2.3	2.4	2.5	2.6	2.7	2.8	2.9	2.9	3.0
3.2	3.3	3.5	3.6	3.7	3.9	4.0	4.1	4.3	4.4
2.3	2.4	2.5	2.6	2.7	2.8	2.8	2.9	3.0	3.1
2.4	2.5	2.6	2.7	2.8	2.9	3.0	3.1	3.2	3.3
5.5	5.7	5.9	6.2	6.4	6.6	6.9	7.1	7.3	7.5
5.0	5.2	5.4	5.6	5.8	6.0	6.2	6.4	6.7	6.9
5.5	5.8	6.0	6.2	6.5	6.7	6.9	7.2	7.4	7.6
2.5	2.6	2.7	2.8	2.9	3.0	3.1	3.2	3.3	3.4
1.6	12.1	12.6	13.0	13.5	14.0	14.5	15.0	15.5	16.0
9.6	10.0	10.5	10.9	11.3	11.7	12.1	12.5	12.9	13.3
3.7	14.3	14.9	15.4	16.0	16.6	17.2	17.8	18.3	18.9
4.8	15.4	16.0	16.5	17.1	17.7	18.3	18.9	19.4	20.0
6.2	16.8	17.4	17.9	18.5	19.1	19.7	20.3	20.8	21.4
7.9	18.5	19.1	19.6	20.2	20.8	21.4	22.0	22.5	23.1
0.5	21.4	22.3	23.1	24.0	24.9	25.7	26.6	27.5	28.3
4.5	4.7	4.9	5.0	5.2	5.4	5.6	5.8	6.0	6.2
7.7	8.1	8.4	8.7	9.0	9.4	9.7	10.0	10.4	10.7
7.7	8.0	8.3	8.6	9.0	9.3	9.6	9.9	10.3	10.6
3.2	3.3	3.5	3.6	3.7	3.9	4.0	4.1	4.3	4.4

ACTIVITY	kcal·min⁻¹·kg⁻¹	50 110	53 117	56 123	59 130	62 137	65 143	68 150
Sitting quietly	0.021	1.1	1.1	1.2	1.2	1.3	1.4	1.4
Skiing, hard snow								
level, moderate speed	0.119	6.0	6.3	6.7	7.0	7.4	7.7	8.1
level, walking	0.143	7.2	7.6	8.0	8.4	8.9	9.3	9.7
uphill, maximum speed	0.274	13.7	14.5	15.3	16.2	17.0	17.8	18.6
Skiing, soft snow								
leisure (F)	0.111	4.9	5.2	5.5	5.8	6.1	6.4	6.7
leisure (M)	0.098	5.6	5.9	6.2	6.5	6.9	7.2	7.5
Skindiving, as frogman								
considerable motion	0.276	13.8	14.6	15.5	16.3	17.1	17.9	18.8
moderate motion	0.206	10.3	10.9	11.5	12.2	12.8	13.4	14.0
Snowshoeing, soft snow	0.166	8.3	8.8	9.3	9.8	10.3	10.8	11.3
Squash	0.212	10.6	11.2	11.9	12.5	13.1	13.8	14.4
Standing quietly (F)	0.025	1.3	1.3	1.4	1.5	1.6	1.6	1.7
Standing quietly (M)	0.027	1.4	1.4	1.5	1.6	1.7	1.8	1.8
Steel mill, working in								
fettling	0.089	4.5	4.7	5.0	5.3	5.5	5.8	6.1
forging	0.100	5.0	5.3	5.6	5.9	6.2	6.5	6.8
hand rolling	0.137	6.9	7.3	7.7	8.1	8.5	8.9	9.3
merchant mill rolling	0.145	7.3	7.7	8.1	8.6	9.0	9.4	9.9
removing slag	0.178	8.9	9.4	10.0	10.5	11.0	11.6	12.1
tending furnace	0.126	6.3	6.7	7.1	7.4	7.8	8.2	8.6
tipping molds	0.092	4.6	4.9	5.2	5.4	5.7	6.0	6.3
Stock clerking	0.054	2.7	2.9	3.0	3.2	3.3	3.5	3.7
Swimming								
backstroke	0.169	8.5	9.0	9.5	10.0	10.5	11.0	11.5
breast stroke	0.162	8.1	8.6	9.1	9.6	10.0	10.5	11.0
crawl, fast	0.156	7.8	8.3	8.7	9.2	9.7	10.1	10.6
crawl, slow	0.128	6.4	6.8	7.2	7.6	7.9	8.3	8.7
side stroke	0.122	6.1	6.5	6.8	7.2	7.6	7.9	8.3
treading, fast	0.170	8.5	9.0	9.5	10.0	10.5	11.1	11.6
treading, normal	0.062	3.1	3.3	3.5	3.7	3.8	4.0	4.2
Table tennis	0.068	3.4	3.6	3.8	4.0	4.2	4.4	4.6
Tailoring								
cutting	0.041	2.1	2.2	2.3	2.4	2.5	2.7	2.8
hand-sewing	0.032	1.6	1.7	1.8	1.9	2.0	2.1	2.2
machine-sewing	0.045	2.3	2.4	2.5	2.7	2.8	2.9	3.
pressing	0.062	3.1	3.3	3.5	3.7	3.8	4.0	4.
Tennis	0.109	5.5	5.8	6.1	6.4	6.8	7.1	7.
Typing								
electric	0.027	1.4	1.4	1.5	1.6	1.7	1.8	1.
manual	0.031	1.6	1.6	1.7	1.8	1.9	2.0	2.
Volleyball	0.050	2.5	2.7	2.8	3.0	3.1	3.3	3.
Walking, normal pace								
asphalt road	0.080	4.0	4.2	4.5	4.7	5.0	5.2	5.
fields and hillsides	0.082	4.1	4.3	4.6	4.8	5.1	5.3	5.
grass track	0.081	4.1	4.3	4.5	4.8	5.0	5.3	5.
plowed field	0.077	3.9	4.1	4.3	4.5	4.8	5.0	5.
Wallpapering	0.048	2.4	2.5	2.7	2.8	3.0	3.1	3.
Watch repairing	0.025	1.3	1.3	1.4	1.5	1.6	1.6	1.
Window cleaning (F)	0.059	3.0	3.1	3.3	3.5	3.7	3.8	4
Window cleaning (M)	0.058	2.9	3.1	3.2	3.4	3.6	3.8	3.
Writing (sitting)	0.029	1.5	1.5	1.6	1.7	1.8	1.9	2.

| 71 | 74 | 77 | 80 | 83 | 86 | 89 | 92 | 95 | 98 |
157	163	170	176	183	190	196	203	209	216
1.5	1.6	1.6	1.7	1.7	1.8	1.9	1.9	2.0	2.1
8.4	8.8	9.2	9.5	9.9	10.2	10.6	10.9	11.3	11.7
10.2	10.6	11.0	11.4	11.9	12.3	12.7	13.2	13.6	14.0
19.5	20.3	21.1	21.9	22.7	23.6	24.4	25.2	26.0	26.9
7.0	7.3	7.5	7.8	8.1	8.4	8.7	9.0	9.3	9.6
7.9	8.2	8.5	8.9	9.2	9.5	9.9	10.2	10.5	10.9
19.6	20.4	21.3	22.1	22.9	23.7	24.6	25.4	26.2	27.0
14.6	15.2	15.9	16.5	17.1	17.7	18.3	19.0	19.6	20.2
11.8	12.3	12.8	13.3	13.8	14.3	14.8	15.3	15.8	16.3
15.1	15.7	16.3	17.0	17.6	18.2	18.9	19.5	20.1	20.8
1.8	1.9	1.9	2.0	2.1	2.2	2.2	2.3	2.4	2.5
1.9	2.0	2.1	2.2	2.2	2.3	2.4	2.5	2.6	2.6
6.3	6.6	6.9	7.1	7.4	7.7	7.9	8.2	8.5	8.7
7.1	7.4	7.7	8.0	8.3	8.6	8.9	9.2	9.5	9.8
9.7	10.1	10.6	11.0	11.4	11.8	12.2	12.6	13.0	13.4
10.3	10.7	11.2	11.6	12.0	12.5	12.9	13.3	13.8	14.2
12.6	13.2	13.7	14.2	14.8	15.3	15.8	16.4	16.9	17.4
8.9	9.3	9.7	10.1	10.5	10.8	11.2	11.6	12.0	12.3
6.5	6.8	7.1	7.4	7.6	7.9	8.2	8.5	8.7	9.0
3.8	4.0	4.2	4.3	4.5	4.6	4.8	5.0	5.1	5.3
12.0	12.5	13.0	13.5	14.0	14.5	15.0	15.5	16.1	16.6
11.5	12.0	12.5	13.0	13.4	13.9	14.4	14.9	15.4	15.9
11.1	11.5	12.0	12.5	12.9	13.4	13.9	14.4	14.8	15.3
9.1	9.5	9.9	10.2	10.6	11.0	11.4	11.8	12.2	12.5
8.7	9.0	9.4	9.8	10.1	10.5	10.9	11.2	11.6	12.0
12.1	12.6	13.1	13.6	14.1	14.6	15.1	15.6	16.2	16.7
4.4	4.6	4.8	5.0	5.1	5.3	5.5	5.7	5.9	6.1
4.8	5.0	5.2	5.4	5.6	5.8	6.1	6.3	6.5	6.7
2.9	3.0	3.2	3.3	3.4	3.5	3.6	3.8	3.9	4.0
2.3	2.4	2.5	2.6	2.7	2.8	2.8	2.9	3.0	3.1
3.2	3.3	3.5	3.6	3.7	3.9	4.0	4.1	4.3	4.4
4.4	4.6	4.8	5.0	5.1	5.3	5.5	5.7	5.9	6.1
7.7	8.1	8.4	8.7	9.0	9.4	9.7	10.0	10.4	10.7
1.9	2.0	2.1	2.2	2.2	2.3	2.4	2.5	2.6	2.6
2.2	2.3	2.4	2.5	2.6	2.7	2.8	2.9	2.9	3.0
3.6	3.7	3.9	4.0	4.2	4.3	4.5	4.6	4.8	4.9
5.7	5.9	6.2	6.4	6.6	6.9	7.1	7.4	7.6	7.8
5.8	6.1	6.3	6.6	6.8	7.1	7.3	7.5	7.8	8.0
5.8	6.0	6.2	6.5	6.7	7.0	7.2	7.5	7.7	7.9
5.5	5.7	5.9	6.2	6.4	6.6	6.9	7.1	7.3	7.5
3.4	3.6	3.7	3.8	4.0	4.1	4.3	4.4	4.6	4.7
1.8	1.9	1.9	2.0	2.1	2.2	2.2	2.3	2.4	2.5
4.2	4.4	4.5	4.7	4.9	5.1	5.3	5.4	5.6	5.8
4.1	4.3	4.5	4.6	4.8	5.0	5.2	5.3	5.5	5.7
2.1	2.1	2.2	2.3	2.4	2.5	2.6	2.7	2.8	2.8

```
* * * * * * * * * * * * * * * * * * * * * * * * * * * * * * * * * * * * * * * * * * * * * * * * * * * * * * * * * * * * * * * * * * * * * * * * * * *

     1576 Calorie Food Plan
     -----------------------------------

     Nutrient Composition
        Carbohydrate...    261 grams or    64.% of your total calories
        Protein........     71 grams or    17.% of your total calories
        Fat............     35 grams or    19.% of your total calories
```

	Breakfast		Lunch		Dinner
Day 1	Cooked grits 1 1/2 cup Milk, skim 1 cup Cream - light 4 tbsp Apricot juice 1 cup		Bread-any kind 3 slice Milk, skim 1 cup Pork - ham 1 ounce Cauliflower 1/2 cup Raisins 6 tbsp		Candy bar, choc 1 small Mashed potato 1 cup Milk, skim 1 cup Veal - cutlets 2 ounce Rhubarb 1 1/2 cup Radishes no limit Diet Margarine 4 tsp Tangarines 2 medium
	Breakfast		Lunch		Dinner
Day 2	Toast 3 slice Milk, skim 1 cup Bacon - crisp 2 strip Prune juice 1/2 cup		Bread-any kind 3 slice Milk, skim 1 cup Peanut butter 2 tbsp Celery 1/2 cup Oranges 3 small		Beer 6 ounce Baked potato 1 small Milk, skim 1 cup Pork Roast 2 ounce Artichokes 1 1/2 cup Lettuce no limit Diet Margarine 4 tsp Pineapple 1 cup

This is an example of the first two days of a 1,576 calorie food plan. The usual procedure is to generate a 14-day plan; because foods are arranged as exchanges within a given food category, each exchange is assigned a specific calorie value. Therefore, one can exchange any one food within a food category with any other food in that category. In addition, any one complete breakfast, lunch, or dinner can be interchanged for any other breakfast, lunch, or dinner. This makes the number of food combinations for a given day equal to 14 factorial.

```
----------------------------------------------------------------------
STEP  Walk for 2 1/2 miles in 47 minutes 24 seconds(18 min 58 sec/mile)
 9    This exercise burns 280 calories.

      Cycle 3 1/2 miles in 19 minutes 26 seconds(10.80 miles/hour)
      Repeat this 2 times. This exercise burns 229 calories.

      Swim 275 yards in 9 minutes 50 seconds(27.96 yards/min)
      Repeat this 5 times. This exercise burns 290 calories.

      The following alternate activites will expend approximately the
      same number of calories as the aerobic activities above expend.
                   Racquetball      for      51. minutes
                   Circuit Training for      22. minutes
                   Squash           for      38. minutes
                   Badminton        for      92. minutes
                   Basketball       for      34. minutes
                   Downhill Skiing  for      40. minutes
                   Tennis           for      82. minutes
                   Golf             for      47. minutes
                   Aerobic dancing  for      28. minutes
----------------------------------------------------------------------
```

Example for Step 9 of the complementary beginner aerobic exercise plan to ac-
company the daily meal plans. With this program, individuals proceed to the next
week's exercise after they complete their choice of exercise at least 3 times in the
same week. Caloric expenditure represents average values for a particular body
weight.

This kind of computer-generated output gives the person freedom to exchange
activities for any given workout; it offers flexibility and variety in planning
workouts to meet individual preferences. The major advantage, however, is the
maintenance of caloric equivalency between the different activities that is linked
with caloric input from the menus. If inclement weather prohibits jogging or cycling, then swimming or racquetball, for example, can be substituted without altering either the required calorie output (activity) or the required calorie input (food)
side of the energy balance equation. In this way, the individual stays in phase with
his or her tailor made weight loss curve. The exercise prescription is sensitive to
individual differences because it considers age, sex, and current level of physical
activity (relative fitness status).

HOW TO ORDER THE COMPUTERIZED MEAL AND EXERCISE PLAN

1. Send $15 (check, money order, or business, school or university purchase order only) to the following address:

Computer Meal and Exercise Plan
P. O. Box 431
Amherst, Ma 01004

2. Make payable to: FITCOMP
3. Outside continental USA and Canada, add $2 for postage and handling.

Please Note: Questionnaires are processed within 48 hours; you should receive the printout, under normal mail conditions, within 10 days. The $15 cost for the program applies until Dec. 31, 1985. Thereafter, price subject to change and availability. For updated information after this date, write to Computer Plan/Katch, McArdle, Lea & Febiger, 600 Washington Square, Philadelphia, Pa 19106. The computer meal and exercise plan is an exclusive product of Fitcomp®, Fitness Central, Inc., 220 E. 57th St., New York, NY 10021.

More detailed information about the FITCOMP computerized meal and exercise plan can be found in the following article: Katch, F.I. and V.L. Katch. Computer technology to evaluate body composition, nutrition, and exercise. *Preventive Medicine. 12:*619–631, 1983.

COMPUTERIZED MEAL PLAN AND EXERCISE QUESTIONNAIRE

Please print with a ballpoint pen.

1. Name _____
   (First)   (Last)

2. Address _____
   (Street Number and Name)   (Apt. #)

   _____
   City   State   Zip

3. Age _____
   (years)

4. a. _____Female   b. _____Male

5. Current body weight _____
                    (nearest pound)

6. Height (nearest ¼ inch) _____ _____ _____
                          feet   inches fraction

7. How much you would like to weigh_____
                              (nearest pound)

8. Place an **X** next to the exercises you would like for your program. Select at least one from Group 1. Group 2 are optional.

9. Place an **X** next to the *one* section which best describes your current level of daily physical activity:

   a. _____ **Inactive:** You have a sit-down job and no regular physical activity.

   b. _____ **Relatively Inactive:** Three to four hours of walking or standing per day are usual. You have *no* regular organized physical activity during leisure time.

   c. _____ **Light Physical Activity:** You are sporadically involved in recreational activities such as weekend golf or tennis, occasional jogging, swimming or cycling.

   d. _____ **Moderate Physical Activity:** Usual job activities might include lifting or stair climbing, or you participate regularly in recreational/fitness activities such as jogging, swimming or cycling at least three times per week for 30 to 60 minutes each time.

   e. _____ **Very Vigorous Physical Activity:** You participate in *extensive* physical activity for 60 minutes or more at least four days per week.

Group 1. a. _____ Walking, Jogging, Running; b. _____ Swimming; c. _____ Cycling.
Group 2. d. _____ Racquetball; e. _____ Circuit Weight Training; f. _____ Squash; g. _____ Badminton; h. _____ Basketball; i. Downhill Skiing; j. _____ Tennis; k. _____ Golf; l. _____ Aerobic dancing.

FOOD PREFERENCE LIST

Select the foods you want as part of your daily diet from the Food Groups below. Mark an **X** in the box next to the food items you wish within each Group. You *must* select at least *one* item from Groups 1 through 18. To ensure menu variety, be sure to select all the foods you would like to eat. If you omit a choice from one of the required groups, the computer will make a selection for you. *Please Note:* The computer *cannot* make vegetarian menus. You may select none, or as many choices as you wish from Groups 19, 20 and 21—these are optional.

Group 1	**A** ☐ milk, skim	**B** ☐ milk, non-fat	**C** ☐ milk, 2%	
Group 2	**A** ☐ yogurt, skim milk **B** ☐ yogurt, 2% milk	**C** ☐ yogurt, regular milk **D** ☐ yogurt, fruit	**E** ☐ whole milk **F** ☐ choc. milk, non-fat	**G** ☐ buttermilk **H** ☐ ice milk
Group 3	**A** ☐ egg **B** ☐ mozzarella	**C** ☐ ricotta cheese **D** ☐ farmers cheese	**E** ☐ cheddar cheese **F** ☐ american cheese	**G** ☐ swiss cheese **H** ☐ canadian bacon
Group 4	**A** ☐ chicken **B** ☐ turkey **C** ☐ hot dog	**D** ☐ corned beef **E** ☐ salmon, canned **F** ☐ tuna	**G** ☐ crab, canned **H** ☐ oysters	**I** ☐ cottage cheese **J** ☐ peanut butter

(continued on next page)

Group 5	A ☐ chuck steak	D ☐ round steak	G ☐ lamb leg	I ☐ lamb roast
	B ☐ flank steak	E ☐ rump steak	H ☐ lamb chops	J ☐ lamb shoulder
	C ☐ tenderloin	F ☐ sirloin		

Group 6	A ☐ cornish hen	E ☐ ground beef	I ☐ pork chops	M ☐ veal cutlets
	B ☐ fish, fresh and frzn.	F ☐ ground round	J ☐ pork roast	N ☐ veal chops
	C ☐ shrimp	G ☐ pork leg	K ☐ pork shoulder	O ☐ veal roast
	D ☐ scallops	H ☐ pork/ham	L ☐ veal shoulder	

| Group 7 | A ☐ avocado | C ☐ almonds | E ☐ peanuts, dry roast | G ☐ cream cheese |
| | B ☐ olives | D ☐ pecans | F ☐ walnuts | H ☐ bacon, crisp |

| Group 8 | A ☐ diet margarine | | | |

| Group 9 | A ☐ cream, light | C ☐ 1000 island dressing | E ☐ mayonnaise | G ☐ blue cheese dressing |
| | B ☐ french dressing | D ☐ italian dressing | F ☐ sour cream | H ☐ tartar sauce |

Group 10	A ☐ raisin bread	D ☐ toast	G ☐ puffed cereal	I ☐ cooked grits
	B ☐ bagel	E ☐ bran flakes	H ☐ cooked cereal	J ☐ donut, plain
	C ☐ english muffin	F ☐ cereal, dry		

| Group 11 | A ☐ bread, any kind | C ☐ arrowroot crackers | E ☐ matzo | G ☐ plain muffin |
| | B ☐ cooked barley | D ☐ graham crackers | F ☐ soda crackers | H ☐ cooked rice |

Group 12	A ☐ cooked spaghetti	F ☐ corn, off cob	J ☐ peas	N ☐ biscuit
	B ☐ cooked noodles	G ☐ corn, on cob	K ☐ baked potato	O ☐ corn bread
	C ☐ cooked macaroni	H ☐ lima beans	L ☐ mashed potato	P ☐ corn muffins
	D ☐ beans, cooked	I ☐ parsnips	M ☐ squash	Q ☐ yam
	E ☐ lentils, cooked			

Group 13	A ☐ apple juice	D ☐ grapefruit	G ☐ pineapple juice	J ☐ apricot juice
	B ☐ banana	E ☐ grape juice	H ☐ prunes	K ☐ papaya
	C ☐ grapefruit juice	F ☐ orange juice	I ☐ prune juice	

Group 14	A ☐ apple	E ☐ blueberries	I ☐ dates	M ☐ pear
	B ☐ apricot	F ☐ raspberries	J ☐ mango	N ☐ plum
	C ☐ apricot, dried	G ☐ strawberries	K ☐ orange	O ☐ raisins
	D ☐ blackberries	H ☐ cider, any kind	L ☐ peach	

Group 15	A ☐ apple sauce	D ☐ cantaloupe	F ☐ watermelon	H ☐ pineapple
	B ☐ cherries	E ☐ honeydew	G ☐ nectarine	I ☐ tangerine
	C ☐ grapes			

| Group 16 | A ☐ cucumber | C ☐ tomato | E ☐ carrots | G ☐ celery |
| | B ☐ vegetable juice | D ☐ tomato juice | F ☐ green pepper | H ☐ cauliflower |

| Group 17 | A ☐ asparagus | C ☐ beets | E ☐ brussel sprouts | G ☐ eggplant |
| | B ☐ bean sprouts | D ☐ broccoli | F ☐ cabbage | |

Group 18	A ☐ collards	E ☐ turnip greens	H ☐ string beans	K ☐ sauerkraut
	B ☐ kale	F ☐ mushrooms	I ☐ artichokes	L ☐ turnips
	C ☐ mustard greens	G ☐ okra	J ☐ rutabaga	M ☐ zucchini
	D ☐ spinach			

Optional Choices

| Group 19 | A ☐ lettuce | C ☐ chicory | E ☐ escarole | G ☐ watercress |
| | B ☐ radishes | D ☐ endive | F ☐ parsley | |

| Group 20 | A ☐ ale | C ☐ liquor | E ☐ sherry | G ☐ cognac |
| | B ☐ beer | D ☐ port | F ☐ wine, red/white | |

Group 21	A ☐ cake, angel food	D ☐ cupcake, with icing	G ☐ marshmallows, reg.	J ☐ sugar cookies
	B ☐ cake, fruit	E ☐ candy bar, choc.	H ☐ choc. chip cookies	K ☐ pudding
	C ☐ cake, pound	F ☐ chocolate fudge	I ☐ oatmeal cookies	L ☐ popcorn, popped

Index

Page numbers in *italics* indicate figures; page numbers followed by 't' indicate tables.

323

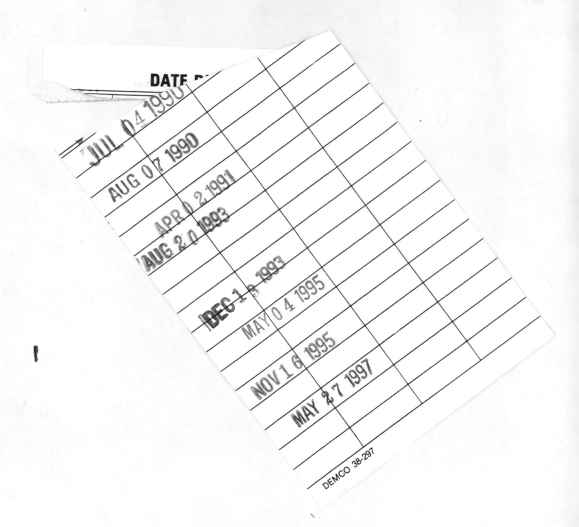